Dual Energy CT and Beyond

Editors

AVINASH KAMBADAKONE
DANIELE MARIN

RADIOLOGIC CLINICS
OF NORTH AMERICA

www.radiologic.theclinics.com

Consulting Editor
FRANK H. MILLER

November 2023 • Volume 61 • Number 6

ELSEVIER

1600 John F. Kennedy Boulevard ● Suite 1800 ● Philadelphia, Pennsylvania, 19103-2899

http://www.theclinics.com

RADIOLOGIC CLINICS OF NORTH AMERICA Volume 61, Number 6
November 2023 ISSN 0033-8389, ISBN 13: 978-0-443-18211-2

Editor: John Vassallo (j.vassallo@elsevier.com)
Developmental Editor: Isha Singh

Radiologic Clinics of North America (ISSN 0033-8389) is published bimonthly by Elsevier Inc., 360 Park Avenue South, New York, NY 10010-1710. Months of issue are January, March, May, July, September, and November. Periodicals postage paid at New York, NY and additional mailing offices. Subscription prices are USD 544 per year for US individuals, USD 1107 per year for US institutions, USD 100 per year for US students and residents, USD 643 per year for Canadian individuals, USD 1415 per year for Canadian institutions, USD 739 per year for international individuals, USD 1415 per year for international institutions, USD 100 per year for Canadian students/residents, and USD 315 per year for international students/residents. To receive student and resident rate, orders must be accompanied by name of affiliated institution, date of term and the signature of program/residency coordinatior on institution letterhead. Orders will be billed at individual rate until proof of status is received. Foreign air speed delivery is included in all *Clinics* subscription prices. All prices are subject to change without notice. **POSTMASTER:** Send address changes to *Radiologic Clinics of North America*, Elsevier Health Sciences Division, Subscription Customer Service, 3251 Riverport Lane, Maryland Heights, MO63043. **Customer Service: Telephone: 1-800-654-2452** (U.S. and Canada); **1-314-447-8871** (outside U.S. and Canada). **Fax: 1-314-447-8029. E-mail: journalscustomerservice-usa@elsevier.com (for print support); journalsonlinesupport-usa@elsevier.com (for online support).**

Reprints. For copies of 100 or more of articles in this publication, please contact the Commercial Reprints Department, Elsevier Inc., 360 Park Avenue South, New York, New York 10010-1710. Tel.: +1-212-633-3874; Fax: +1-212-633-3820; E-mail: reprints@elsevier.com.

Radiologic Clinics of North America also published in Greek Paschalidis Medical Publications, Athens, Greece.

Radiologic Clinics of North America is covered in *MEDLINE/PubMed (Index Medicus), EMBASE/Excerpta Medica, Current Contents/Life Sciences, Current Contents/Clinical Medicine, RSNA Index to Imaging Literature, BIOSIS, Science Citation Index,* and *ISI/BIOMED*.

Contributors

CONSULTING EDITOR

FRANK H. MILLER, MD, FACR, FSAR, FSABI
Lee F. Rogers, MD, Professor of Medical
Education, Chief, Body Imaging Section,
Medical Director, MRI, Professor, Department
of Radiology, Northwestern Memorial Hospital,
Northwestern University Feinberg School of
Medicine, Chicago, Illinois, USA

EDITORS

**AVINASH KAMBADAKONE, MD, DNB,
FRCR, FSABI, FSAR**
Division Chief, Abdominal Imaging, Associate
Professor, Harvard Medical School, Director,
Center for Research and Innovation in
Abdominal Imaging, Department of Radiology,
Massachusetts General Hospital, Boston,
Massachusetts, USA

DANIELE MARIN, MD, FSABI
Associate Professor, Medical Director, Multi-D
Lab, Department of Radiology, Duke University
Medical Center, Durham, North Carolina, USA

AUTHORS

LAKSHMI ANANTHAKRISHNAN, MD
Department of Radiology, UT Southwestern
Medical Center, Dallas, Texas, USA

BENJAMIN BÖTTCHER, MD
Division of Cardiothoracic Imaging,
Department of Radiology and Imaging
Sciences, Emory University Hospital, Atlanta,
Georgia, USA; Institute of Diagnostic and
Interventional Radiology, Pediatric Radiology
and Neuroradiology, University Medical Centre
Rostock, Rostock, Germany

PRIYA BHOSALE, MD
Department of Diagnostic Radiology, Division
of Diagnostic Imaging, The University of Texas
MD Anderson Cancer Center, Houston, Texas,
USA

JINJIN CAO, MD
Department of Radiology, Massachusetts
General Hospital, Harvard Medical School,
Boston, Massachusetts, USA

DARREN CHAN, MBBS
Vancouver General Hospital, University of
British Columbia, Vancouver, British Columbia,
Canada

RYAN CHUNG, MD
Department of Radiology, Massachusetts
General Hospital, Boston, Massachusetts,
USA

BARI DANE, MD
Department of Radiology, NYU Langone
Medical Center, NYU Langone Health, New
York, New York, USA

CARLO N. DE CECCO, MD, PhD
Associate Professor of Radiology and
Biomedical Informatics, Division of
Cardiothoracic Imaging, Nuclear Medicine and
Molecular Imaging, Department of Radiology
and Imaging Sciences, Emory University
Hospital, Emory Healthcare, Inc, Atlanta,
Georgia, USA

SUBBA R. DIGUMARTHY, MD
Division of Thoracic Imaging and Intervention, Massachusetts General Hospital, Harvard Medical School, Boston, Massachusetts, USA

JOEL G. FLETCHER, MD
Department of Radiology, Mayo Clinic, Rochester, Minnesota, USA

SEBASTIAN GALLO-BERNAL, MD
Research Fellow, Division of Pediatric Imaging, Department of Radiology, Massachusetts General Hospital, Department of Radiology, Harvard Medical School, Boston, Massachusetts, USA

MICHAEL S. GEE, MD, PhD
Principal Investigator, Division of Pediatric Imaging, Department of Radiology, Massachusetts General Hospital, Department of Radiology, Harvard Medical School, Boston, Massachusetts, USA

RAJIV GUPTA, MD, PhD
Department of Radiology, Massachusetts General Hospital, Harvard Medical School, Boston, Massachusetts, USA

ZACHARY J. HARTLEY-BLOSSOM, MD, MBA
Division of Thoracic Imaging and Intervention, Massachusetts General Hospital, Harvard Medical School, Boston, Massachusetts, USA

NATTHAWUT JARUNNARUMOL, MD
Department of Diagnostic and Therapeutic Radiology, Ramathibodi Hospital, Mahidol University, Bangkok, Thailand; Department of Radiology, Massachusetts General Hospital, Harvard Medical School, Boston, Massachusetts, USA

SANJEEVA P. KALVA, MD
Department of Radiology, Massachusetts General Hospital, Boston, Massachusetts, USA

SHAHMIR KAMALIAN, MD
Department of Radiology, Massachusetts General Hospital, Harvard Medical School, Boston, Massachusetts, USA

AVINASH KAMBADAKONE, MD, DNB, FRCR, FSABI, FSAR
Division Chief, Abdominal Imaging, Associate Professor, Harvard Medical School, Director, Center for Research and Innovation in Abdominal Imaging, Department of Radiology, Massachusetts General Hospital, Boston, Massachusetts, USA

NAVEEN KULKARNI, MD
Department of Radiology, Medical College of Wisconsin, Milwaukee, Wisconsin, USA

SHUAI LENG, PhD
Department of Radiology, Mayo Clinic, Rochester, Minnesota, USA

MICHAEL H. LEV, MD
Department of Radiology, Massachusetts General Hospital, Harvard Medical School, Boston, Massachusetts, USA

LUDOVICA LOFINO, MD
Duke University Medical Center, Durham, North Carolina, USA

DANIELE MARIN, MD, FSABI
Associate Professor, Medical Director, Multi-D Lab, Department of Radiology, Duke University Medical Center, Durham, North Carolina, USA

CRAIG MAY, MD
Chief Resident, Department of Radiology, Brigham and Women's Hospital, Boston, Massachusetts, USA

EMTENEN MEER, MBBS
Vancouver General Hospital, University of British Columbia, Vancouver, British Columbia, Canada; King Faisal Specialist Hospital and Research Centre, Jeddah, Saudi Arabia

FELIX G. MEINEL, MD, EBCR, EBIR, FCIRSE
Professor of Radiology, Institute of Diagnostic and Interventional Radiology, Pediatric Radiology and Neuroradiology, University Medical Centre Rostock, Rostock, Germany

ACHILLE MILETO, MD
Department of Radiology, Virginia Mason Medical Center, Seattle, Washington, USA

DESIREE E. MORGAN, MD
Department of Radiology, The University of Alabama at Birmingham, Birmingham, Alabama, USA

AVINASH K. NEHRA, MD
Department of Radiology, Mayo Clinic,
Rochester, Minnesota, USA

SAVVAS NICOLAOU, FRCPC
Vancouver General Hospital, University of
British Columbia, Vancouver, British Columbia,
Canada

MITULKUMAR PATEL, MD
Vancouver General Hospital, University of
British Columbia, Vancouver, British Columbia,
Canada

VALERIA PEÑA-TRUJILLO, MD
Research Fellow, Division of Pediatric Imaging,
Department of Radiology, Massachusetts
General Hospital, Department of Radiology,
Harvard Medical School, Boston,
Massachusetts, USA

PRABHAKAR S. RAJIAH, MBBS, MD, FRCR
Department of Radiology, Mayo Clinic,
Rochester, Minnesota, USA

DUSHYANT V. SAHANI, MD
Department of Radiology, University of
Washington, Seattle, Washington,
USA

**UWE JOSEPH SCHOEPF, MD, FACR, FAHA,
FNASCI, FSCBT-MR, FSCCT**
Professor of Radiology, Division of
Cardiovascular Imaging, Department of
Radiology and Radiological Science, Medical
University of South Carolina, Charleston, South
Carolina, USA

ADNAN M. SHEIKH, MD
Vancouver General Hospital, University of
British Columbia, Vancouver, British Columbia,
Canada

AARON SODICKSON, MD, PhD
Division Chief of Emergency Radiology,
Department of Radiology, Brigham and
Women's Hospital, Boston, Massachusetts,
USA

SHRAVYA SRINIVAS-RAO, MD
Department of Radiology, Massachusetts
General Hospital, Harvard Medical School,
Boston, Massachusetts, USA

PATRICK SUTPHIN, MD
Department of Radiology, Massachusetts
General Hospital, Boston, Massachusetts,
USA

ARAN TOSHAV, MD
Department of Radiology, Southeast Louisiana
Veterans Healthcare System, LSUHSC, New
Orleans, Louisiana, USA

ERIK L. TUNG, MD
Chief Resident, Department of Radiology,
Massachusetts General Hospital, Department
of Radiology, Harvard Medical School, Boston,
Massachusetts, USA

MARLY VAN ASSEN, MSc, PhD
Assistant Professor, Division of Cardiothoracic
Imaging, Department of Radiology and
Imaging Sciences, Emory University Hospital,
Atlanta, Georgia, USA

**AKOS VARGA-SZEMES, MD, PhD, FNASCI,
FSCMR**
Associate Professor of Radiology, Division of
Cardiovascular Imaging, Department of
Radiology and Radiological Science, Medical
University of South Carolina, Charleston, South
Carolina, USA

MAYUR K. VIRARKAR, MD
Department of Radiology, University of Florida
College of Medicine, Clinical Center,
Jacksonville, Florida, USA

SAI SWARUPA R. VULASALA, MD
Department of Radiology, University of Florida
College of Medicine, Clinical Center,
Jacksonville, Florida, USA

BENJAMIN M. YEH, MD
Department of Radiology and Biomedical
Imaging, University of California, San
Francisco, San Francisco, California, USA

EMESE ZSARNOCZAY, MD
Division of Cardiovascular Imaging,
Department of Radiology and Radiological
Science, Medical University of South Carolina,
Charleston, South Carolina, USA; MTA-SE
Cardiovascular Imaging Research Group,
Medical Imaging Center Semmelweis
University, Budapest, Hungary

Contents

Computed tomography (CT) has seen remarkable developments in the past several decades, radically transforming the role of imaging in day-to-day clinical practice. Dual-energy CT (DECT), an exciting innovation introduced in the early part of this century, has widened the scope of CT, opening new opportunities due to its ability to provide superior tissue characterization. The introduction of photon-counting CT (PCCT) heralds a paradigm shift in CT scanner technology representing another significant milestone in CT innovation. PCCT offers several advantages over DECT, such as improved spectral resolution, enhanced tissue characterization, reduced image artifacts, and improved image quality.

Compared to conventional single-energy CT (SECT), dual-energy CT (DECT) provides additional information to better characterize imaged tissues. Approaches to DECT acquisition vary by vendor and include source-based and detector-based systems, each with its own advantages and disadvantages. Despite the different approaches to DECT acquisition, the most utilized DECT images include routine SECT equivalent, virtual monoenergetic, material density (eg, iodine map), and virtual noncontrast images. These images are generated either through reconstructions in the projection or image domains. Designing and implementing an optimal DECT workflow into routine clinical practice depends on radiologist and technologist input with special considerations including appropriate patient and protocol selection and workflow automation. In addition to better tissue characterization, DECT provides numerous advantages over SECT such as the characterization of incidental findings and dose reduction in radiation and iodinated contrast.

Optimization of dual-energy CT (DECT) workflow is critical for successful integration of DECT into practice. Patient selection strategies differ by scanner type and may be based on patient size, exam indication, or both. All stakeholders involved in patient scheduling and scan acquisition should be involved in patient triage to DECT. Automation of DECT postprocessing frees up technologist and radiologist time, but care must be taken to avoid sending unnecessary reconstructions to PACS. DECT use in the Emergency Department aids in incidentaloma characterization and improves reader diagnostic confidence, and results in quantifiable cost savings by eliminating the need for follow-up exams.

Computed tomography (CT) imaging has become an essential diagnostic tool for most emergent clinical conditions, owing to its speed, accuracy, cost, and few contraindications, compared with MR imaging cross-sectional imaging. Spectral CT, which includes dual, multienergy, and photon-counting CT, is superior to conventional single-energy CT (SECT) in many respects. Spectral information enables differentiation between materials with similar Hounsfield Unit attenuations on SECT; examples include but are not limited to "virtual noncontrast," "virtual noncalcium," and most notably for neuro applications, "hemorrhage versus iodine." This article expands on the many possible benefits of spectral CT in neuroimaging.

This article examines the intrathoracic applications for dual-energy computed tomography (DECT), focusing on lung cancer. The topics covered include the image data sets, methods for iodine quantification, and clinical applications. The applications of DECT are to differentiate benign and malignant lung nodules, determining the grade of lung cancer and expression of ki-67 expression. Iodine quantification has role in assessment of treatment response in both the primary tumor and nodal metastases.

Dual-energy computed tomography (DECT) acquires images using two energy spectra and offers a variation of reconstruction techniques for improved cardiac imaging. Virtual monoenergetic images decrease artifacts improving coronary plaque and stent visualization. Further, contrast attenuation is increased allowing significant reduction of contrast dose. Virtual non-contrast reconstructions enable coronary artery calcium scoring from contrast-enhanced scans. DECT provides advanced plaque imaging with detailed analysis of plaque components, indicating plaque stability. Extracellular volume assessment using DECT offers noninvasive detection of myocardial fibrosis. This review aims to outline the current cardiac applications of DECT, summarize recent literature, and discuss their findings.

Dual- or multi-energy CT imaging provides several advantages over conventional CT in the context of vascular imaging. Specific advantages include the use of low-energy virtual monoenergetic images (VMIs) to boost iodine attenuation to salvage suboptimal enhanced studies, perform low-contrast material dose studies, and increase conspicuity of small vessels and lesions. Alternatively, high-energy VMIs reduce artifacts caused by some metals, endoprosthesis, calcium blooming, and beam hardening. Virtual non-contrast (VNC) images reduce radiation dose by eliminating the need for a true non-contrast acquisition in multiphasic CT studies. Iodine maps can be used to evaluate perfusion of tissues and lesions.

The use of dual-energy computed tomography (CT) allows for reconstruction of energy- and material-specific image series. The combination of low-energy monochromatic images, iodine maps, and virtual unenhanced images can improve lesion detection and disease characterization in the gastrointestinal tract in comparison with single-energy CT.

By virtue of material differentiation capabilities afforded through dedicated postprocessing algorithms, dual-energy CT (DECT) has been shown to provide benefit in the evaluation of various diseases. In this article, we review the diagnostic use of DECT in the assessment of genitourinary diseases, with emphasis on its role in renal stone characterization, incidental renal and adrenal lesion characterization, retroperitoneal trauma, reduction of radiation, and contrast dose and cost-effectiveness potential. We also discuss future perspectives of the DECT scanning mode, including the use of novel contrast injection strategies and photon-counting detector computed tomography.

There is renewed interest in novel pediatric dual-energy computed tomography (DECT) applications that can image awake patients faster and at low radiation doses. DECT enables the simultaneous acquisition of 2 data sets at different energy levels, allowing for better material characterization and unique image reconstructions that enhance image analysis and provide quantitative and qualitative information about tissue composition. Pediatric DECT reduces radiation doses further while accelerating image acquisition and improving motion robustness. Current applications include the improved evaluation of congenital and acquired cardiovascular anomalies, lung perfusion and ventilation, renal stone composition, tumor extension and treatment response, and gastrointestinal diseases.

Dual-energy computed tomography affords emergency radiologists with important tools to aid in the detection and discrimination of commonly encountered ED pathologies. In doing so, it can increase the speed of diagnosis and diagnostic certainty while sparing patients potentially unnecessary downsteam workups and radiation exposure. This article demonstrates these clinical benefits through a case-based approach.

Traditional monoenergetic computed tomography (CT) scans in musculoskeletal imaging provide excellent detail of bones but are limited in the evaluation of soft tissues. Dual-energy CT (DECT) overcomes many of the traditional limitations of CT and offers anatomical details previously seen only on MR imaging. In addition, DECT has benefits in the evaluation and characterization of arthropathies, bone marrow edema, and collagen applications in the evaluation of tendons, ligaments, and vertebral discs. There is current ongoing research in the application of DECT in arthrography and bone mineral density calculation.

Photon Counting Computed Tomography–Applications   1111

Ludovica Lofino and Daniele Marin

Photon-counting detector CT (PCCT) is a new technology that has recently emerged as a powerful tool for a more precise, patient-centered imaging. Ever since the FDA approved the first Photon-counting system on September 30, 2021, this new technology raised much interest all over the scientific community and numerous studies have been published in a short period of time. By the end of 2022, the first results of phantom and in-vivo studies started showing the great potential of this new imaging modality, with benefits that range from neuroradiology to abdominal imaging and the promise to push previous limits of both patient size and age as well as image resolution. In this article, we will provide a brief explanation of how commercially available photon-counting detector CTs work and how they differ from energy-integrating detector CT systems. Then we will focus on the different clinical applications of this new technology with an in-depth systematic approach based on the most recent evidence. Because nearly every subspecialty of radiology has had impressive results, we will delve into each of these subspecialties and explain how every single domain can undergo significant transformation. This includes a wide range of possibilities, from the opportunistic screening of many different pathologies to the ability of seeing small structures with unprecedented precision, as well as a new kind of multi-energy imaging that can provide much more information on tissue characteristics, all while maintaining a lighter workflow and post-processing burden compared to what has been observed in the past.

PROGRAM OBJECTIVE
The objective of the *Radiologic Clinics of North America* is to keep practicing radiologists and radiology residents up to date with current clinical practice in radiology by providing timely articles reviewing the state of the art in patient care.

TARGET AUDIENCE
Practicing radiologists, radiology residents, and other healthcare professionals who provide patient care utilizing radiologic findings.

LEARNING OBJECTIVES
Upon completion of this activity, participants will be able to:
1. Describe how Dual-energy CT (DECT) has widened the scope of CT and opened new opportunities.
2. Discuss the most utilized DECT images and how they aid radiologists in detecting and discriminating commonly encountered pathologies.
3. Recognize various strategies for successfully integrating a DECT program into practice and acquiring support regarding its value.

ACCREDITATION
The Elsevier Office of Continuing Medical Education (EOCME) is accredited by the Accreditation Council for Continuing Medical Education (ACCME) to provide continuing medical education for physicians.

The EOCME designates this journal-based CME activity for a maximum of 13 *AMA PRA Category 1 Credit*(s)™. Physicians should claim only the credit commensurate with the extent of their participation in the activity.

All other healthcare professionals requesting continuing education credit for this enduring material will be issued a certificate of participation.

DISCLOSURE OF CONFLICTS OF INTEREST
The EOCME assesses conflict of interest with its instructors, faculty, planners, and other individuals who are in a position to control the content of CME activities. All relevant conflicts of interest that are identified are thoroughly vetted by EOCME for fair balance, scientific objectivity, and patient care recommendations. EOCME is committed to providing its learners with CME activities that promote improvements or quality in healthcare and not a specific proprietary business or a commercial interest.

The planning committee, staff, authors, and editors listed below have identified no financial relationships or relationships to products or devices they or their spouse/life partner have with commercial interest related to the content of this CME activity:

Lakshmi Ananthakrishnan, MD; Priya Bhosale, MD; Benjamin Böttcher, MD; Jinjin Cao, MD; Darren Chan, MBBS; Ryan Chung, MD; Joel G. Fletcher, MD; Sebastian Gallo Bernal, MD; Michael S. Gee, MD, PhD; Rajiv (Raj) Gupta, PhD, MD; Zachary J. Hartley-Blossom, MD, MBA; Natthawut Jarunnarumol, MD; Sanjeeva P. Kalva, MD; Shahmir Kamalian, MD; Kothainayaki Kulanthaivelu, BCA, MBA; Naveen Kulkarni, MD; Shuai Leng, PhD; Michael Lev, MD; Michelle Littlejohn; Ludovica Lofino, MD; Daniele Marin, MD; Craig May, MD; Emtenen Meer, MBBS; Achille Mileto, MD; Avinash K. Nehra, MD; Mitul Kumar Patel, MD; Valeria Peña-Trujillo, MD; Prabhakar Shantha Rajiah, MBBS, MD, FRCR; Adnan M. Sheikh, MD; Shravya Srinivas-Rao, MD; Patrick Sutphin, MD; Erik L. Tung, MD; Mayur K. Virarkar, MD; Sai Swarupa R. Vulasala, MD; Emese Zsarnoczay, MD

The planning committee, staff, authors, and editors listed below have identified financial relationships or relationships to products or devices they or their spouse/life partner have with commercial interest related to the content of this CME activity:

Bari Dane, MD: Speaker and Researcher: Siemens

Carlo N. De Cecco, MD, PhD: Researcher: Bayer, Siemens

Subba R. Digumarthy, MD: Independent Contractor: Merck, Pfizer, Bristol Myers Squibb, Novartis, Roche, Polaris, Cascadian, Abbvie, Gradalis, Bayer, Zai laboratories, Biengen, Resonance, Analise; Researcher: Lunit Inc, GE, Qure AI, Vuno Inc.; Speaker: Siemens

Avinash Kambadakone, MD, DNB, FRCR: Researcher: Philips Healthcare, GE Healthcare, PanCAN, Bayer; Consultant: Bayer Advisory Board

Felix G. Meinel, MD: Speaker: GE Healthcare; Researcher: GE Healthcare, Circle Cardiovascular Imaging, Bayer Vital

Desiree E. Morgan, MD: Researcher: GE Healthcare

Savvas Nicolaou, FRCPC: Researcher: Siemens

Dushyant V. Sahani, MD: Consultant: GE Healthcare, Canon Medical Systems, Philips Healthcare; Advisor: Bayer

U. Joseph Schoepf, MD: Researcher: Bayer, Bracco, Elucid Bioimaging, Guerbet, HeartFlow, Inc., Keya Medical, Siemens

Aaron Sodickson, MD PhD: Researcher: Siemens

Aran Toshav, MD: Speaker: Philips Healthcare

Marly van Assen, MSc, PhD: Researcher: Siemens

Akos Varga-Szemes, MD, PhD: Researcher: Bayer, Elucid Bioimaging, Siemens

Benjamin M. Yeh, MD: Researcher: GE Healthcare, Philips Healthcare, Canon Medical Systems; Speaker: GE Healthcare, Philips Healthcare; Shareholder: Nextrast, Inc

UNAPPROVED/OFF-LABEL USE DISCLOSURE
The EOCME requires CME faculty to disclose to the participants:
1. When products or procedures being discussed are off-label, unlabelled, experimental, and/or investigational (not US Food and Drug Administration [FDA] approved); and
2. Any limitations on the information presented, such as data that are preliminary or that represent ongoing research, interim analyses, and/or unsupported opinions. Faculty may discuss information about pharmaceutical agents that is outside of FDA-approved labelling. This information is intended solely for CME and is not intended to promote off-label use of these medications. If you have any questions, contact the medical affairs department of the manufacturer for the most recent prescribing information.

TO ENROLL
To enroll in the *Radiologic Clinics of North America* Continuing Medical Education program, call customer service at 1-800-654-2452 or sign up online at http://www.theclinics.com/home/cme. The CME program is available to subscribers for an additional annual fee of USD 340.00.

METHOD OF PARTICIPATION
In order to claim credit, participants must complete the following:
1. Complete enrolment as indicated above.
2. Read the activity.
3. Complete the CME Test and Evaluation. Participants must achieve a score of 70% on the test. All CME Tests and Evaluations must be completed online.

CME INQUIRIES/SPECIAL NEEDS
For all CME inquiries or special needs, please contact elsevierCME@elsevier.com.

RADIOLOGIC CLINICS OF NORTH AMERICA

THE CLINICS ARE AVAILABLE ONLINE!
Access your subscription at:
www.theclinics.com

Preface

Unveiling the Spectrum: Dual-Energy Computed Tomography and Beyond!

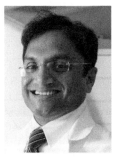

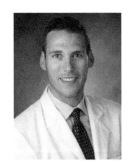

Avinash Kambadakone, MD, DNB, FRCR, FSABI, FSAR

Daniele Marin, MD, FSABI

Editors

The field of Computed Tomography (CT) has witnessed incredible technological advancements in the past several decades ever since its introduction in the 1970s. These advancements have led to a paradigm shift in the field of evidence-based medicine with enormous impact in day-to-day clinical practice. In this era of precision medicine with rising emphasis on multidisciplinary care and with the availability of a wide range of novel therapeutic agents, advanced imaging tools that provide superior tissue characterization are imperative. While conventional single-energy CT provides tissue characterization, the advent of Dual-Energy Computed Tomography (DECT) heralded a new era in determination of tissue composition and multimaterial imaging. Ever since, many innovations in the realm of spectral CT, including the recent introduction of Photon-Counting Computed Tomography (PCCT), promises a fascinating future ahead for the role of CT in the ever increasing complex multidisciplinary care of patients. The utilization of multienergy CT scanners is still growing, and their implementation in clinical practice is

gradually finding wider acceptance. As the field of spectral CT continues to grow, we are delighted to be provided with the opportunity to present this exciting issue exploring the various aspects of this remarkable technology, which is close to our hearts. This issue serves as a comprehensive guide, delving into the principles, applications, and future prospects of both DECT and PCCT, and is designed to broaden your understanding of this groundbreaking technology.

We would like to extend our sincere gratitude and appreciation to Frank Miller, consulting editor of *Radiologic Clinics of North America*, for believing in us to lead this important effort. We are also immensely thankful to John Vassallo and the amazing staff at Elsevier for making this endeavor an enjoyable experience. A special mention to Karen Dino and Isha Singh for their tremendous patience during the entire process and for keeping us on track. As we get busier on the clinical front, their kind and persistent prodding was just the push we needed to make this happen in a timely manner. This unbelievable effort would

Radiol Clin N Am 61 (2023) xv–xvi
https://doi.org/10.1016/j.rcl.2023.07.005
0033-8389/23/© 2023 Published by Elsevier Inc.

certainly not have been possible without the incredibly generous experts in the field of spectral imaging who contributed to this issue. We are honored to have a very distinguished panel of innovators and physician-scientists from across the various imaging subspecialities who have contributed to create this, detailed, technically focused, and practically oriented amalgamation of articles on DECT and PCCT. Each of the articles in this section have been carefully designed and tailored as a practical guide to meet the demands of clinical radiologists in integrating this technology in their busy clinical practice, ultimately adding value and enhancing patient care. We would like to thank each of the exceptional contributing authors for their hard work, dedication, and commitment to this project. We would also like to acknowledge the incredible efforts of countless physicists, scientists, technologists, and radiologists over the past two decades who have helped refine the multienergy CT technology. Equally important have been the collaboration and partnership with vendors who have contributed to the success of this technology. We hope that this issue is a useful addition to a radiologist's library of DECT and that the readers find it useful in clinical practice to help deliver high-quality imaging care to our referring providers and patients.

Avinash Kambadakone, MD, DNB, FRCR, FSABI, FSAR
Harvard Medical School
Department of Radiology
Massachusetts General Hospital
55 Fruit Street, White 270
Boston, MA 02114, USA

Daniele Marin, MD, FSABI
Multi-D Lab
Department of Radiology
Duke University Medical Center
1. Duke University
Durham, NC 27710, USA

E-mail addresses:
akambadakone@mgh.harvard.edu
(A. Kambadakone)
daniele.marin@duke.edu (D. Marin)

Dual-Energy Computed Tomography to Photon Counting Computed Tomography: Emerging Technological Innovations

Shravya Srinivas-Rao, MD[a], Jinjin Cao, MD[a], Daniele Marin, MD[b],
Avinash Kambadakone, MD, DNB, FRCR, FSABI, FSAR[a,*]

KEYWORDS

- Dual-energy CT • Spectral CT • Photon-counting CT

KEY POINTS

- Dual-energy computed tomography (DECT) permits improved characterization of tissues and allows superior material differentiation.
- Integrating DECT into clinical practice has enabled higher confidence in radiologists, improved diagnostic performance, and provided opportunities to reduce radiation and contrast media doses.
- Photon-counting CT has immense potential and offers several advantages over DECT, including improved spectral resolution, enhanced tissue characterization, reduced image artifacts, and improved image quality.

INTRODUCTION

Tremendous strides have been made in imaging, from two-dimensional projection radiography to modern cross-sectional three- and four-dimensional high-resolution imaging capabilities.[1] Alessandro Vallebona, an Italian radiologist, developed computed tomography (CT) using radiographic film to view a single slice of the body in the early 1900s.[2] Sir Godfrey Hounsfield, who is said to have received funding from the Beatles song sales, developed the first CT scanner in 1967 using x-ray technology and the first brain CT was scanned in Wimbledon, England in 1971.[2,3] Ever since then, there have been numerous technological advancements in CT which have paralleled a significant increase in CT utilization from 3 million to 68 million scans annually between 1980 and 2005.[2] The increased utilization of CT has been enabled by developments in CT scanner technology including spiral CT, multi-detector CT, and various types of dual-energy CT (DECT) or multi-energy CT. This has provided the impetus for other phenomenal innovations in CT, such as novel reconstruction algorithms enabling radiation dose reduction, volumetric techniques, newer contrast agents with better safety profile, and various quantitative imaging tools. Faster scanning time and widespread availability have made CT a workhorse of any imaging facility with a wide gamut of clinical applications ranging from stroke evaluation to cancer detection. The U.S. Food and Drug Administration (FDA) approval of photon-counting CT (PCCT) in 2021 heralds a paradigm shift in the realm of CT and opens new horizons to enable delivering high-quality patient care in this era of precision medicine.

[a] Department of Radiology, Massachusetts General Hospital, Harvard Medical School, 55 Fruit Street, White 270, Boston, MA 02114-2696, USA; [b] Department of Radiology, Duke University Medical Center, Box 3808 Erwin Road, Durham, NC 27710, USA
* Corresponding author.
E-mail address: akambadakone@mgh.harvard.edu

Radiol Clin N Am 61 (2023) 933–944
https://doi.org/10.1016/j.rcl.2023.06.015

Among the various CT innovations, the introduction of DECT or multi-energy CT represented an important milestone as it enabled better tissue characterization based on the principle of interaction of matter with x-ray photons. Although the initial conceptualization of DECT was made in 1973, the first dual-source DECT system was FDA-approved for clinical use in 2006.[3] Ever since then, there has been a rapid growth in this sphere with the development of various types of DECT scanner technologies and related innovations. DECT offers multiple different types of image data sets such as virtual monoenergetic or monochromatic images (VME or VMC), effective atomic number maps (Z_{eff}), virtual non-contrast images (VNC), virtual non-calcium images, iodine maps, uric acid images, and so forth, which have found increasing applications in day-to-day clinical practice. PCCT uses a different approach to spectral imaging with the use of a photon-counting detector (PCD) instead of the conventionally used energy-integrating detector (EID). This novel detector counts and measures the energies of distinct x-ray photons rather than averaging them.[4] PCDs offer several benefits in CT imaging, including a significant reduction in image noise, reduced radiation dose, improved spatial resolution, and the ability to perform K-shell binding energy (K-edge) imaging to quantify the concentration of specific elements.[5] In these subsequent sections, the authors provide a broad overview of the two fascinating CT innovations, DECT, and PCCT describing their basic principles, benefits, clinical applications, and challenges in routine practice which are explained in detail in the subsequent articles.

DUAL-ENERGY COMPUTED TOMOGRAPHY
Basic Principles

Conventional CT scanners use a single x-ray beam to provide a polychromatic x-ray spectrum (peak energy 80–140 kVp) for patient scanning. DECT exploits the fact that different materials absorb x-rays differently as a function of x-ray energy and uses the differential behavior of various tissues at different energy levels to enable material separation and differentiation. DECT uses multiple energy levels to gather additional information about the attenuation characteristics of structures by analyzing the attenuation spectra at different energies. The difference in attenuation between the low- and high-energy spectra depends on the effective atomic number of materials which allows the differentiation of materials with higher atomic numbers from those with lower atomic numbers. The ability of DECT to characterize

materials is based on the capability to discern such variations in attenuation.[6] Earlier versions of DECT scanners allowed generation of additional information for material differentiation by simultaneously acquiring two sets of data at different energy levels (high- and low-energy) by using two polychromatic beams. The acquired data sets are then processed to generate various images, including material-specific and virtual spectral images.[7] Subsequent versions of multi-energy CT scanners enabled spectral separation at the detector level.

DECT Scanner Technology

Since the introduction of the first dual-source DECT scanner in 2006, various types of technical approaches to spectral scanning are available, which include temporal sequential scanning of entire scan volume, temporal sequential scanning of single axial rotation, rapid kilovolt peak (kVp)–switching DECT, multi-layer detector, split-filter DECT, and slow kVp–switching DECT.[8,9] The dual-source DECT (ds-DECT) technology uses two x-ray sources and two data acquisition systems positioned perpendicular to each other on the same gantry to enable scanning at low and high energies.[3] Rapid kVp-switching DECT (rs-DECT) technology uses fast switching of x-ray tube potential (kVp) between high and lower energies to enable near-simultaneous acquisition of high- and low-energy data sets.[10] The dual-layer/dual-detector technique DECT (dl-DECT) involves the utilization of a single x-ray tube and a scintillation detector with two layers. The inner layer detects the low-energy data set, whereas the outer layer detects the high-energy data set. A detailed description of the different DECT technologies is provided in Chapter 3.

DECT allows generation of multiple image data sets that provide material-specific and material-nonspecific energy-dependent information allowing qualitative and quantitative evaluation of tissues. Qualitative evaluation includes monoenergetic imaging, effective atomic map (Z_{eff}), and electron density map. Quantitative assessment includes material decomposition, material labeling, and material highlighting.[11] VME/VMC are synthesized using image-domain and projection-domain methods.[12] VMC images are specific to DECT technology and are available from 40 to 200 keV.[9] Monoenergetic images at lower keV (45–65 keV) provide higher image contrast, whereas VME at higher keV (>90 keV) reduces metal artifacts. Depending on the DECT technology, 70 to 77 keV VMC images have imaging appearance and characteristics similar to 120 kVp images.[9] With minor errors, 1.7% and 4.1%, effective atomic number (Z_{eff}) map and electron density map (ρ_e), respectively, can also be obtained.[13] Z_{eff} analyzes attenuation changes as a function of energy where Z_{eff} of water is 7.4 to 7.5. Perfusion defects can be more clearly identified on the Z_{eff} map than on the iodine map.

Material decomposition using DECT technology can be three-material or two-material-based. Material decomposition allows the creation of material-specific images, such as iodine images and virtual unenhanced (VUE) images. Iodine images or maps depict the distribution of iodine within tissues and allows qualitative and quantitative assessment of tissue enhancement which is a surrogate for tissue vascularity. VUE or VNC images are generated by removing iodine from imaging acquired at multiple energies. VUE images act as a surrogate for true non-contrast (TNC) images, thereby providing opportunity for reduction in radiation dose due to elimination of TNC images and reducing the need for additional follow-up imaging such as for renal lesion characterization. However, the attenuation value of VUE might be different from TNC images.[14] Material differentiation or labeling is by principle that two materials having two different dual-energy slopes, which are due to different photoelectric effects, can be separated by a line. This has applications in nephrolithiasis, gout imaging, dual-energy bone removal, and vessel analysis. Material highlighting allows better visualization of tendons and ligaments owing to the difference in atomic numbers between the structure and its surroundings.

Clinical Applications

In routine clinical practice, DECT has found increasing applications across various body regions and has replaced single-energy CT (SECT) as the most preferred imaging technique for several indications.[14] DECT image acquisition allows generation of multiple different types of image data sets, which have been shown to have numerous applications in routine clinical practice. The image data sets which are routinely useful in day-to-day clinical practice include VUE, VME, and iodine images. VUE images generated from a contrast-enhanced acquisition have been used as a replacement for TNC images in patients undergoing renal mass protocol CT or CT angiography studies thereby reducing radiation dose. A combination of VUE and iodine images aid in differentiating hemorrhage from enhancing masses, which has significant problem-solving capabilities in patients with incidental adrenal nodules, renal lesions, vascular emergencies, and GI bleed, mitigating the need for additional imaging studies or intervention. Post-processed DECT images allow for the characterization of stone composition in patients with urolithiasis enabling determination of treatment strategies as well as in identification and quantification of monosodium urate crystals in joints in patients with gout. Low keV VME images (40-55 KeV) allow optimization of contrast in CT angiographic (CTA) studies as they accentuate iodine attenuation and have been used to reduce the dose of iodinated contrast and salvage CTA scans with suboptimal vascular enhancement, which is especially valuable in patients with borderline renal dysfunction. In oncology, DECT has multiple applications, such as improving lesion detection, lesion characterization, assessment of treatment response, and in prediction of patient outcome. In the following paragraphs, the authors provide a broad overview of the range of clinical applications of DECT, which are described in detail in various chapters in this section.

In the gastrointestinal system, DECT allows improved diagnosis and lesion characterization in both solid and hollow visceral structures. In the liver and pancreas, low keV (45–65 keV) monoenergetic and iodine images have been shown to allow improved detection of hyper vascular lesions such as hepatocellular carcinoma, hepatic metastases from hyper vascular primary tumors (melanoma, renal cell carcinoma (RCC), neuroendocrine tumors, papillary carcinoma of thyroid), and pancreatic neuroendocrine tumor (**Fig. 1**). In patients with pancreatic ductal adenocarcinoma, low-keV monoenergetic and iodine images have been shown by several investigators to improve confidence in the detection of hypo-enhancing tumors by providing improved conspicuity against the background enhancing pancreatic parenchyma (**Fig. 2**).[15–17] DECT also allows better identification of calcium, hemorrhage, iron, and fat within liver lesions.[18] Liver iron quantification with DECT using VUE has been shown to be comparable to MR imaging.[19] By enabling the depiction of enhancement within focal hepatic lesions, iodine-specific images allow differentiation of non-enhancing hepatic cysts from enhancing hepatic lesions or complex cysts.[20] In patients with inflammatory bowel disease, Dane and colleagues showed that iodine images allow improved depiction of bowel wall enhancement and quantitative iodine estimation enables the determination of disease activity and response to therapy.[21] In patients with acute abdomen, iodine images improve differentiation of ischemic bowel wall from normal enhancing mucosa. DECT processed VUE and low-keV monoenergetic images also enable improved visualization of gallstones which are not seen on conventional SECT.[22]

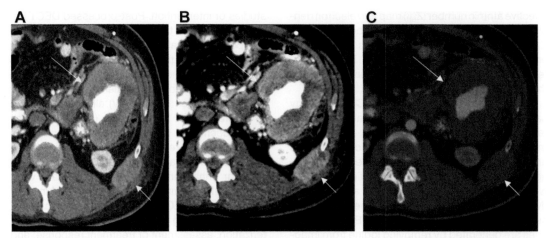

Fig. 1. Improved visualization of melanoma metastasis on ds-DECT in a 58-year-old man. (*A*) Axial contrast-enhanced blended 120 kVp equivalent image shows an enhancing jejunal mass (*top left arrow*) and enhancing metastases in the posterior abdominal wall musculature (*bottom right arrow*). Axial contrast-enhanced 50 keV monoenergetic (*B*) and color-coded iodine map (*C*) allows improved visualization of abdominal wall metastasis (*bottom right arrow*).

In the genitourinary system, DECT enables more robust determination of stone composition, particularly differentiating between uric acid and non-uric acid stones, thereby impacting various treatment approaches. In patients with incidental renal lesions, a combination of iodine and VUE images has been shown to allow the differentiation of simple cysts, hyperdense cysts (proteinaceous or hemorrhagic cysts) from enhancing masses (**Fig. 3**). In patients with renal cell neoplasms, quantitative iodine metrics have been shown to allow differentiation of clear cell from chromophobe and papillary RCC.[23–25]

In patients with lung nodules, DECT has been found to be useful in differentiating benign from malignant pulmonary nodules.[26] Iodine maps also allow improved identification of enhancing and non-enhancing components of heterogenous lesions to better target appropriate area for biopsy and reduce biopsy failure. Iodine overlay maps have been shown to provide additional information by highlighting perfusion abnormalities associated with pulmonary pathology, as in cases such as COVID-19 pneumonia and pulmonary embolism.[27] Iodine maps also enable the characterization of mediastinal masses, such as differentiating thymic cysts from epithelial tumors.[28]

In cardiac imaging, iodine maps facilitate detection of myocardial infarction and myocardial perfusion defects.[29] Iodine maps improve the detection of myocardial fibrosis, myocardial late enhancement, and myocardial enhancement patterns and allow detection of minor perfusion defect in pulmonary embolism.[30] Low-keV monoenergetic images (40–60 keV) allow performance of CT angiography with low contrast media dose, which is beneficial in patients with

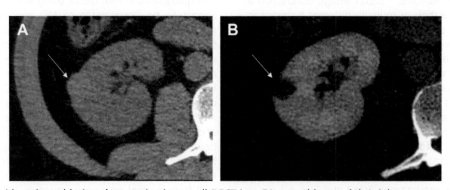

Fig. 2. Incidental renal lesion characterization on dl-DECT in a 51-year-old man. (*A*) Axial true non-contrast CT image shows a hyperattenuating (60HU) lesion in the interpolar aspect of the RIGHT kidney. (*B*) Axial gray scale iodine image generated from the contrast-enhanced dl-DECT image shows absence of iodine uptake in the renal lesion (*arrow*). Diagnosis: Hemorrhagic cyst.

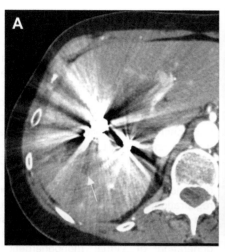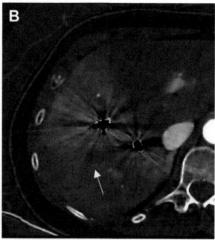

Fig. 3. Improved characterization of hypodense hepatic metastasis in presence of metal related artifacts in a 63-year-old man. (*A*) Axial contrast-enhanced 120 kVp equivalent CT image shows extensive streak artifacts from the portal vein embolization coils which limits visualization of hypodense hepatic metastasis in the vicinity of the coils (*arrow*). (*B*) Axial grayscale iodine image shows improved visualization of hypodense hepatic metastasis (*arrow*) due to mitigation of the artifacts related to the hyperdense coils.

borderline renal insufficiency.[31] VUE images, even though noisier than unenhanced images, allow detection of intramural hematoma and intimal calcifications in aortic and lower limb angiography, thereby mitigating the need for a TNC scan and reducing radiation dose.[32] Colored iodine overlay of DECT is useful in detecting endoleak after aneurysmal repair.[33] DECT is also helpful in CT venography where VME at 40 keV is useful in assessing poorly opacified liver veins in patients with cirrhosis, assessment of portal vein thrombosis and deep vein thrombosis.[34]

DECT-enabled detection of monosodium urate crystals has had a significant impact on diagnosis of patients with hyperuricemia and gout.[35] Virtual non-calcium imaging can be used to evaluate bone marrow lesions, marrow edema, and occult fractures, which cannot be easily assessed on conventional CT.[36] VUE can be used in CT arthrography to identify synovial hemosiderin deposits in pigmented villonodular synovitis.[37] In patients with metal implants, VMC images allow for better visualization of anatomy and pathology due to reduced beam hardening, partial volume, and aliasing artifacts.[38]

Iodine map is useful for detecting tumoral hemorrhage and intracerebral hemorrhage.[39] It is also helpful to differentiate contrast extravasation from intracerebral hemorrhage after intra-arterial revascularization for acute ischemic stroke.[40] In CT cerebral angiography, VME at 40 to 60 keV allows angiographic evaluation of carotid and cerebral arteries with reduced beam-hardening artifacts of the base of skull.[32]

Challenges and Pitfalls

DECT provides many benefits over conventional SECT technology such as higher radiologist confidence, improved diagnostic performance and provides opportunities to reduce radiation and contrast media doses. Despite its advantages, DECT has its limitations. This technology is expensive, requiring special hardware and software tools. Successful integration of DECT into clinical practice requires technologist training, as they are involved in several key steps including postprocessing of data to generate the various DECT image data sets. Depending on the DECT technology, there are limitations in scanning patients with large body habitus, which impedes its universal application.[41] The radiologists need training on the use of various image data sets generated to appreciate the diagnostic value of additional images. The lack of realization of its true impact on clinical practice can lead to underutilization. DECT allows generation of a large number of different types of images which provide varying information. To reduce radiologist burden and limit interpretation time, it is critical to limit the number of images sent to picture archiving and communication system (PACS) such that minimum number of high-quality diagnostic images providing the most material-specific information are available for interpretation.[41] Although there is extensive literature exploring the clinical benefit of DECT in various day-to-day clinical applications, there are limited data establishing its cost-effectiveness.[42,43] In addition, there are several pitfalls in the qualitative and quantitative interpretation of various images generated from the DECT scanners.[9,44] For example, calcium in tissues might appear smaller on VUE images than in TNC imaging; hence small calcifications/calculi can be overlooked.[24] In patients with chronic parenchymal liver disease, the presence of liver fat can confound quantification of liver iron deposition.[9,44] Another major limitation of DECT is the variation in the technology, terminology, and image data sets depending on the vendor. This limits the standardization of quantitative metrics and hinders multicenter research studies as comparison between different technologies can be challenging. Collaborative efforts involving stakeholders in CT including physicists, physician investigators, technology leaders, and vendors are crucial to achieve standardization.

PHOTON-COUNTING COMPUTED TOMOGRAPHY

DECT systems have been available commercially for over a decade and these scanners use detectors that are similar to those in conventional CT. Therefore, they have similar limitations, such as noise, resolution, contrast, and dose efficiency.[4] The introduction of PCDs in spectral imaging has marked the beginning of a new era in CT technology. The PCDs, unlike EIDs, detect individual photons and generate signals.[45] In the past, PCDs have been used in various settings such as single-photon emission CT and PET imaging, and until recently, their use in CT was limited due to the higher count rate for photons required for CT scanning.[46] With the development of detector materials with higher atomic numbers and high spatial resolution fast application-specific integrated circuits (ASICs), PCDs are now introduced into CT practice.[47]

Basic Principles

PCDs are commonly composed of semiconductors such as cadmium telluride or cadmium zinc telluride, whereas materials such as silicon or gallium arsenide are also being investigated. The detector elements of PCD are smaller and lack the septa between individual elements contributing to higher spatial resolution.[48] When incident photons penetrate the semiconductor, they generate electron–hole pairs, resulting in the formation of a sizable electron cloud. The electrons are then attracted toward the anode, generating an electronic pulse that is subsequently converted into electrical energy through an ASIC. The produced electrical signal is directly correlated to the energy of the incident photon. The electronic system uses distinct threshold levels to segregate the signal based on pulse height (**Fig. 4**).[49] This process of segregation of signals based on their energies is called energy binning. We can thus manage the data more efficiently that is generated in the system. This allows spectral imaging, noise filtering, and improved material decomposition.[50] PCD CT technology allows for the simultaneous acquisition of multiple energy CT images, surpassing the traditional two-acquisition limit. This enables the use of a single x-ray tube potential, a single acquisition, and a single filter for multi-energy CT. With a single detector layer, the acquired multi-energy data achieve impeccable temporal and spatial registration, effectively eliminating numerous sources of artifacts. Advanced data processing techniques can then be applied, including the generation of virtual monoenergetic images, VNC, and automated bone removal in the resulting images.

Advantages

PCCT offers several advantages over DECT. The elimination of very low amplitude signals from the energy bin, especially in low-flux imaging in infants, children, and obese individuals, allows for reduction of image noise.[51] Smaller detector elements with lack of septa between individual elements in PCDs produce smaller pixel elements making it easier to count a small number of photons per element, thereby increasing the spatial resolution.[52]

The signals from low-energy photons are detected more efficiently by x-ray detector elements. However, the signal from such low-energy photons is eclipsed by that from high-energy photons EID. PCCT applies different weights to different energy bins during image formation, thereby improving contrast and contrast-to-noise ratio.[53] While using PCCT, the anti-scatter grid can be removed, thus improving dose efficiency as 100% of the detector face is used for detection.[54]

Owing to the separation of photons into different energy bins, an energy bin image can be reconstructed with the use of higher energy photons, thereby reducing beam-hardening artifacts in areas around dense bones (calcium blooming).[55] The data set in each energy bin can be used to generate energy-weighted and postprocessed images such as DECT. Material maps thus produced contain spatial information and concentration of target materials and therefore offer several spectral applications.[56]

Current Clinical Applications

The clinical applications of PCCT are emerging in various body parts. The improvement of anatomic

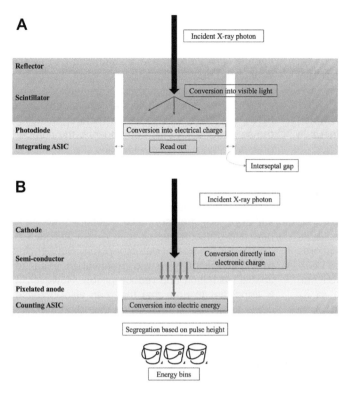

Fig. 4. (A) Energy integrating detector (EID) where incident x-ray photon is converted into visible light by the scintillator and a photodiode converts it into an electric charge which is read out by integrating ASIC. (B) Photon-counting detector (PCD) where incident x-ray photon is converted directly into electronic charge by a semiconductor and a counting ASIC converts it into electric energy which is segregated into different energy bins based on pulse height.

detail due to higher spatial resolution and reduced noise spectrum due to higher image reconstruction strength allows improved diagnosis of various abdominal pathologies in the liver, pancreas, and peritoneum using monoenergetic images.[57] Low-dose non-contrast abdominal PCCT has been shown to offer higher SNR and image quality compared with low-dose EID-CT (Fig. 5).[58]

Similar to DECT, PCCT allows assessment of lung parenchyma and surrounding low-contrast structures using blood volume maps.[59] Dose reduction is valuable in patients with interstitial disease or those undergoing lung cancer screening and low-dose high-resolution PCCT provides great opportunities in these groups of patients.[59] High-quality VUE reconstructions can be used for emphysema evaluation and can replace TNC scans. Ultra-high-resolution (UHR) PCCT imaging can also be optimal for evaluating lung nodules and interstitial lung disease.[60]

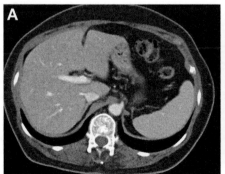
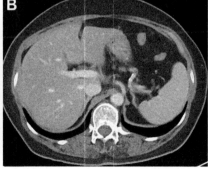

Fig. 5. Reduced image noise and radiation dose in PCCT compared to EID-CT in the same patient. (A) Axial portal venous phase CT image on PCCT shows less image noise with lower patient radiation dose (CTDIvol 6.39mGy). (B) Axial portal venous phase CT image on conventional EID-CT shows comparatively higher image noise with higher patient radiation dose (CTDIvol 8.12mGy). Figure courtesy: Bari Dane, MD, Department of Radiology, NYU Grossman School of Medicine.

Si-Mohamed and colleagues found that PCCT allowed improved subjective visualization of small arteries, stents, calcifications, and non-calcified plaques in coronary CT angiogram compared with EID-CT.[61] By using UHR acquisition, partially calcified plaques could be depicted sharply, and the difference between calcium and non-calcified components could be made, which potentially improves the detection of vulnerable plaques.[62] By increasing the amount of iodine contrast, it is possible to reduce the dose of iodine that is administered while still maintaining the visibility of small, low-contrast structures. For coronary artery calcium score, low-dose PCCT can be used to calculate Agatston scores.[63] However, images reconstructed without iodinated contrast signals can be used to calculate calcium scores in coronary CT angiography scans, thereby obviating the need for a TNC scan. UHR PCCT can be used in coronary stent imaging due to its reduced blooming artifacts resulting in accurate measurements.[64] Few studies show that extracellular volume quantification, myocardial texture assessment, quantification of epicardial adipose tissue attenuation, and myocardial perfusion assessment can be done using PCCT.

In neuroimaging, PCCT allows better differentiation between gray and white matter.[65] High monoenergetic levels can reduce beam-hardening artifacts commonly encountered in head CT. UHR-PCCT can be beneficial in the evaluation of anatomic structures in temporal bone imaging by producing sharp images with a reduced partial volume effect.[66] PCCT allows visualizing trabecular bone, benign focal changes, and small metastases by UHR images.[67] Evaluation of implant–bone interface, periprosthetic fractures, and implant loosening is possible with PCCT.[68]

Challenges with Potential Solutions

Despite the promise of PCCT, it is a new technology and further multicenter large cohort research studies are necessary before its integration into routine clinical practice as the CT modality of choice. The achievable image quality is limited by the x-ray tube that has a maximum filament current, maximum power, and inadequate focal spot size.[5] In an ideal scenario, PCDs would exhibit exceptional dose efficiency and spectral separation. However, in practice, these desirable characteristics come with certain limitations.[5] Photon starvation is one of them. It refers to a situation where the number of detected photons is insufficient for accurate image reconstruction.[53] Another limitation is the occurrence of cross talk, where detector elements incoherently record incident photons, leading to undesired signal interference. Pileup, where photons may be missed if their influx exceeds the counting speed of the detector, is another limitation. These phenomena negatively impact the spatial resolution, spectral resolution, and noise performance of PCCT systems.[5]

The level of cross talk and pileup effects in PCCT is influenced by various factors, including the speed of electronic components, the number of energy bins, the used flux, and the size of the detector pixel element.[4] To ensure proper functionality at the desired flux level, it is crucial to design a system with an appropriate number of energy bins and detector element size, allowing for sufficient spectral separation between different bins and detector elements.[4,5] A key objective is optimizing the size of detector pixels. Smaller detector elements have the potential to enhance spatial resolution and reduce pileup. However, it is important to note that they can also increase cross talk, leading to spectral distortion and energy contamination.[4,69] This also lowers the quality of material decomposition. Finding the right balance between improved spatial resolution, reduced pileup, and minimizing cross talk is essential to achieve optimal spatial resolution while managing pileup and maintaining accurate material identification.

Future Developments

The emergence of machine learning and deep learning-based techniques has augmented the capabilities of spectral CT imaging.[70] Deep learning-based reconstruction algorithms have the potential to lower image noise on different postprocessed DECT data sets, thereby facilitating radiation dose reduction. These algorithms have been demonstrated to improve image quality, assess liver fat quantification, liver iron quantification, and low-contrast detectability of lesions.[70] Furthermore, the development of tools and techniques to reduce artifacts in VMC, material density, and VUE images is necessary for appropriate and accurate interpretation of images.[44] PCDs are compatible with high flux rates, and newer PCCTs can use this. PCCT also offers reduced charge sharing, which can negatively affect conventional CT images due to the double counting of photons and is particularly problematic for material decomposition images. However, charge summing and digital schemes, and few such corrections, will benefit material decomposition applications such as imaging of K-edge agents.[47] A dual-source PCCT would provide better spectral contrast and allow improved temporal resolution for cardiac scans.[71] In the future, we anticipate significant advancements in the spectral capabilities of PCCT.[4] This will lead to better iodine imaging, allowing for contrast-enhanced imaging with lower radiation or iodine doses.[71] In addition, the improvements in spectral imaging will help in the detection of newer contrast agents, specifically K-edge contrast agents and non-iodinated contrast media.[72] Nevertheless, the major obstacle to adopting these new contrast agents is their toxicity at doses necessary for accurate diagnosis. Additional research is needed to investigate the role of artificial intelligence based tools in PCCT.

SUMMARY

Tremendous technical advances in CT have radically transformed role of imaging in patient care. Over the past 2 decades, DECT has established its value in clinical practice through its advantages over SECT. Although DECT is still being widely integrated into clinical practice, PCCT is an emerging technology that has several potential new exciting opportunities. This technology is currently undergoing validation and standardization efforts as it gets installed at various clinical practices. Extensive multicenter research efforts encompassing collaborations among engineers, physicists, and clinicians are ongoing to understand and harness the complete capabilities of PCCT. The transition from DECT to PCCT holds the promise of revolutionizing radiological imaging and propelling radiology into a new era of precision and accuracy.

CLINICS CARE POINTS

- DECT allows material differentiation and quantification of unique substances such as iodine, calcium, fat, and iron.
- Post-processed low keV iodine, VUE, and monoenergetic images are especially useful in routine clinical practice for the detection and characterization of incidental renal lesions, hepatocellular carcinoma, pancreatic ductal adenocarcinoma and determination of renal stone composition.
- VUE images serve as a substitute for TNC images eliminating the need of pre-contrast scanning and reducing radiation dose.
- Low keV VME images facilitate reduction of iodinated contrast volume without compromising vascular enhancement and is beneficial in patients with borderline renal dysfunction.
- Inter-vendor and inter-scanner variability in material-specific decomposition methods due to vendor-specific proprietary algorithms creates challenges for standardization of quantitative DECT metrics such as attenuation values on VUE images and measurement of iodine concentration. This can lead to difficulty in comparison of quantitative results across scanners and monitoring response in patients getting scanned on different DECT technologies in multi-vendor practice.
- PCCT is a novel promising technology which offers higher SNR and image quality with reduced radiation dose and iodine dose.

CONFLICTS OF INTEREST

None.

FUNDING

None.

REFERENCES

1. Singh R, Wu W, Wang G, et al. Artificial intelligence in image reconstruction: The change is here. Phys Med 2020;79:113–25.
2. Half A Century In CT: How Computed Tomography Has Evolved — ISCT. Available at: https://www.isct.org/computed-tomography-blog/2017/2/10/half-a-century-in-ct-how-computed-tomography-has-evolved. Accessed May 7, 2023.
3. Flohr TG, McCollough CH, Bruder H, et al. First performance evaluation of a dual-source CT (DSCT) system. Eur Radiol 2006;16(2):256–68.
4. Samei E, Rajagopal J, Jones E. Hallway Conversations in Physics. AJR Am J Roentgenol 2020;215(5):50–2.
5. Willemink MJ, Persson M, Pourmorteza A, et al. Photon-counting CT: Technical principles and clinical prospects. Radiology 2018;289(2):293–312.
6. Kaza RK, Ananthakrishnan L, Kambadakone A, et al. Update of Dual-Energy CT Applications in the Genitourinary Tract. AJR Am J Roentgenol 2017;208(6):1185–92.
7. Lennartz S, Hokamp NG, Kambadakone A. Dual-Energy CT of the Abdomen: Radiology In Training. Radiology 2022;305(1):19–27.
8. McCollough CH, Leng S, Yu L, et al. Dual- and multi-energy CT: Principles, technical approaches, and clinical applications. Radiology 2015;276(3):637–53.
9. Parakh A, Lennartz S, An C, et al. Dual-energy CT images: Pearls and pitfalls. Radiographics 2021;41(1):98–119.
10. Kalender WA, Perman WH, Vetter JR, et al. Evaluation of a prototype dual-energy computed tomographic apparatus. I. Phantom studies. Med Phys 1986;13(3):334–9.

11. Goo HW, Goo JM. Dual-Energy CT: New Horizon in Medical Imaging. Korean J Radiol 2017;18(4):555.

12. Yu L, Leng S, McCollough CH. Dual-Energy CT–Based Monochromatic Imaging. AJR Am J Roentgenol 2012;199(5 Suppl):S9–15.

13. Garcia LIR, Azorin JFP, Almansa JF. A new method to measure electron density and effective atomic number using dual-energy CT images. Phys Med Biol 2016;61(1):265–79.

14. Hamid S, Nasir MU, So A, et al. Clinical Applications of Dual-Energy CT. Korean J Radiol 2021;22(6):970.

15. Mroueh N, Cao J, Kambadakone A. Dual-Energy CT in the Pancreas. Journal of Gastrointestinal and Abdominal Radiology 2022;05(02):114–20.

16. George E, Wortman JR, Fulwadhva UP, et al. Dual energy CT applications in pancreatic pathologies. Br J Radiol 2017;90(1080). https://doi.org/10.1259/BJR.20170411.

17. Liang H, Zhou Y, Zheng Q, et al. Dual-energy CT with virtual monoenergetic images and iodine maps improves tumor conspicuity in patients with pancreatic ductal adenocarcinoma. Insights Imaging 2022;13(1):1–12.

18. Mileto A, Ananthakrishnan L, Morgan DE, et al. Clinical Implementation of Dual-Energy CT for Gastrointestinal Imaging. AJR Am J Roentgenol 2020;217(3):651–63.

19. Luo XF, Xie XQ, Cheng S, et al. Dual-Energy CT for Patients Suspected of Having Liver Iron Overload: Can Virtual Iron Content Imaging Accurately Quantify Liver Iron Content? Radiology 2015;277(1):95–103.

20. Sanghavi PS, Jankharia BG. Applications of dual energy CT in clinical practice: A pictorial essay. Indian J Radiol Imaging 2019;29(3):289.

21. Dane B, Kernizan A, ODonnell T, et al. Crohn's disease active inflammation assessment with iodine density from dual-energy CT enterography: comparison with endoscopy and conventional interpretation. Abdom Radiol (NY) 2022;47(10):3406–13.

22. Lee HA, Lee YH, Yoon KH, et al. Comparison of Virtual Unenhanced Images Derived From Dual-Energy CT With True Unenhanced Images in Evaluation of Gallstone Disease. AJR Am J Roentgenol 2016;206(1):74–80.

23. Pourvaziri A, Parakh A, Cao J, et al. Comparison of Four Dual-Energy CT Scanner Technologies for Determining Renal Stone Composition: A Phantom Approach. Radiology 2022;304(3):580–9.

24. Cao J, Lennartz S, Pisuchpen N, et al. Renal Lesion Characterization by Dual-Layer Dual-Energy CT: Comparison of Virtual and True Unenhanced Images. AJR Am J Roentgenol 2022;219(4):614–23.

25. Manoharan D, Netaji A, Diwan K, et al. Normalized Dual-Energy Iodine Ratio Best Differentiates Renal Cell Carcinoma Subtypes Among Quantitative Imaging Biomarkers From Perfusion CT and Dual-Energy CT. AJR Am J Roentgenol 2020;215(6):1389–97.

26. Sudarski S, Hagelstein C, Weis M, et al. Dual-energy snap-shot perfusion CT in suspect pulmonary nodules and masses and for lung cancer staging. Eur J Radiol 2015;84(12):2393–400.

27. Lang M, Som A, Mendoza DP, et al. Hypoxaemia related to COVID-19: vascular and perfusion abnormalities on dual-energy CT. Lancet Infect Dis 2020;20(12):1365–6.

28. Yan WQ, Xin YK, Jing Y, et al. Iodine Quantification Using Dual-Energy Computed Tomography for Differentiating Thymic Tumors. J Comput Assist Tomogr 2018;42(6):873.

29. Arnoldi E, Lee YS, Ruzsics B, et al. CT detection of myocardial blood volume deficits: dual-energy CT compared with single-energy CT spectra. J Cardiovasc Comput Tomogr 2011;5(6):421–9.

30. Pontana F, Faivre JB, Remy-Jardin M, et al. Lung perfusion with dual-energy multidetector-row CT (MDCT): feasibility for the evaluation of acute pulmonary embolism in 117 consecutive patients. Acad Radiol 2008;15(12):1494–504.

31. Martin SS, Wichmann JL, Scholtz JE, et al. Noise-Optimized Virtual Monoenergetic Dual-Energy CT Improves Diagnostic Accuracy for the Detection of Active Arterial Bleeding of the Abdomen. J Vasc Interv Radiol 2017;28(9):1257–66.

32. Wichmann JL, Gillott MR, De Cecco CN, et al. Dual-Energy Computed Tomography Angiography of the Lower Extremity Runoff: Impact of Noise-Optimized Virtual Monochromatic Imaging on Image Quality and Diagnostic Accuracy. Invest Radiol 2016;51(2):139–46.

33. Ascenti G, Mazziotti S, Lamberto S, et al. Dual-energy CT for detection of endoleaks after endovascular abdominal aneurysm repair: usefulness of colored iodine overlay. AJR Am J Roentgenol 2011;196(6):1408–14.

34. Weiss J, Schabel C, Othman AE, et al. Impact of dual-energy CT post-processing to differentiate venous thrombosis from iodine flux artefacts. Eur Radiol 2018;28(12):5076–82.

35. Christiansen SN, Muller FC, Østergaard M, et al. Dual-energy CT in gout patients: Do all colour-coded lesions actually represent monosodium urate crystals? Arthritis Res Ther 2020;22(1):1–11.

36. Wang CK, Tsai JM, Chuang MT, et al. Bone marrow edema in vertebral compression fractures: detection with dual-energy CT. Radiology 2013;269(2):525–33.

37. Omoumi P, Becce F, Racine D, et al. Dual-Energy CT: Basic Principles, Technical Approaches, and Applications in Musculoskeletal Imaging (Part 1). Semin Musculoskelet Radiol 2015;19(5):431–7.

38. Vellarackal AJ, Kaim AH. Metal artefact reduction of different alloys with dual energy computed tomography (DECT). Sci Rep 2021;11(1):1–11.

39. Kim SJ, Lim HK, Lee HY, et al. Dual-energy CT in the evaluation of intracerebral hemorrhage of unknown origin: differentiation between tumor bleeding and

pure hemorrhage. AJNR Am J Neuroradiol 2012;
33(5):865–72.

40. Tijssen MPM, Hofman PAM, Stadler AAR, et al. The
role of dual energy CT in differentiating between
brain haemorrhage and contrast medium after mechanical revascularisation in acute ischaemic
stroke. Eur Radiol 2014;24(4):834–40.

41. Megibow AJ, Kambadakone A, Ananthakrishnan L.
Dual-Energy Computed Tomography: Image Acqui-
sition, Processing, and Workflow. Radiol Clin North
Am 2018;56(4):507–20.

42. Patel BN, Boltyenkov AT, Martinez MG, et al. Cost-
effectiveness of dual-energy CT versus multiphasic
single-energy CT and MRI for characterization of
incidental indeterminate renal lesions. Abdom Radiol (NY) 2020;45(6):1896–906.

43. Atwi NE, Sabottke CF, Pitre DM, et al. Follow-up
Recommendation Rates Associated With Spectral
Detector Dual-Energy CT of the Abdomen and
Pelvis: A Retrospective Comparison to Single-
Energy CT. J Am Coll Radiol 2020;17(7):940–50.

44. Parakh A, An C, Lennartz S, et al. Recognizing and
Minimizing Artifacts at Dual-Energy CT. Radiographics 2021;41(2):509–23.

45. Pourmorteza A, Symons R, Sandfort V, et al. Abdominal imaging with contrast-enhanced photon-counting CT: First human experience. Radiology 2016;
279(1):239–45.

46. Iwanczyk JS, Nygard E, Meirav O, et al. Photon
counting energy dispersive detector arrays for X-ray
imaging. IEEE Trans Nucl Sci 2009;56(3):535–42.

47. Leng S, Bruesewitz M, Tao S, et al. Photon-counting
detector CT: System design and clinical applications
of an emerging technology. Radiographics 2019;
39(3):729–43.

48. Flohr T, Petersilka M, Henning A, et al. Photon-counting CT review. Phys Med 2020;79:126–36.

49. Taguchi K, Iwanczyk JS. Vision 20/20: Single photon
counting x-ray detectors in medical imaging. Med
Phys 2013;40(10):100901.

50. Danielsson M, Persson M, Sjolin M. Photon-counting
x-ray detectors for CT. Phys Med Biol 2021;66(3):
03TR01.

51. Yu Z, Leng S, Kappler S, et al. Noise performance of
low-dose CT: comparison between an energy integrating detector and a photon counting detector using a whole-body research photon counting CT
scanner. J Med Imaging 2016;3(4):043503.

52. Leng S, Rajendran K, Gong H, et al. 150-μm Spatial
Resolution Using Photon-Counting Detector
Computed Tomography Technology: Technical Performance and First Patient Images. Invest Radiol
2018;53(11):655–62.

53. Gutjahr R, Halaweish AF, Yu Z, et al. Human imaging
with photon counting-based computed tomography
at clinical dose levels: Contrast-to-noise ratio and
cadaver studies. Invest Radiol 2016;51(7):421–9.

54. Symons R, Pourmorteza A, Sandfort V, et al. Feasibility
of dose-reduced chest CT with photon-counting detectors: Initial results in humans. Radiology 2017;285(3):
980–9.

55. Bennett JR, Opie AMT, Xu Q, et al. Hybrid spectral
micro-CT: System design, implementation, and preliminary results. IEEE Trans Biomed Eng 2014;
61(2):246–53.

56. Leng S, Zhou W, Yu Z, et al. Spectral performance of
a whole-body research photon counting detector
CT: quantitative accuracy in derived image sets.
Phys Med Biol 2017;62(17):7216.

57. Sartoretti T, Landsmann A, Nakhostin D, et al. Quantum
Iterative Reconstruction for Abdominal Photon-
counting Detector CT Improves Image Quality. Radiology 2022;303(2):339–48.

58. Decker JA, Bette S, Lubina N, et al. Low-dose CT of
the abdomen: Initial experience on a novel photon-
counting detector CT and comparison with energy-
integrating detector CT. Eur J Radiol 2022;148:
110181.

59. Graafen D, Emrich T, Halfmann MC, et al. Dose
Reduction and Image Quality in Photon-counting
Detector High-resolution Computed Tomography of
the Chest: Routine Clinical Data. J Thorac Imaging
2022;37(5):315–22.

60. Inoue A, Johnson TF, White D, et al. Estimating the
Clinical Impact of Photon-Counting-Detector CT in
Diagnosing Usual Interstitial Pneumonia. Invest Ra-
diol 2022;57(11):734–41.

61. Si-Mohamed SA, Boccalini S, Lacombe H, et al. Coronary CT Angiography with Photon-counting CT:
First-In-Human Results. Radiology 2022;303(2):
303–13.

62. Mergen V, Sartoretti T, Baer-Beck M, et al. Ultra-
High-Resolution Coronary CT Angiography With
Photon-Counting Detector CT: Feasibility and Image
Characterization. Invest Radiol 2022;57(12):780–8.

63. Eberhard M, Mergen V, Higashigaito K, et al. Coronary Calcium Scoring with First Generation Dual-
Source Photon-Counting CT—First Evidence from
Phantom and In-Vivo Scans. Diagnostics 2021;
11(9):1708.

64. Boccalini S, Si-Mohamed SA, Lacombe H, et al. First
In-Human Results of Computed Tomography Angi-
ography for Coronary Stent Assessment With a
Spectral Photon Counting Computed Tomography.
Invest Radiol 2022;57(4):212.

65. Pourmorteza A, Symons R, Reich DS, et al. Photon-
Counting CT of the Brain: In Vivo Human Results and
Image-Quality Assessment. Am J Neuroradiol 2017;
38(12):2257–63.

66. Benson JC, Rajendran K, Lane JI, et al. A New Frontier in Temporal Bone Imaging: Photon-Counting Detector CT Demonstrates Superior Visualization of
Critical Anatomic Structures at Reduced Radiation
Dose. Am J Neuroradiol 2022;43(4):579–84.

67. Wehrse E, Sawall S, Klein L, et al. Potential of ultra-high-resolution photon-counting CT of bone metastases: initial experiences in breast cancer patients. NPJ Breast Cancer 2021;7(1):1–8.

68. Zhou W, Bartlett DJ, Diehn FE, et al. Reduction of Metal Artifacts and Improvement in Dose Efficiency Using Photon-Counting Detector Computed Tomography and Tin Filtration. Invest Radiol 2019;54(4):204–11.

69. Taguchi K, Stierstorfer K, Polster C, et al. Spatio-energetic cross-talk in photon counting detectors: Numerical detector model (PcTK) and workflow for CT image quality assessment. Med Phys 2018;45(5): 1985–98.

70. Noda Y, Kawai N, Nagata S, et al. Deep learning image reconstruction algorithm for pancreatic protocol dual-energy computed tomography: image quality and quantification of iodine concentration. Eur Radiol 2022;32(1):384–94.

71. Hsieh SS, Leng S, Rajendran K, et al. Photon Counting CT: Clinical Applications and Future Developments. IEEE Trans Radiat Plasma Med Sci 2021; 5(4):441.

72. Amato C, Klein L, Wehrse E, et al. Potential of contrast agents based on high-Z elements for contrast-enhanced photon-counting computed tomography. Med Phys 2020;47(12):6179–90.

Dual-Energy Computed Tomography: Technological Considerations

Ryan Chung, MD[a],*, Bari Dane, MD[b], Benjamin M. Yeh, MD[c],
Desiree E. Morgan, MD[d], Dushyant V. Sahani, MD[e],
Avinash Kambadakone, MD, DNB, FRCR, FSABI, FSAR[a]

KEYWORDS

- Dual-energy CT • DECT • Spectral CT • Multi-energy CT • Technological considerations
- Image reconstruction

KEY POINTS

- DECT systems can be source-based (dual-source, rapid kVp switching, dual-spin, and split beam) or detector-based (dual-layer).
- DECT image reconstruction is either in the projection (pre-reconstruction) or image (post-reconstruction) domains.
- The most utilized DECT images include routine SECT equivalent, virtual monoenergetic, material density (eg, iodine map), and virtual non-contrast images.
- Important DECT acquisition considerations include patient body size, protocol selection, and workflow integration into routine clinical practice.

INTRODUCTION

Over the past five decades, computed tomography (CT) has evolved dramatically and simultaneously revolutionized the practice of medicine and the understanding of patient anatomy and pathophysiology.[1] Technological advancements in CT scanner technology, including helical and multidetector CT, enabled CT to become widely adopted for a multitude of clinical scenarios (eg, stroke, infection, vascular abnormalities, trauma, cancer). Dual-energy CT (DECT) or multi-energy CT introduced in 2006, provides enhanced tissue characterization due to superior material separation due to the acquisition of high- and low-energy data. Our article reviews the current DECT technologies in clinical practice, DECT nomenclature, basic principles of DECT image reconstruction, commonly utilized DECT images, and workflow considerations including patient and protocol selection. Additional details regarding subspecialty-specific DECT applications in radiology and photon-counting detector CT are discussed later within this issue.

DUAL-ENERGY COMPUTED TOMOGRAPHY: PHYSICS AND TECHNICAL PRINCIPLES

In conventional or single energy CT (SECT), a single x-ray source produces a polyenergetic x-ray beam that interacts with the patient before it is detected by a single layered detector. This polyenergetic

a Department of Radiology, Massachusetts General Hospital, 55 Fruit Street, White 270, Boston, MA 02114, USA; b Department of Radiology, NYU Langone Health, 660 1st Avenue, New York, NY 10016, USA; c Department of Radiology and Biomedical Imaging, University of California – San Francisco, 505 Parnassus Avenue, M391, Box 0628, San Francisco, CA 94143-0628, USA; d Department of Radiology, University of Alabama at Birmingham, 619 19th Street, South JTN 456, Birmingham, AL 35249-6830, USA; e Department of Radiology, University of Washington, 1959 Northeast Pacific Street, RR220, Seattle, WA 98112, USA
* Corresponding author. Department of Radiology, Massachusetts General Hospital, 55 Fruit Street, White 270, Boston, MA 02114.
E-mail address: rchung5@mgh.harvard.edu

Radiol Clin N Am 61 (2023) 945–961
https://doi.org/10.1016/j.rcl.2023.05.002

x-ray beam is composed of a spectrum of photons with energies up to a maximum energy or peak kilovoltage (kVp), most commonly 120 kVp.[2] The mean energy of a 120 kVp beam is usually 60-90 kiloelectron volts (keV). The attenuation of tissues as indicated by their linear attenuation coefficient or CT number in Hounsfield units (HU) depends on the x-ray beam energy and the tissue characteristics (density and atomic number).[3–5]

Interactions between the x-ray and the tissues predominantly occur through Compton scatter and the photoelectric effect.[3] Compton scatter is the dominant interaction in CT and occurs when an incident x-ray transfers some energy to an electron in the outermost electron shell of an atom. This interaction results in a subsequent change in the wavelength of the incident x-ray. Compton scatter is mostly dependent on electron density, which correlates with tissue mass density. In contrast, the photoelectric effect occurs in a smaller proportion of interactions in CT when the incident x-ray transfers enough energy to dislodge an electron from the innermost electron shell of an atom (k-shell electron). The resultant void in the k-shell is filled by an electron from a higher electron shell which results in the release of a photon. The photoelectric effect is dependent on the tissue atomic number and the x-ray energy. Current CT contrast agents are based on iodine and barium, which have k-edges of 33 and 37 keV, respectively. At the lower end of the energy spectra typical in medical imaging, the photoelectric effect dominates with the peak attenuation of the x-ray occurring at the k-edge of the material (the energy level just above the k-shell binding energy at which peak attenuation occurs). At higher energies, both interactions decrease, with photoelectric effect decreasing more rapidly than Compton scatter.[3,4]

At SECT, tissues with different atomic numbers (eg, iodine and calcium) may be indistinguishable at a given single energy spectrum due to similar mass densities which result in similar attenuation measurements.[6] The principle of DECT relies on imaging these same tissues at a second energy spectrum, which results in attenuation measurements that now differ from one another. Combining the information obtained by imaging the tissues at two distinct energy levels (high- and low-energy spectra) allows DECT to distinguish these tissues based on attenuation measurements at each energy spectrum as well as the known change in attenuation measurements between energy spectra.[3,6] DECT can also isolate and quantify different materials, providing material specific data sets which is explained later within this article. Additionally, DECT can provide energy-specific data

sets that can optimize contrast visualization, increase lesion conspicuity, reduce contrast dose, or reduce metallic artifact. The abundance of additional data provided by DECT surpasses that of SECT and can aid in diagnosis.

TECHNOLOGY AND NOMENCLATURE

The concept of DECT was first theorized and described in the 1970s[5] but only became a practical reality in the early 2000s because of technological advancements. Today, the different CT vendors have devised several approaches to acquiring DECT images which are divided into source-based and detector-based techniques. The source-based techniques include dual-source, rapid kVp switching, dual-spin, and twin-beam systems while the detector-based techniques include the dual-layer and photon-counting systems.[4] The photon-counting system will be discussed in more detail elsewhere within this issue.

The dual-source system (dsDECT) uses two sets of x-ray tubes and detectors off-set by 90-95 degrees (Fig. 1A). There are currently three generations of the dsDECT system. One source produces a high-energy beam (140–150 kVp) and the other produces a low-energy beam (70–100 kVp). Spectral data are acquired simultaneously; however, the field of view (FOV) of the low-energy tube is 50 cm whereas the FOV of the high-energy tube is between 26 and 36 cm (depending on scanner generation), which limits dual-energy data acquisition in patients with anatomy outside of the overlapping FOVs, for example, in those with large body circumference.[4,7] The main advantage of this system is the flexibility to modulate the tube parameters and filters of the two x-ray tubes independently according to patient body habitus and clinical indication.[4] The main disadvantages of this system include the limited dual-energy FOV, image domain reconstruction, and a need to prospectively select the dual-energy mode.

The rapid kVp switching system (rsDECT) utilizes a single x-ray source that rapidly switches (0.25 msec) between low (80 kVp) and high (135–140 kVp) energies as the gantry rotates around the patient during image acquisition with a single detector layer that receives data from the two different energy beams (Fig. 1B). This means that dual-energy data is acquired near simultaneously allowing for high spatial and temporal resolution of the two energies. This implementation allows for image reconstruction in the projection domain and provides flexibility in material decomposition and the ability to correct for beam hardening artifact.[7] Additionally, the full FOV is available for

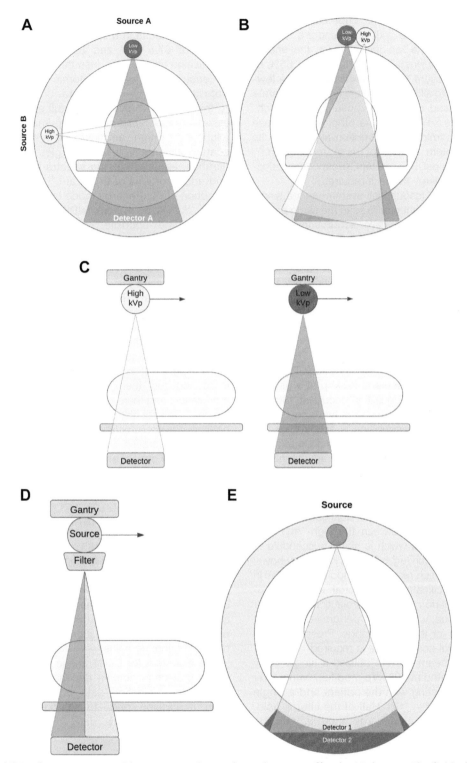

Fig. 1. (*A*) Dual-source system with two x-ray tubes and two detectors offset by 95 degrees. The field-of-view of detector A is 50 cm whereas the field-of-view of detector B is 36 cm. (*B*) Rapid kVp switching system with a single x-ray tube and single layer detector. The x-ray tube rapidly switches from low (*blue*) and high (*yellow*) kV beams as the gantry rotates around the patient. (*C*) Dual-spin system scans the entire patient volume twice, once at low-energy (*yellow*) and once at high-energy (*blue*). Each scan is performed at half the dose of a conventional single energy CT to avoid doubling the dose. (*D*) Twin-beam system uses a filter split into two-halves; a gold filter which

dual-energy reconstruction.[4] Tube current modulation is not possible with one vendor's rsDECT system due to the rapidity at which the energy states alternate. Instead, approximately 65% of the total exposure time is performed in the low-energy state to allow for reduced noise at this state and decreased radiation exposure at the high-energy state.[4] However, the other vendor's use of a deep learning reconstruction algorithm in its rsDECT system allows for dose modulation.[8,9] Similar to the dsDECT system, prospective selection of dual-energy mode is required.

The dual-spin (sequential) system uses a single x-ray source and detector to scan the same patient volume in two consecutive acquisitions at two different energy levels (Fig. 1C). The system operates in either an axial or helical mode. In the axial mode, two gantry rotations (one at each energy level) are obtained at each table position prior to table movement in the z-axis dimension.[6] In the helical mode, the entire scan volume is scanned with a helical acquisition at one energy level followed immediately by a helical acquisition of the same scan volume at another energy level. The scans are performed at an overlapped pitch. Typically, the first acquisition occurs at 80 kVp at a pitch of 0.6 and the second acquisition occurs at 130-140 kVp at a pitch of 1.2. Because two acquisitions are obtained, each acquisition is acquired at half the dose of a conventional 120 kVp scan to avoid increased radiation exposure.[2] The advantages to this system include the ability to optimize tube current modulation and filters at each voltage, a full spectral FOV, and the absence of cross scatter. The main disadvantage to the dual-spin system is the temporal delay between the high- and low-energy acquisitions which is highly susceptible to motion degradation (eg, respiratory, cardiac, bowel motion) and which results in temporal variations in contrast opacification.[2,4] Spectral image reconstruction is performed in the projection domain for the axial mode, whereas it is performed in the image domain for the helical mode. Prospective selection of dual-energy mode is required.

The twin-beam system utilizes a single x-ray source operated at 120 kVp modified with a filter prior to interacting with the patient and a single layer detector (Fig. 1D). Half of the filter is gold, which filters out high-energy photons, and the other half is tin, which filters out low-energy photons. This results in a split beam with mean energies of 67.5 keV and 85.3 keV.[4] A helical acquisition with a pitch less than 0.5 is required to ensure adequate anatomic coverage for both high- and low-energy data.[2,4] An advantage to the twin-beam system is a full spectral FOV. Disadvantages include suboptimal temporal alignment of high- and low-energy data, cross-scatter, inherently lower energies due to the filtration, and overlapping spectra in the central and edge portions of the beam.[4,10] Prospective selection of dual-energy mode is required.

The dual-layer system (dlDECT) has a single x-ray source opposite two layered detectors (Fig. 1E). The inner (top) yttrium-based layer absorbs low-energy photons but allows high-energy photons to pass through. The outer (bottom) gadolinium-based layer absorbs these high-energy photons. The differential absorption of low- and high-energy photons by the two layers is best at 120 and 140 kVp.[7] Because spectral data processing occurs at the detector level, there is excellent spatial and temporal registration. In addition, the prospective selection of dual-energy mode is not required, there are no limitations to dose modulation, and there are no dual-energy FOV limitations.[4] Several disadvantages include cross-talk between the detector layers, occasional inaccurate spectral separation, and a truncated z-axis coverage of 4 cm.[11] Table 1 summarizes and compares the features of each DECT system.

DUAL-ENERGY COMPUTED TOMOGRAPHY IMAGE POSTPROCESSING/RECONSTRUCTION

DECT data contain a wealth of information about the presence and concentration of different materials within imaged tissues and takes advantage of the fact that unique materials have different attenuation values at varying energy levels. DECT image postprocessing either occurs in the projection (pre-reconstruction) or image (post-reconstruction) domains.

The algorithm for DECT image postprocessing in the projection domain depends on high- and low-energy projection data obtained from the scan acquisition prior to tomographic image reconstruction (ie, raw data).[4,12] This requires

---

filters out high-energy photons (*yellow*) and a tin filter which filters out low-energy photons (*blue*). (*E*) Dual-layer system with a single x-ray tube and two layered detectors composed of an inner yttrium layer and an outer gadolinium layer. Low energy photons are absorbed by the inner layer whereas higher energy photons pass through the inner layer and are absorbed by the outer layer. Dual energy information is only available for the anatomy exposed by both beams in the dual-source system (*A*) whereas it is available in all exposed anatomy in the rapid kVp switching, dual-spin, twin-beam, and dual-layer systems (*B–E*).

Table 1
Comparison of technical specifications for DECT scanners

Specification	Source-Based Technique					Detector-Based Technique
	Dual-Source[b]	Rapid kVp Switching[b,c]	Rapid kVp Switching	Dual-Spin[c]	Twin-Beam	Dual-Layer
Vendor	Siemens Healthineers	GE Healthcare	Canon Medical Systems	Canon Medical Systems	Siemens Healthineers	Philips Healthcare
Number of x-ray sources	2	1	1	1	1	1
Number of detectors	2	1	1	1	1	1
DECT acquisition	Prospective	Prospective	Prospective	Prospective	Prospective	Retrospective
Peak tube voltage (kVp)[a]	1. 80/140 2. 80, 100/140 Sn 3. 70, 80, 90, 100/150 Sn	1. 80/140 2. 70/140	80/135	80/135	120 Au Sn	120, 140
Maximum tube current (mA)[a]	1. 500/571 2. 650, 650/714 3. 1300, 1300, 1300, 1200/800	1. 630 2. 570	900	580	800	1000, 750
Dose modulation	1. Yes 2. Yes 3. Yes	1. No 2. No	Yes	Yes	Yes	Yes
Focal spot size (mm)	1. 0.8 × 0.9 2. 0.9 × 1.1 3. 0.8 × 1.1	1. 1.0 × 0.7 2. 1.0 × 0.7	0.9 × 0.8	0.4 × 0.5	0.9 × 1.1	0.6 × 0.7
Field of view (cm)	1. 50/26 2. 50/33 3. 50/35.5	1. 50 2. 50	50	50	50	50
Z-axis coverage (mm)	1. 19.2 2. 38.4 3. 57.6	1. 40 2. 40 or 80 (H); 120, 140, or 160 (A)	160	40–160	38.4	40
Pitch	1. 0.2–1.2 2. 0.2–1.2 3. 0.3–1.2	1. 0.5–1.375 2. 0.5–1.5	Up to 1.575	Up to 1.5	0.25–0.45	0.1–1.8

(continued on next page)

Table 1
(continued)

	Source-Based Technique					Detector-Based Technique
Fastest rotation time (msec)	1. 330 2. 280 3. 250	1. 500 2. 280	275	270	280	270
Temporal offset (msec)	1. 83 2) 75 3. 66	1. 0.25 2. 0.25	<1	270 (A) >1 scan time (H)	310–560	None
Reconstruction domain	Image	Projection	Projection	Projection (A) Image (H)	Image	Projection
Reconstruction method	Iterative	Iterative	Deep Learning	Iterative	Iterative	Iterative

Note—All listed parameters reflect the options available for DECT acquisition only. Sn–tin filter, Au–gold filter.
[a] For dual-source DECT, the "/" separates the kVp and mA settings for the low- and high-energy tubes.
[b] For the dual-source and rapid kVP switching (GE) systems, the "1)," "2)," and "3)" denote the 1st, 2nd, and 3rd generation scanners, respectively.
[c] For the rapid kVp switching (GE) and dual-spin systems, "H" refers to helical mode and "A" refers to axial mode.
Adapted from Parakh A, An C, Lennartz S, et al. Recognizing and Minimizing Artifacts at Dual-Energy CT. *RadioGraphics 2021; 41:509-523;* with permission.

high spatial and temporal registration of both energy datasets which is possible with the rsDECT, dlDECT, and axial dual-spin systems. This technique is less susceptible to beam hardening artifacts.

Image reconstruction in the image domain occurs after the high- and low-energy datasets have been separately reconstructed into high- and low-energy polychromatic images. This occurs in the other DECT systems (dsDECT, twin-beam, and helical dual-spin systems). DECT image postprocessing occurs after the reconstruction of the high- and low-energy images and is more susceptible to beam hardening artifacts, although these can be reduced with improved iterative reconstruction techniques.[13]

TYPES OF IMAGE RECONSTRUCTIONS

All DECT systems can produce multiple image reconstruction types including routine SECT equivalent, virtual monoenergetic, material density (eg, iodine map), and virtual non-contrast (VNC) image reconstructions.[6] **Table 2** summarizes the commonly utilized DECT image reconstructions and their clinical value.

Images appearing similar to those produced by conventional SECT are generally obtained by use of a combination of the high- and low-energy DECT data. In the dsDECT, dual-spin, and twin-beam systems, blended images of approximately 60% low-energy and 40% high-energy data produce images with comparable contrast and noise to SECT images.[4,7] In the rsDECT system, virtual monoenergetic images of approximately 70-77 keV are analogous to the 120-kVp images from SECT.[2] In the dlDECT system, the two detector layers function as a single detector combining both the high- and low-energy data and produce conventional 120-kVp or 140 kVp images directly.[14]

Virtual monoenergetic (monochromatic) images are reconstructed images that would theoretically

Table 2
Dual-energy CT image reconstructions

Image Reconstruction	Clinical Value
Routine SECT equivalent • dsDECT – blended image of low and high kVp data • rsDECT – 70–77 keV monoenergetic image • dlDECT – 120 or 140 kVp image	Routine interpretation
Virtual monoenergetic – low keV (<60 keV)	Increase conspicuity of enhanced structures Reduce required contrast dose
Virtual monoenergetic – high keV (>95 keV)	Reduce metal artifact Reduce image noise
Material density – iodine[a]	Increase conspicuity of enhanced structures Reduce iodinated contrast dose
Material density – uric acid	Characterize urinary tract stone composition Detect possible gouty joint deposits
Material density – calcium	Characterize urinary tract stone composition Distinguish calcium from hemorrhage Detect calcium within bone and plaque
Virtual non-contrast (VNC, VUE)	Determine enhancement Assess for presence of non-enhancing hyperdense material (eg, calcium, hemorrhage) Assess non-contrast attenuation (eg, adrenal nodule or renal lesion characterization) Reduce metal artifact
Effective atomic number (Z effective)	Assess whether a radiodense structure is enhancing (eg, confirm absence of iodine, assess relative atomic number of a given object)

Abbreviations: dlDECT, dual-layer dual-energy CT; dsDECT, dual-source dual-energy CT; keV, kiloelectron volt; kVp, kilovoltage peak; rsDECT, rapid kVp switching dual-energy CT; VNC, virtual non-contrast; VUE, virtual unenhanced.

[a] Pitfall: Bright radiodensities seen on material density iodine reconstructions are not necessarily due to iodine or barium, and might be due to calcium or other radiodense metals. The presence of contrast may be confirmed by showing absence of high density on the virtual non-contrast reconstructions.

be produced from a true monoenergetic x-ray source denoted by its energy in keV.[2] These images are produced from 35 to 200 keV depending on the vendor.[2] Low-energy virtual monoenergetic images (<60 keV) increase the attenuation of iodine because the energy is close to the k-edge of iodine (33 keV). As a result, iodine-containing structures such as contrast-opacified vasculature and hypervascular tumors are more conspicuous with low keV images at the cost of increased noise (Fig. 2). This aids in lesion detection and allows for a reduction in the administered volume of intravenous iodinated contrast.[15] For example, without sacrificing diagnostic quality, iodinated contrast dose reductions of up to 50% are achievable when using 40- and 50-keV monoenergetic images in CT angiography of the abdominal aorta (Fig. 3).[16–19] Iodinated contrast dose reductions of 50% in CT urography[20] and 40% in coronary CT angiography[21] are also possible. High-energy virtual monoenergetic images (>95 keV) have less contrast, but also less noise, and are useful for beam-hardening and metal artifact reduction (Fig. 4).[4]

Material density images are generated from either two-material or three-material decomposition. The two-material decomposition approach is used in single-source DECT systems by selecting two materials (basis pairs) that have two different attenuation characteristics at different energy levels, typically iodine and water. The three-material decomposition approach uses three basis pairs and is used in the dsDECT system and one vendor's rsDECT system. This requires an additional constraint (mass conservation) which assumes that the mass fraction of the three materials adds up to one.[22] Material density images

generated by these methods can produce iodine-only images (iodine maps) which are used for the qualitative and quantitative assessment of iodine uptake/enhancement (Fig. 5).[4] Other material density images, such as uric acid images (for example, to characterize urinary stone composition or possible gouty joint deposits) or calcium images (for example, to detect calcium within vascular plaque and differentiate calcium from hemorrhage within the brain) are also commonly utilized.[4]

VNC images are generated by using iodine-water decomposition to remove the iodine content within tissues. These are qualitatively similar to true non-contrast images at conventional SECT and are useful for assessing the presence of hemorrhage, calcium, and enhancement within structures (see Fig. 5; Fig. 6). Because VNC images are generated from data obtained during a DECT acquisition rather than a separate true non-contrast acquisition, they are free from misregistration that might occur from motion between acquisitions (see Fig. 6). In addition, VNC images avoid additional time and radiation dose incurred when obtaining a separate true non-contrast acquisition. These benefits occur during commonly performed multiphasic studies where a true non-contrast acquisition may be eliminated, for example, CT angiography, CT urography, or multiphasic liver CT with radiation dose reductions between 19 and 60% depending on protocol.[4,23–27]

However, there are differences in quantitative analysis based on scanner geometry and method of VNC image generation, notably the three-material decomposition in dsDECT and the two-material decomposition in rsDECT and dlDECT.[28] In the dsDECT and dlDECT systems, attenuation measurements in HU can be measured directly

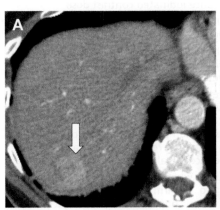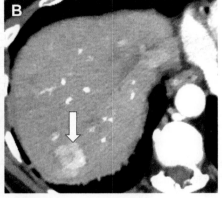

Fig. 2. 61-year-old woman with hepatocellular carcinoma imaged on a dual-layer dual-energy CT scanner. (A) Routine SECT equivalent image at 120 kilovoltage peak and (B) virtual monoenergetic image at 50 kiloelectron volts (keV) in the arterial phase demonstrate a 2.3 cm segment 7 mass with arterial hyperenhancement (arrow). Mass conspicuity is increased on the (B) 50 keV virtual monoenergetic image due to increased attenuation of iodine.

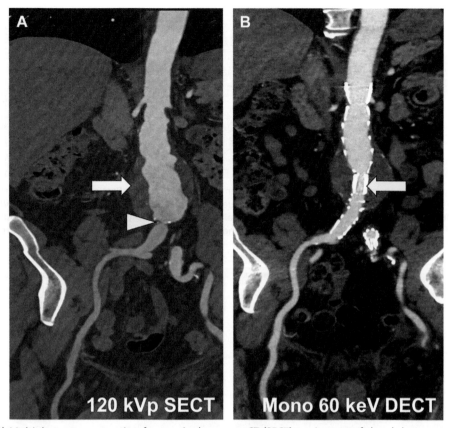

Fig. 3. (A) Multiplanar reconstruction from a single energy CT (SECT) angiogram of the abdomen and pelvis at 120 kilovoltage peak (kVp) with standard iodine dose (33 g) demonstrates a fusiform infrarenal abdominal aortic aneurysm (*white arrow*) and right common iliac artery stenosis (*white arrowhead*). Patient subsequently underwent endovascular aneurysm repair. (B) Multiplanar reconstruction virtual monoenergetic image at 60 kiloelectron volts (keV) from a follow-up dual-energy CT (DECT) angiogram of the abdomen and pelvis performed on a rapid kVp switching system with 50% iodinated contrast dose (16 g) shows a patent endovascular graft (*yellow arrow*). The contrast dose is optimized with 50% reduction in volume with the use of the 60 keV virtual monoenergetic image which allows for diagnostic quality attenuation of the opacified aorta.

on the VNC images. In the rsDECT system, attenuation measurements in HU can be assessed on the virtual unenhanced (VUE) images which are equivalent to the VNC images from the other vendors. However, HU measurements cannot be measured on water images with suppressed iodine (ie, "water (iodine)") image as the values in these images do not represent x-ray attenuation, but instead represent the fractional volume of water within the voxel.[29] Minor quantitative

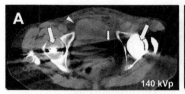
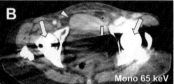
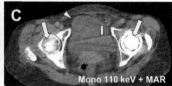

Fig. 4. 57-year-old woman with breast cancer imaged on a rapid kVp switching dual-energy CT scanner. (A) Routine SECT equivalent image at 140 kilovoltage peak, (B) virtual monoenergetic image at 65 kiloelectron volts (keV), and (C) virtual monoenergetic image at a 110 keV with metal artifact reduction algorithm (MAR) demonstrate bilateral metallic hip hardware (*yellow arrows*). Dark bands from beam hardening artifact (*white arrow*) partially obscure the bladder (*white arrowhead*) and other pelvic organs in (A), with increased artifact at low keV (65 keV) in (B) and markedly reduced artifact at high keV (110 keV) with MAR in (C) where there is improved visualization of pelvic organs.

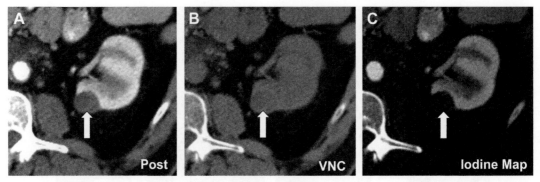

Fig. 5. 68-year-old man imaged on a dual-layer dual-energy CT scanner. (*A*) Post-contrast and (*B*) virtual non-contrast (VNC) images demonstrate a 2.0 cm hypoattenuating left posterior interpolar renal lesion (*white arrow*) with attenuation measurements of 34 and 25 Hounsfield units, respectively. (*C*) Iodine map demonstrates the absence of iodine within the renal lesion. Imaging findings are compatible with a non-enhancing renal cyst with hemorrhagic/proteinaceous contents.

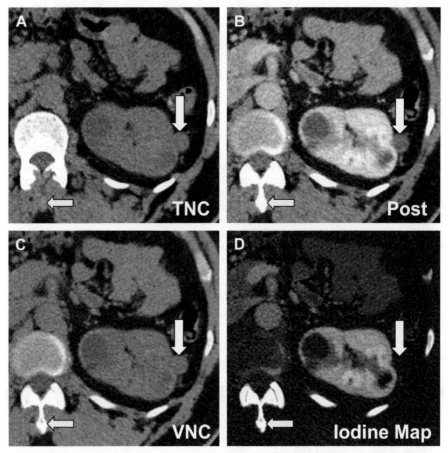

Fig. 6. 55-year-old man imaged on a dual-source dual-energy CT scanner. (*A*) True non-contrast (TNC), (*B*) nephrographic phase (post), and (*C*) virtual non-contrast (VNC) images demonstrate a 1.5 cm hypoattenuating left lateral interpolar renal lesion (*white arrow*) with attenuation measurements of 32, 28, and 25 Hounsfield units, respectively. (*D*) Iodine map demonstrates absence of iodine within the renal lesion (*white arrow*). Imaging findings are compatible with a non-enhancing renal cyst with hemorrhagic/proteinaceous contents. The spinous process of the vertebral body (*yellow arrow*) is absent in the TNC image (*A*) and present in the post, VNC, and iodine map images (*B–D*). There is slight misregistration in the z-axis dimension between the TNC and post images because they are two separate acquisitions. However, there is perfect registration between the latter three images because they are derived from the same data obtained from a single acquisition.

differences in attenuation measurements varies across vendor systems, organ of interest, phase of contrast, and radiation dose which should all be taken into consideration when evaluating the diagnostic value of a given attenuation measurement.[28,29] The attenuation measurements on VNC images obtained on a dsDECT scanner compared to those obtained on true non-contrast images were within 15 HU in one patient study,[30] and the HU obtained on rsDECT and dlDECT system were within 10 HU of the expected values for soft tissue and unenhanced blood in a phantom study.[29]

WORKFLOW CONSIDERATIONS
Patient Selection

Apart from the dlDECT system, the remainder of the DECT systems require a prospective selection of dual-energy mode. However, it is of the authors' opinions that patients should be scanned with DECT whenever possible because of the added information provided by DECT acquisitions. This is particularly helpful when encountering incidental findings, such as adrenal and renal masses, which may otherwise require additional imaging for further characterization if identified in a single phase SECT acquisition (**Fig. 7**).[31–35] As mentioned previously, scanning on DECT scanners can also reduce the volume of intravenously administered iodinated contrast and can provide substantial radiation dose reduction.[15] Scanning patients on DECT scanners whenever possible obviates the need to select patients for dual-energy mode and instead allows the technologist or radiologist to reserve the right to select patients for SECT when DECT is not feasible or appropriate, such as in large patients.

Large patient size can erode image quality, increase artifacts, and potentially compromise diagnosis.[36] This is a result of increased image noise and photon starvation that is more likely to occur at a low kVp setting (for example, 80 kVp in the rsDECT system or 70–80 kVp in the dsDECT system) when there is greater photon attenuation by increased patient thickness and fewer photons reaching the detector.[7,10,37–39] This has been shown to reduce the detection accuracy and characterization of urinary tract stones < 3 mm in size but not in clinically significant stones > 3 mm in size.[37,40–42] Of note, each DECT system has its own way of mitigating the impact of increased image noise from the low kVp source.

When imaging larger patients with the dsDECT system, the low-energy source is set at 90-100 kVp instead of 80 kVp for improved x-ray penetration.[40,43] The disadvantage to the use of a 100 kVp low-energy source is increased radiation dose and spectral overlap with the high-energy beam. To mitigate this, a tin filter is applied to the high-energy source to remove low-energy photons which contribute to radiation dose and spectral overlap. Tube current modulation is also available in the dsDECT system which helps further reduce radiation dose. As mentioned previously, a major drawback in the dsDECT system is the smaller FOV of the second source-detector set which limits the overlapping dual-energy FOV. As a result, proper positioning of the patient to include the area of interest within the overlapping FOV is critical to harnessing the advantage of DECT in this system. Although this may be difficult to determine prospectively, the dual-energy FOV is located centrally and encompasses the internal organs while excluding the skin, subcutaneous fat, and musculature in most patients. Occasionally, particularly in larger patients, this may exclude peripherally located organs of interest, for example, peripheral portions of the liver, spleen, and colon (**Fig. 8**).

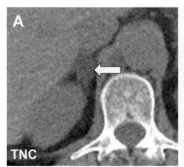 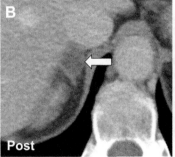 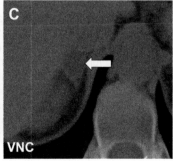

Fig. 7. 59-year-old woman imaged on a rapid kVp switching dual-energy CT scanner. (*A*) True non-contrast (TNC), (*B*) portal venous phase, and (*C*) virtual non-contrast (VNC) images demonstrate a 1.5 cm homogeneous hypoattenuating right adrenal nodule (*white arrow*) with attenuation measurements of −8, 20, and 6 Hounsfield units, respectively. The findings confirm an enhancing right adrenal nodule with a non-contrast attenuation of ≤10 Hounsfield units (both on TNC and VNC images) which is compatible with an adrenal adenoma.

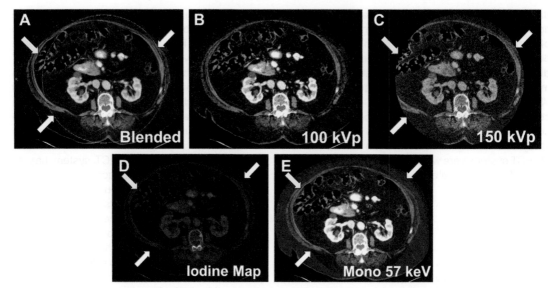

Fig. 8. 85-year-old woman with lung cancer imaged on a dual-source dual-energy CT scanner. (*A*) Blended routine SECT equivalent, (*B*) low-energy source (100 kVp), (*C*) high-energy source (150 kVp), (*D*) iodine map, and (*E*) 57 kiloelectron volt (keV) virtual monoenergetic images. Dual-energy data is only available in the overlapping fields of view with the yellow circle in (*A*) (*white arrow*) denoting the field of view of the high energy source with a corresponding artifact on the iodine map and monoenergetic image reconstructions. Tissues such as portions of the right colon (*yellow arrow*) and subcutaneous fat are excluded from dual-energy characterization.

Because the low-energy source is fixed at 80 kVp in the rsDECT system, other methods are required to mitigate increased noise in large patients. For example, higher tube current, slower rotation time, and lower pitch increase the photon flux to improve image quality at the cost of higher radiation dose.[36] In contrast to the dsDECT system, tube current modulation to help reduce radiation dose is not possible with the rsDECT system.

In dlDECT, body habitus did not impact image quality or material decomposition when 70 keV virtual monoenergetic images were compared with conventional 120 kVp images.[44] However, the x-ray source in dlDECT can be increased from 120 kVp to 140 kVp as needed to improve image quality and spectral separation.[45]

Additionally, deep learning reconstruction techniques in one vendor's rsDECT system and iterative reconstruction techniques in the other systems can further improve image quality. Despite these above-described mitigation techniques, many institutions exclude the use of DECT in patients with large body habitus defined as >260 lbs (118 kg) or 38-46 cm in maximal transverse dimension and instead scan these patients on SECT mode.[7,46]

The technologist plays a critical role in protocol optimization, appropriate patient selection, and the acquisition of diagnostic images. The technologist must be aware of the above-described limitations for each system, for example, to ensure proper patient positioning in the dsDECT system because of spectral FOV limitations, to select 90-100 kVp instead of 80 kVp for the low-energy source in the dsDECT system, to adjust other scan parameters to maintain adequate image quality in the rsDECT system due to the restricted 80 kVp low-energy acquisition, and to opt for SECT scanning in patients not suitable for DECT scanning.[7,15]

Protocol Selection

In addition to patient selection, the process of protocol selection plays a direct role in the workflow. To optimize workflow efficiency and simplicity, particularly at initial implementation, the determination of DECT acquisition is best determined at the protocol level (eg, multiphasic liver CT) rather than the indication level (eg, cirrhosis) which avoids the need to sort through indications to determine whether DECT is appropriate.[46] Finer customization of DECT protocols also involves determining which phase(s) of contrast in multiphasic studies should be performed with DECT. A consensus panel on DECT recommends DECT acquisition in the arterial phase of multiphasic abdominal examinations, nephrographic phase of CT urograms, and for certain single-phase and renal stone examinations.[46]

Additional considerations for the DECT protocol design include reductions in radiation and iodinated contrast doses. Depending on department preference, a DECT protocol may eliminate true non-contrast acquisitions and instead replace them with VNC images to substantially reduce radiation dose without compromising diagnosis. As previously discussed, iodinated contrast dose reductions of up to 50% without sacrificing diagnostic quality are achievable by using low keV monoenergetic images.[16–21] Routine creation of low keV monoenergetic reconstructions for certain protocols (eg, CT angiography) may allow for lower iodinated contrast volumes in patients with or without renal dysfunction.

Image Transfer and Interpretation

There are three main methods for generating dual-energy images from the CT data. The first method involves the creation of the images at a dedicated vendor-specific workstation. After the CT data is pushed to the workstation, an individual with appropriate expertise, (eg, technologist, radiologist) processes the data to create the desired images and then pushes them to the picture archiving and communications system (PACS).[47] This method requires manual post-processing which is time and labor intensive, requires proficiency with the workstation, and is limited by the physical location of the workstation. Furthermore, interruptions (eg, phone call, emergency) experienced by the user during post-processing can disrupt workflow and result in variability in the quality and availability of images.

An alternative method of DECT image postprocessing utilizes a thin-client server. The vendor-specific thin-client software can be installed on any computer and accesses the server that processes the data. It provides comparatively better access than the standalone workstation and can be used on the same PACS workstation used for interpretation for improved workflow integration.[47] However, like the standalone workstation, CT data must first be pushed to the thin-client server before post-processing is performed, and it requires manual post-processing by an individual proficient with the software. Once the images are generated, the user can then push the images to the PACS. The third method of generating DECT images occurs directly at the CT console and avoids many of the previous methods' disadvantages, notably the dependence on manual post-processing. Following the acquisition of the CT data, a standard set of images (depending on scanner vendor, imaging protocol, and departmental preference) are automatically generated at the CT console which can be predetermined during initial DECT workflow implementation.

Standardizing the image sets helps automate the image reconstruction process and allows the technologist to carry out other tasks (eg, helping the patient off the scan table, preparing the scanner for the next patient) while the images are reconstructed. Once complete, the postprocessed images are automatically sent to the PACS without additional post-processing required by the radiologist. The CT data is also often sent to the vendor-specific workstation or thin-client server for archival purposes or for additional postprocessing which provides flexibility on top of standardization.

Regardless of the approach by which DECT images are created and transferred to the PACS, an important consideration is the greater volume of data produced by DECT acquisitions compared to that produced by SECT acquisitions and its effect on data transfer and storage.[7,48] A single DECT acquisition generates many times the number of images (eg, blended, high-energy, low-energy, and VNC images in the dsDECT system) as a SECT examination. When implementing and maintaining a DECT system, a department must consider the strategies required to avoid burdening the system. For example, purchasing additional server space and being selective about which DECT images are created under each protocol while reserving additional post-processing for troubleshooting.[7,48]

The DECT images generated by the CT data and sent to PACS vary by vendor, imaging protocol, and departmental preference. Routine SECT equivalent images (blended images in dsDECT, 70–77 keV monoenergetic images in rsDECT, and 120 or 140 kVp equivalent images in dlDECT) along with their multiplanar reconstructions are routinely generated by the scanners and sent to PACS for interpretation. Additional DECT images such as iodine maps, monoenergetic images at various keV, and VNC images can be created and sent to PACS, based on departmental preference. As discussed previously, low keV monoenergetic images can help accentuate hypervascular tumors, contrast-opacified vasculature, or sources of gastrointestinal bleeding and high keV monoenergetic images can reduce metallic artifacts. Iodine maps can increase radiologist confidence in differentiating cysts or hemorrhage from enhancing tumors particularly in the setting of incidental findings, and VNC images can replace true non-contrast images in various protocols, resulting in significant radiation dose reduction. Any image set not initially created can be reconstructed at a later time on the dedicated workstation or with the thin-client server. **Fig. 9** is a schematic summary of a DECT workflow.

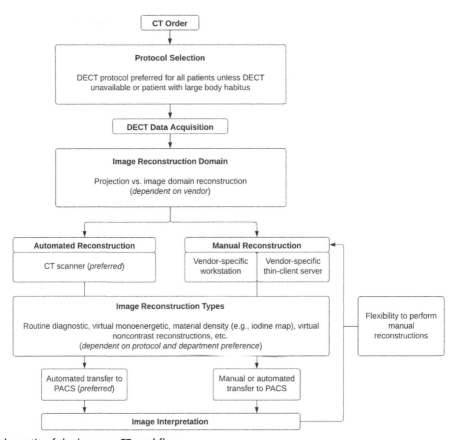

Fig. 9. Schematic of dual-energy CT workflow.

Artificial Intelligence

Artificial intelligence (AI) and its subsets of machine learning and deep learning play a current and future role in optimizing CT and DECT workflow (eg, order entry, scan acquisition, image reconstruction, image interpretation, report generation).[49–51] For example, one CT vendor's infrared camera and trained AI algorithm optimizes radiation dose by automatically positioning the patient at the isocenter which substantially decreases positioning errors when compared to manual patient positioning.[52,53] Appropriate patient positioning optimizes the automatic exposure control which adjusts the tube current at different body regions as the gantry rotates around the patient. Deep learning algorithms improve image reconstructions by reducing noise and artifacts.[50,51] One vendor's rsDECT system uses a deep learning reconstruction algorithm to generate DECT images. This algorithm exploits the fact that there is redundant anatomic information between the low- and high-energy data sets and transforms views of one energy into the other to create "Deep Learning Views."[8,9] Information provided in the "Deep Learning Views" and the actual

measured views creates a complete sinogram at each energy level which is further reconstructed into the desired DECT images and optimized with additional reconstruction techniques. With all vendors, automated DECT image generation and transfer to the PACS is currently available and should be adjusted by protocol and department preference to provide seamless optimized DECT image interpretation. Furthermore, AI has the potential to improve lesion detection, characterization, and segmentation, and process large volumes of parametric data present in DECT datasets which can further improve DECT workflow.[49,54]

SUMMARY

Compared to conventional SECT, DECT provides additional information to better characterize imaged tissues. Approaches to DECT acquisition vary by vendor and include source-based and detector-based systems, each with its own advantages and disadvantages. Despite the different approaches to DECT acquisition, the most utilized DECT images include routine SECT equivalent, virtual monoenergetic, material density (eg, iodine map), and VNC images. These images are generated either through reconstructions in the projection or image domains. Designing and implementing an optimal DECT workflow into routine clinical practice depends on radiologist and technologist input with special considerations including appropriate patient and protocol selection and workflow automation. In addition to better tissue characterization, DECT provides numerous advantages over SECT such as the characterization of incidental findings and dose reductions in radiation and iodinated contrast. Further discussion on subspecialty specific uses of DECT technology and the concept of photon-counting detectors is discussed later within this issue.

DISCLOSURES

R. Chung: No relevant disclosures. B. Dane: Speaker honorarium and research support from Siemens Healthineers, Germany. B.M. Yeh: Research grants from GE Healthcare, Philips Healthcare, and Canon Medical Systems. Speaker for GE Healthcare, United States and Philips Healthcare. Shareholder of Nextrast, Inc. Book royalties from Oxford University Press. Patent royalties from the University of California, San Francisco. D.E. Morgan: UAB receives research support (equipment) from GE Healthcare used by Dr Morgan to carry out DECT investigations. D.V. Sahani: Consultant for GE Healthcare, Canon Medical Systems, Japan, and Philips Healthcare. Advisory board member for Bayer, Germany. A. Kambadakone: Research grants from Philips Healthcare, GE Healthcare, PanCAN, United States, and Bayer. Consultant for Bayer Advisory Board.

ACKNOWLEDGMENTS

The authors would like to thank Nayla Mroueh for her assistance in gathering images for this article.

REFERENCES

1. Rubin GD. Computed tomography: revolutionizing the practice of medicine for 40 years. Radiology 2014;273(2 Suppl):S45–74.
2. Siegel MJ, Kaza RK, Bolus DN, et al. White paper of the society of computed body tomography and magnetic resonance on dual-energy CT, part 1: technology and terminology. J Comput Assist Tomogr 2016;40(6):841–5.
3. Omoumi P, Becce F, Racine D, et al. Dual-energy CT: basic principles, technical approaches, and applications in musculoskeletal imaging (part 1). Semin Muscoskel Radiol 2015;19(5):431–7.
4. Rajiah P, Parakh A, Kay F, et al. Update on multienergy CT: physics, principles, and applications. Radiographics 2020;40(5):1284–308.
5. Hounsfield GN. Computerized transverse axial scanning (tomography). 1. Description of system. Br J Radiol 1973;46(552):1016–22.
6. McCollough CH, Leng S, Yu L, et al. Dual- and multienergy CT: principles, technical approaches, and clinical applications. Radiology 2015;276(3):637–53.
7. Megibow AJ, Kambadakone A, Ananthakrishnan L. Dual-energy computed tomography: image acquisition, processing, and workflow. Radiol Clin North Am 2018;56(4):507–20.
8. Boedeker K, Hayes M, Zhou J, et al. Deep learning spectral CT - faster, easier and more intelligent [White Paper]. Canon Medical Systems; 2019.
9. Kojima T, Shirasaka T, Kondo M, et al. A novel fast kilovoltage switching dual-energy CT with deep learning: accuracy of CT number on virtual monochromatic imaging and iodine quantification. Phys Med 2021;81:253–61.
10. Parakh A, An C, Lennartz S, et al. Recognizing and minimizing artifacts at dual-energy CT. Radiographics 2021;41(3):E96.
11. Almeida IP, Schyns LE, Ollers MC, et al. Dual-energy CT quantitative imaging: a comparison study between twin-beam and dual-source CT scanners. Med Phys 2017;44(1):171–9.
12. Patino M, Prochowski A, Agrawal MD, et al. Material separation using dual-energy CT: Current and Emerging Applications. Radiographics 2016;36(4):1087–105.
13. Kyriakou Y, Meyer E, Prell D, et al. Empirical beam hardening correction (EBHC) for CT. Med Phys 2010;37(10):5179–87.
14. Rassouli N, Etesami M, Dhanantwari A, et al. Detector-based spectral CT with a novel dual-layer technology: principles and applications. Insights Imaging 2017;8(6):589–98.
15. Megibow AJ, Sahani D. Best practice: implementation and use of abdominal dual-energy CT in routine patient care. AJR Am J Roentgenol 2012;199(5 Suppl):S71–7.
16. Agrawal MD, Oliveira GR, Kalva SP, et al. Prospective comparison of reduced-iodine-dose virtual monochromatic imaging dataset from dual-energy CT angiography with standard-iodine-dose single-energy CT angiography for abdominal aortic aneurysm. AJR Am J Roentgenol 2016;207(6):W125–32.
17. Pinho DF, Kulkarni NM, Krishnaraj A, et al. Initial experience with single-source dual-energy CT abdominal angiography and comparison with single-energy CT angiography: image quality, enhancement, diagnosis and radiation dose. Eur Radiol 2013;23(2):351–9.
18. Patino M, Parakh A, Lo GC, et al. Virtual monochromatic dual-energy aortoiliac CT angiography with

reduced iodine dose: a prospective randomized study. AJR Am J Roentgenol 2019;212(2):467–74.

19. Shuman WP, Chan KT, Busey JM, et al. Dual-energy CT aortography with 50% reduced iodine dose versus single-energy CT aortography with standard iodine dose. Acad Radiol 2016;23(5):611–8.

20. Shuman WP, Mileto A, Busey JM, et al. Dual-energy CT Urography with 50% reduced iodine dose versus single-energy CT urography with standard iodine dose. AJR Am J Roentgenol 2019;212(1):117–23.

21. Rotzinger DC, Si-Mohamed SA, Yerly J, et al. Reduced-iodine-dose dual-energy coronary CT angiography: qualitative and quantitative comparison between virtual monochromatic and polychromatic CT images. Eur Radiol 2021;31(9):7132–42.

22. Liu X, Yu L, Primak AN, et al. Quantitative imaging of element composition and mass fraction using dual-energy CT: three-material decomposition. Med Phys 2009;36(5):1602–9.

23. Baliyan V, Shaqdan K, Hedgire S, et al. Vascular computed tomography angiography technique and indications. Cardiovasc Diagn Ther 2019;9(Suppl 1):S14–27.

24. Sun H, Hou XY, Xue I ID, et al. Dual-source dual-energy CT angiography with virtual non-enhanced images and iodine map for active gastrointestinal bleeding: image quality, radiation dose and diagnostic performance. Eur J Radiol 2015;84(5):884–91.

25. Stolzmann P, Frauenfelder T, Pfammatter T, et al. Endoleaks after endovascular abdominal aortic aneurysm repair: detection with dual-energy dual-source CT. Radiology 2008;249(2):682–91.

26. Chandarana H, Godoy MC, Vlahos I, et al. Abdominal aorta: evaluation with dual-source dual-energy multidetector CT after endovascular repair of aneurysms–initial observations. Radiology 2008;249(2):692–700.

27. Ho LM, Yoshizumi TT, Hurwitz LM, et al. Dual energy versus single energy MDCT: measurement of radiation dose using adult abdominal imaging protocols. Acad Radiol 2009;16(11):1400–7.

28. Lennartz S, Pisuchpen N, Parakh A, et al. Virtual unenhanced images: qualitative and quantitative comparison between different dual-energy CT scanners in a patient and phantom study. Invest Radiol 2022;57(1):52–61.

29. Li B, Pomerleau M, Gupta A, et al. Accuracy of dual-energy CT virtual unenhanced and material-specific images: a phantom study. AJR Am J Roentgenol 2020;215(5):1146–54.

30. Toepker M, Moritz T, Krauss B, et al. Virtual non-contrast in second-generation, dual-energy computed tomography: reliability of attenuation values. Eur J Radiol 2012;81(3):e398–405.

31. Gnannt R, Fischer M, Goetti R, et al. Dual-energy CT for characterization of the incidental adrenal mass: preliminary observations. AJR Am J Roentgenol 2012;198(1):138–44.

32. Ho LM, Marin D, Neville AM, et al. Characterization of adrenal nodules with dual-energy CT: can virtual unenhanced attenuation values replace true unenhanced attenuation values? AJR Am J Roentgenol 2012;198(4):840–5.

33. Graser A, Johnson TR, Hecht EM, et al. Dual-energy CT in patients suspected of having renal masses: can virtual nonenhanced images replace true nonenhanced images? Radiology 2009;252(2):433–40.

34. Kaza RK, Caoili EM, Cohan RH, et al. Distinguishing enhancing from nonenhancing renal lesions with fast kilovoltage-switching dual-energy CT. AJR Am J Roentgenol 2011;197(6):1375–81.

35. Meyer M, Nelson RC, Vernuccio F, et al. Virtual unenhanced images at dual-energy CT: influence on renal lesion characterization. Radiology 2019;291(2):381–90.

36. Fursevich DM, LiMarzi GM, O'Dell MC, et al. Bariatric CT imaging: challenges and solutions. Radiographics 2016;36(4):1076–86.

37. Primak AN, Fletcher JG, Vrtiska TJ, et al. Noninvasive differentiation of uric acid versus non-uric acid kidney stones using dual-energy CT. Acad Radiol 2007;14(12):1441–7.

38. Guimaraes LS, Fletcher JG, Harmsen WS, et al. Appropriate patient selection at abdominal dual-energy CT using 80 kV: relationship between patient size, image noise, and image quality. Radiology 2010;257(3):732–42.

39. Jepperson MA, Cernigliaro JG, Sella D, et al. Dual-energy CT for the evaluation of urinary calculi: image interpretation, pitfalls and stone mimics. Clin Radiol 2013;68(12):e707–14.

40. Qu M, Jaramillo-Alvarez G, Ramirez-Giraldo JC, et al. Urinary stone differentiation in patients with large body size using dual-energy dual-source computed tomography. Eur Radiol 2013;23(5):1408–14.

41. Kordbacheh H, Baliyan V, Singh P, et al. Rapid kVp switching dual-energy CT in the assessment of urolithiasis in patients with large body habitus: preliminary observations on image quality and stone characterization. Abdom Radiol (NY) 2019;44(3):1019–26.

42. Kordbacheh H, Baliyan V, Uppot RN, et al. Dual-source dual-energy CT in detection and characterization of urinary stones in patients with large body habitus: observations in a large cohort. AJR Am J Roentgenol 2019;212(4):796–801.

43. Baliyan V, Kordbacheh H, Serrao J, et al. Dual-source dual-energy CT portal venous phase abdominal CT scans in large body habitus patients: preliminary observations on image quality and material decomposition. J Comput Assist Tomogr 2018;42(6):932–6.

44. Atwi NE, Smith DL, Flores CD, et al. Dual-energy CT in the obese: a preliminary retrospective review to evaluate quality and feasibility of the single-source dual-detector implementation. Abdom Radiol (NY) 2019;44(2):783–9.

45. van Ommen F, Bennink E, Vlassenbroek A, et al. Image quality of conventional images of dual-layer SPECTRAL CT: a phantom study. Med Phys 2018; 45(7):3031–42.

46. Patel BN, Alexander L, Allen B, et al. Dual-energy CT workflow: multi-institutional consensus on standardization of abdominopelvic MDCT protocols. Abdom Radiol (NY) 2017;42(3):676–87.

47. Tamm EP, Le O, Liu X, et al. "How to" incorporate dual-energy imaging into a high volume abdominal imaging practice. Abdom Radiol (NY) 2017;42(3): 688–701.

48. Mileto A, Ananthakrishnan L, Morgan DE, et al. Clinical Implementation of dual-energy CT for gastrointestinal imaging. AJR Am J Roentgenol 2021; 217(3):651–63.

49. Hosny A, Parmar C, Quackenbush J, et al. Artificial intelligence in radiology. Nat Rev Cancer 2018; 18(8):500–10.

50. McCollough CH, Leng S. Use of artificial intelligence in computed tomography dose optimisation. Ann ICRP 2020;49(1_suppl):113–25.

51. Lell MM, Kachelriess M. Recent and upcoming technological developments in computed tomography: high speed, low dose, deep learning, multienergy. Invest Radiol 2020;55(1):8–19.

52. Saltybaeva N, Schmidt B, Wimmer A, et al. Precise and automatic patient positioning in computed tomography: avatar modeling of the patient surface using a 3-dimensional camera. Invest Radiol 2018;53(11):641–6.

53. Booij R, Budde RPJ, Dijkshoorn ML, et al. Accuracy of automated patient positioning in CT using a 3D camera for body contour detection. Eur Radiol 2019;29(4):2079–88.

54. Su KH, Kuo JW, Jordan DW, et al. Machine learning-based dual-energy CT parametric mapping. Phys Med Biol 2018;63(12):125001.

Dual-Energy Computed Tomography: Integration Into Clinical Practice and Cost Considerations

Lakshmi Ananthakrishnan, MD[a],*, Naveen Kulkarni, MD[b], Aran Toshav, MD[c]

KEYWORDS

- Multi-energy CT • Workflow optimization • Dual-energy CT • Efficiency • Spectral

KEY POINTS

- A workflow to direct appropriate patients for scanning on DECT is needed. This workflow may incorporate patient size, indication for the exam, or both.
- An automated workflow in which pre-selected reconstructions are automatically postprocessed and sent to PACS is preferred to decrease post-processing burden for technologists and radiologists.
- If distant future postprocessing of MECT data is desired, image archiving modifications are needed to permanently store spectral data for future use.
- MECT use in the Emergency Department can be used for incidentaloma characterization with resultant cost and time savings, as well as improved reader diagnostic confidence.

INTRODUCTION

Although the various scanner implementations of dual-energy CT (DECT) have different methods of obtaining DECT reconstructions, a common theme to successful implementation of DECT into practice is recognizing and addressing workflow modifications for all stakeholders. In this article, the authors outline various strategies for successful integration of a DECT program into practice, including patient selection strategies, automating creation of reconstructions, and getting buy-in from the health care system regarding the value of DECT.

Patient Selection

Most radiology practices have a mix of both single-energy and DECT scanners. Therefore, strategies are needed to identify patients who would benefit from DECT and triage those patients to the appropriate scanners. There is no single strategy for patient selection for DECT, but general trends have emerged over the years.[1] Strategies may be based on patient size, indication, or both.

Strategies Based on Patient Size

Dual-source dual-energy CT

For dual-source DECT (Siemens Healthineers, Erlangen, Germany), a size-based patient selection strategy is needed when scanning in dual-energy mode, as a field-of-view limitation exists due to a discrepancy in the detector array size of tubes A (50 cm) and B (33 cm for second-generation scanner, 35 cm for third-generation scanner). This discrepancy could result in important anatomy being excluded from the DECT field of view (FOV) (Fig. 1). Some institutions may choose to create a weight- or transverse

[a] Department of Radiology, UT Southwestern Medical Center, 5323 Harry Hines Boulevard, Dallas, TX 75390, USA; [b] Department of Radiology, Medical College of Wisconsin, 9200 West Wisconsin Avenue, Milwaukee, WI 53226, USA; [c] Department of Radiology, Southeast Louisiana Veterans Healthcare System, LSUHSC, New Orleans, LA 70119, USA
* Corresponding author.
E-mail address: lakshmi.ananthakrishnan@utsouthwestern.edu

Radiol Clin N Am 61 (2023) 963–971
https://doi.org/10.1016/j.rcl.2023.05.003
0033-8389/23/© 2023 Elsevier Inc. All rights reserved.

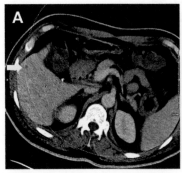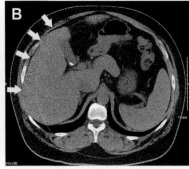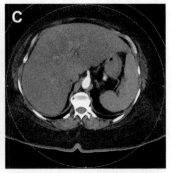

Fig. 1. Field of view (FOV) concerns with dual-source DECT. (*A*) Patient scanned on a second-generation dual-source DECT scanner (33 cm FOV) was not appropriately centered in the gantry, resulting in a lesion (*arrow*) being partially obscured by the circle (which delineates the anatomy included in the FOV of both x-ray sources). There is a FOV discrepancy between the two detector arrays of a dual source DECT, so appropriate positioning of the anatomy in the center of the gantry is vital. This is less of an issue with the later generation scanners with a larger DECT FOV. (*B*) Patient scanned on a second-generation dual-source DECT scanner, where the smaller detector array has a 33-cm FOV. Exclusion of less critical anatomy such as subcutaneous fat is a common occurrence for patients of larger body habitus scanned on dual-source DECT. However, in this patient who weighed 285 pounds (body mass index 38.7), portions of the liver were excluded from the full DECT FOV. To avoid this pitfall, many institutions use a size-based cutoff for imaging patients in DECT mode. (*C*) Patient weighing 280 pounds scanned on a third-generation dual-source DECT scanner (35 cm DECT field of view) with a 3D isocenter camera. Important anatomy was included in the field of view.

diameter-based cutoff for scanning in DECT mode on a dual-source scanner,[1] whereas others rely on technologist judgment.[2] In the author's practice, patients less than 280 pounds are scanned in dual-energy mode on a dual-source scanner to facilitate inclusion of important anatomy in the DECT field of view. Newer generation scanners are now equipped with a 3D isocenter camera (FAST 3D Camera, Siemens Healthineers, Erlangen, Germany) positioned above the CT table. This camera creates a 3D avatar of the patient and then uses that avatar along with a single topogram to automatically isocenter the patient in the CT gantry.[3] Dane and colleagues found that the use of the isocenter camera resulted in approximately 9.5 mm improvement in isocentering the patient in the gantry, with a resultant 21% to 31% decrease in radiation dose, depending on the anatomy scanned.[4] However, although the isocenter camera improves overall patient centering in the gantry (see Fig. 1C), its effect on centering relevant anatomy within the DECT FOV is unclear.

Rapid kV-switching dual-energy CT

In earlier rapid kV-switching CT systems (GE Healthcare, Milwaukee, WI), tube current modulation was not possible, impacting dose efficiency. Further, because the low-energy acquisition is restricted to 80 kVp, image noise is a concern, especially when scanning chest and abdomen/pelvis in large patients: if parameters were to be adjusted to increase photon flux, this would come at the cost of excess radiation dose to the patient.[5,6] Therefore, in the authors' experience, selecting patients with a weight of less than 250 pounds for imaging on rapid kV switching DECT provides the radiologist with optimal image quality. Patients weighing more than 250 pounds are generally not selected for dual-energy scanning due to image noise concerns, although on newer generation scanners (Revolution CT/Revolution Apex, GE Healthcare) patients up to 300 pounds for abdomen/pelvis and 350 pounds for chest indications can be scanned after careful patient selection. Unlike fixed mA on older rapid kV-switching DECT systems, Revolution Apex with the newer Quantix x-ray tube (GE Healthcare, Milwaukee, WI) offers synchronized kV and mA switching that allows increased flux associated with low-kV projections to match high-kV views.[7] This feature improves the image noise of low-kiloelectron volts (keV) and iodine images by over 10% compared with conventional technology and facilitates scanning larger patients (Fig. 2). Deep learning reconstruction now offered on the rapid kV-switching system can further decrease image noise.[8,9] There is no field of view limitation on the rapid kV-switching system because a single detector is used to acquire projections from both data sets, and therefore full 50 cm effective dual-energy FOV is feasible. Single-tube design with a lack of kV combinations other than 80 and 140 and inability to modulate tube current limits rapid kV-switching DECT applications in the pediatric age group.[10]

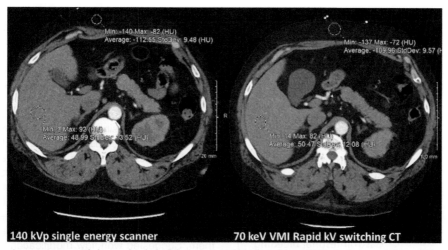

140 kVp single energy scanner | **70 keV VMI Rapid kV switching CT**

Fig. 2. Imaging patients with larger body habitus on rapid kV-switching DECT. Patient weighing 332 pounds was imaged on a single-energy scanner at 140 kVp (*left*) and on a rapid kV-switching DECT scanner (*right*) with a higher output Quantix tube (GE Healthcare). Image noise (standard deviation in subcutaneous fat) is comparable between the two scans. Increased photon flux from the higher output x-ray tube allows for imaging patients with larger body habitus who otherwise could have been precluded from DECT imaging.

Dual-layer detector dual-energy CT

For the dual-layer detector CT scanner (Philips Healthcare, Einthoven, the Netherlands), Atwi and colleagues demonstrated the feasibility and maintained image quality in patients greater than 270 pounds.[11] As the spectral separation is performed at the detector level, the conventional images appear similar in image quality to images from a comparable single-energy CT scanner, and monoenergetic reconstructions can be used to decrease image noise on all patients regardless of size (**Fig. 3**). No weight or size cutoff is used on a dual-layer detector scanner in the authors' practice.

Indication-Based Strategies

Practices may choose to send patients to a DECT scanner based on the indication for the examination. For outpatient examinations in the oncology setting, certain malignancies may be preferentially routed to DECT. A multi-institutional consensus study involving major academic centers published institutional practices and preferences regarding which phases of a multiphase examination where DECT was highest yield. Participating institutions supported the use of dual-energy mode in the arterial phase for multiphase examinations (liver and pancreas indications) and nephrographic

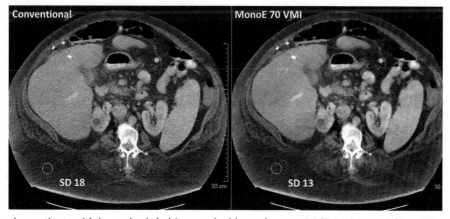

Conventional | MonoE 70 VMI
SD 18 | SD 13

Fig. 3. Imaging patients with larger body habitus on dual-layer detector DECT. Patient weighing 420 pounds was imaged on a dual-layer detector DECT scanner. Image noise on the conventional image (*left*) was comparable to noise when the patient was imaged on a single-energy scanner (not shown). Image noise can further be improved by use of VMI (*right*).

Table 1 Current indications for dual-energy CT scanning	
Body Region	**Suggested Indications for DECT**
Chest	Pulmonary angiogram Oncology (contrast-enhanced)
Abdomen	Liver mass Pancreatic mass Renal mass Enterography Renal stone characterization
Vascular	Thoracoabdominal aorta Gastrointestinal bleeding Venogram
Neuro	Head and neck angiogram Myelogram Bleed vs contrast
Musculoskeletal	Gout Fracture detection

phase for genitourinary indications.[1] McNamara and colleagues showed improved subjective conspicuity and improved contrast-to-noise ratio of the tumor to surrounding tissues using rapid kV-switching DECT for pancreatic masses,[12] and Quiney and colleagues demonstrated improved reader confidence in pancreatic lesion detection with DECT.[13] Alternatively, practices may choose to route particular protocols or anatomy to DECT. For example, one author's practice preferentially scans musculoskeletal CTs on the DECT scanner. Suggested indications to preferentially image with DECT are listed in Table 1 and are delineated in more detail in future chapters.

For emergency department and inpatient examinations, patient selection strategies are generally more straightforward. Simple instructions of preferentially scanning contrast-enhanced CTs with DECT are easily implemented by technologists. Specific indications can also be routed to DECT when possible, including CT angiograms to evaluate for gastrointestinal bleeding and pulmonary embolism and musculoskeletal CT for fracture evaluation.

Radiology practices vary in whether a radiologist or technologist selects the CT protocol, and a radiology practice may read imaging performed at a variety of geographic locations and scanners. This then poses the question of who ultimately makes the decision of routing a patient to a location with a DECT scanner and scanning in DECT mode. It is important to involve all stakeholders involved in

this process. One author's practice follows a hybrid approach: technologists are given generalized guidelines with both specific indications and examination types to preferentially route to DECT. In addition, any radiologist or technologist may choose to route a patient to a DECT scanner at the examination when the examination is protocolled in the electronic medical record (EMR). An added benefit of using the EMR to route patients to DECT is that schedulers can also see this information and help ensure the patient's examination is scheduled in the correct location. This is particularly important for larger health systems with scanners in multiple geographic locations. Ultimately, it is important to keep the selection strategies simple and streamlined so all stakeholders can follow them. Suggested workflow modifications to incorporate triaging the appropriate patients to DECT scanners are outlined in **Fig. 4.**

Reconstructing and Reviewing Dual-Energy CT Data

After patient selection, the next major consideration is implementing a workflow for image reconstruction that reduces the strain on busy radiologists and CT technologists. DECT protocols need to be tailored toward the clinical question and incorporate only the necessary data sets without overloading the radiologists with unnecessary images.

When DECT was first introduced nearly 2 decades ago, postprocessing was performed in a more manual fashion and was more time- and labor-intensive. All DECT vendors have made significant strides toward a more automated workflow from all scanner implementations. Automated postprocessing can be performed at the scanner console, with user-selected reconstructions sent directly to picture archiving and communication system (PACS). Sending the most pertinent reconstructions to PACS can cut down on the need for radiologists to access a separate thin client.[14] These selections are built into the individual protocol examination cards on the scanner itself, so the radiologist must therefore preselect which reconstructions to send to PACS for each imaging protocol. Automating this process can be facilitated by application specialists during scanner installation, and many DECT practices train a "super tech" as a point person for DECT protocol building and optimization.

The process of sending selected reconstructions automatically to PACS lessens the barrier to the radiologist reviewing the data, as these reconstructions are available for the radiologist in PACS at the time of image interpretation.[15] On-

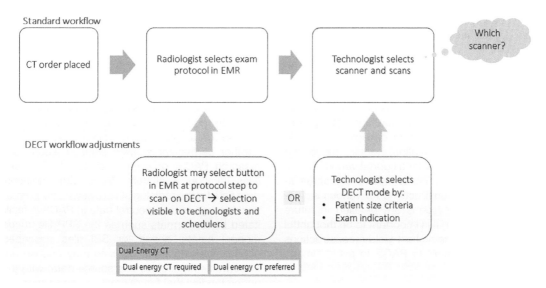

Fig. 4. Workflow modifications for patient triage to DECT. Patient selection and triage to DECT should involve all stakeholders, including radiologists, technologists, and schedulers. EMR, electronic medical record.

demand postprocessing can be performed on an ad hoc basis on stand-alone workstations or thin client–servers, but their day-to-day use in a busy practice is challenging.[16,17] This is related to several factors including availability of workstations and training on the software, but the main barrier is simply interruption of the radiologist reading workflow. Progress is being made with integrating thin clients into PACS systems, making the thin client easier for the radiologist to access. For example, with dual-layer detector computed tomography (CT) technology, an on-the-fly analysis tool integrated into PACS (Spectral Magic Glass, Philips Healthcare) can mitigate some of these limitations.[2]

Most Commonly Used Reconstructions Are Described Below

Routine diagnostic images

All dual-energy systems can generate single-energy equivalent images that are routinely sent to PACS as the primary series used for image interpretation. While the dual-layer detector DECT scanner creates conventional polychromatic 120-kVp images, other DECT systems synthesize images analogous to conventional 120-kVp series. In dual-source CT, this is achieved by linear blending of high- and low-energy images (blending ratio will vary depending on kVp selection and user preference).[2,18] In the rapid KV-switching DECT technology, virtual monochromatic image (VMI) generated at 70 keV energy level serve as 120-kVp equivalent surrogate.[19]

Virtual monochromatic images

VMIs are synthetic data sets that simulate what the image would look like if it had been created using a monochromatic x-ray beam (keV) instead of a polychromatic x-ray beam (kVp). VMIs are generated by linear combination of material basis pair images at varying proportion and energy level measured in keV. Depending on the vendor, VMI can be reconstructed over a range from 40 to 200 keV. VMI reconstructions in the lower energy range are used to increase conspicuity of high Z materials, including iodinated contrast. Low-keV VMI reconstructions can be used to increase lesion conspicuity. Conversely, VMI at high-energy level can minimize streak and beam-hardening artifacts, for example, with metal prostheses or in areas affected by dense contrast material such as axilla or subclavian veins.[20,21]

Material decomposition images

Material decomposition images are created when a preselected basis pair of materials are selectively identified using material decomposition algorithms, then either highlighted or suppressed in the reconstructed image. The most common example is use of the iodine–water basis pair to create iodine quantification images (often generically termed "iodine maps") and virtual non-contrast images. Other applications of material decomposition images include evaluation of renal stones and gout (calcium–uric acid basis pair) and bone marrow edema (calcium–water basis pair). It should be noted that iodine maps sent to PACS are typically evaluated qualitatively; quantitative measurements (eg, iodine concentration within an indeterminate renal lesion) often necessitate additional postprocessing in the thin client.

Ultimately, the reconstructions selected to routinely send to PACS vary by the indication for the examination, the anatomy being imaged, and user preference.[1,14] For oncologic examinations, the authors prefer 50 keV monoenergetic reconstructions to improve lesion conspicuity.[22–26] At another author's institution, iodine maps are routinely sent to PACS for all portal venous phase imaging to assist with incidentaloma characterization. Preferred reconstructions for various indications and organ systems are detailed in future chapters. However, it is important to be thoughtful in selecting only the highest yield reconstructions to automatically send to PACS to avoid "image overload."

Image Archiving

With dual-source DECT, data from two different x-ray sources (tubes A and B) and detector arrays are combined to create a 120-kVp equivalent image (linear blended). Information from these two data sets can be then used to create various material decomposition or virtual monoenergetic reconstructions, created in the image space, after image reconstruction.[2,27] The data from each x-ray source (tube A and tube B data) have historically been needed for future spectral postprocessing (SPP), and therefore, tube A and tube B data are sent to the thin client server (Syngo Via, Siemens Healthineers) at 0.6 mm thickness. However, a new file format (termed SPP file) is now available; this single series can be created at a maximal slice thickness of 2 mm and retains the spectral information for future postprocessing. This SPP file can be sent in a format that can be interpreted (eg, a VMI image) and can therefore replace an existing reconstruction sent to PACS.

On the rapid kV-switching DECT, 80 and 140 kV data sets are reconstructed in the projection space to create VMI, material density, and any other desired images based on the protocol. The spectral information can be retained within the reconstructed VMI series (known as mega monochromatic series) which can be used for postprocessing off the scanner. For dual-layer detector CT, the spectral information can be stored in a file termed the spectral base image (SBI); this file is created at the scanner console and is needed for future postprocessing.[2] The SBI file can be created at any slice thickness, but if multiplanar postprocessing is needed, thinner slices are recommended.

For all vendors, the spectral data are typically sent from the scanner console to a thin client server for temporary storage. The thin client has finite storage space, and older examinations are automatically deleted when the server is full. If the permanent storage of these data sets is desired for the future use (preoperative planning, research purposes), a radiology practice may choose to archive these source data sets in another permanent storage solution (such as a research PACS) or even in clinical PACS itself (less ideal as it clutters PACS with additional data sets for the radiologist to review). This permanent storage of the spectral data in PACS is facilitated by file formats such as the SPP file, mega monochromatic series, or SBI files described above. Alternatively, a practice may choose not to permanently archive this source data, with the understanding that future creation of additional reconstructions will not be feasible.

Cost–Benefit Analysis

When making the decision to purchase a DECT scanner, many factors must be taken into consideration, including but not limited to patient population (eg, oncology center vs trauma center), location of the scanner (outpatient, inpatient, emergency department), and cost. One of the first areas investigated in DECT cost–benefit analysis was the effect of DECT on follow-up recommendation rates. Atwi and colleagues retrospectively reviewed 3221 abdominopelvic CT scans from both single-energy and DECT scanners and compared follow-up recommendation rates.[15] Recommendation rates were separated into three categories: conventional single-energy CT, DECT with no iodine maps automatically sent to PACS, and DECT where iodine maps were automatically sent to PACS as part of the automated workflow. They found that follow-up recommendations because of incomplete diagnosis were significantly lower in studies for which an iodine map was automatically sent over (9.1%) than in conventional single energy CTs (11.9%, $P < .01$). Follow-up recommendations for MR imaging and PET/CT were significantly lower when iodine maps were automatically sent (9.6%) compared with conventional single-energy CTs (13.0%, $P < .003$). They also noted the increased diagnostic confidence of the radiologists interpreting the DECT scans.[15,28]

Cost–benefit analysis of more specific categories is described below. Although these categories have some overlap, together they provide more tangible data supporting DECT use in various care settings.

Incidental lesions

DECT characterization of incidentally detected abnormalities also holds much promise. Itani and colleagues retrospectively reviewed 69 patients who underwent single-phase post-contrast abdominal DECT studies.[29] Incidental abdominal findings needing further imaging were identified. They found 34 incidental findings including renal, adrenal, and pancreatic lesions. Of the 34 incidental findings, DECT data sets were able to characterize 27 incidental findings in 15 patients and accounted for cost savings of 15 additional imaging examinations. Wortman and colleagues reviewed 2729 CT scans on 2406 unique patients and found that 5.2% of patients had an indeterminate renal lesion, and over half of those indeterminate lesions could be definitively characterized as benign Bosniak II cysts using DECT.[30] The implication is that additional CT scans were not required because the DECT data set resolved the incidental finding without requiring additional imaging.[28]

Emergency Department imaging

DECT imaging may have the most potential impact in emergent imaging.[30–36] The ability to characterize a finding at the time of its discovery can not only cut down on additional imaging but also save time. The application of DECT described above is particularly pertinent in the emergency department, and DECT has the added benefit of improving conspicuity of pathology as well. Wong and colleagues retrospectively reviewed 3159 cases performed on DECT in the emergency department at a single institution to determine how often DECT altered the interpreting physician's report.[37] They found that DECT led to findings potentially altering management in 298 (9.4%) cases, increased diagnostic confidence in 455 (14.4%) cases, provided relevant information in 174 (5.6%) cases, and helped characterize an incidental finding in 44 (1.4%) cases. They further calculated the potential downstream benefits by determining the difference in follow-up studies between conventional CT and DECT. They found that DECT findings avoided 162 to 191 recommended follow-up MR imaging examinations, 21 to 28 CT examinations, and 2 to 25 ultrasound examinations compared with conventional CT alone, with a net cost reduction of $52,991.53-61,598.44. In addition to the benefit of cost reduction, it is also important to note the increased radiologist confidence where their interpretations are critical for timely management of emergency department patients.[28]

Management of organ-specific diseases

Several studies have looked at the cost differences associated with management of organ-specific diseases on conventional CT versus DECT.[15,28,29,36–38] Characterization of renal lesions with DECT is a prime example of this principle.[30,37,38] Patel and colleagues evaluated the cost-effectiveness of DECT versus multiphasic CT and MR imaging for characterizing small incidentally detected indeterminate renal lesions.[38] They found that expected mean costs per patient undergoing characterization of incidental renal lesions were $2567 for single-phase DECT, $3290 for multiphasic CT, and $3751 for multiphasic MR imaging. Associated quality-adjusted life-years were the highest for single-phase DECT at 0.962, for multiphasic MR imaging it was 0.940, and was the lowest for multiphasic CT at 0.925.

Dual-Energy CT: Improving Utilization

Cost benefits of DECT are described above, and the organ-specific evidence supporting DECT to improve diagnostic capabilities will be discussed in more detail in future chapters. Despite this, DECT remains underused. Many of the perceived barriers that radiologists describe when explaining their concerns with adopting DECT existed when DECT was first introduced but have since been improved on. For example, a perceived concern of "too much postprocessing time" is markedly decreased by the more automated postprocessing workflow used by most DECT practices. Increasing radiologists' comfort level with DECT interpretation will help radiologists incorporate DECT into their search patterns. This can be achieved by sharing cases where DECT adds value (making a diagnosis with more confidence, characterizing an incidentaloma) in journal clubs or other forums. It is important to also acknowledge that the concerns about adding more images to review are valid. DECT champions can combat this by being cognizant of how many reconstructions are automatically sent to PACS and by sharing data on how DECT helps both the radiologist and the patient. Andersen and colleagues reviewed 503 CT scans of the chest, abdomen, and pelvis, with and without the spectral data available.[39] They found that while interpretation time increased by 82 seconds per scan, significantly more cancer findings were detected (89 vs 77% sensitivity for scans with vs without spectral information). Perceived diagnostic confidence for cystic lesions was increased from 30% to 96% with spectral information available and fewer follow-up recommendations when using spectral data. Radiology trainees can be included in these discussions as well, as trainees are often more easily able to adapt to changes their interpretation patterns.

SUMMARY

Workflow strategies addressing patient selection can aid integration of DECT into a busy clinical practice. Automating postprocessing steps is critical to minimize interruptions into the radiologist and technologist workflow. Selecting DECT reconstructions to automatically send to PACS is ultimately based on user preference. DECT can be of value in the emergency department; in addition to the cost benefit of incidentaloma characterization, there is an increase in diagnostic confidence when using DECT. Radiologist adoption of DECT can be enabled by making radiologists more comfortable with DECT interpretation and data sets, optimizing workflow and avoiding "image overload," and sharing data on the benefits of DECT for both the radiologist and the patient.

CLINICS CARE POINTS

- Patient selection workflow for DECT should incorporate all stakeholders involved in selecting CT exam parameters and scheduling. This workflow may differ depending on which DECT scanner is used. Strategies for patient selection may be based on patient size and exam indication.

- Reconstructions to send to PACS depend on the anatomy being scanned and radiologist preference; care must be taken to avoid "image overload". Automated postprocessing saves time for both radiologists and technologists.

- DECT use in the Emergency Department results in quantifiable cost savings by avoiding further workup of incidentalomas and other abnormalities.

DISCLOSURES

A. Toshav is a member of the Philips Healthcare speakers bureau. L. Ananthakrishnan and N. Kulkarni have no relevant financial disclosures.

REFERENCES

1. Patel BN, Alexander L, Allen B, et al. Dual-energy CT workflow: multi-institutional consensus on standardization of abdominopelvic MDCT protocols. Abdom Radiol (NY) 2017;42(3):676–87.
2. Megibow AJ, Kambadakone A, Ananthakrishnan L. Dual-Energy Computed Tomography: Image Acquisition, Processing, and Workflow. Radiol Clin 2018; 56(4):507–20.
3. Saltybaeva N, Schmidt B, Wimmer A, et al. Precise and Automatic Patient Positioning in Computed Tomography: Avatar Modeling of the Patient Surface Using a 3-Dimensional Camera. Invest Radiol 2018;53(11):641–6.
4. Dane B, O'Donnell T, Liu S, et al. Radiation dose reduction, improved isocenter accuracy and CT scan time savings with automatic patient positioning by a 3D camera. Eur J Radiol 2021;136:109537.
5. Grajo JR, Sahani DV. Dual-Energy CT of the Abdomen and Pelvis: Radiation Dose Considerations. J Am Coll Radiol : JACR 2018;15(8):1128–32.
6. McCollough CH, Leng S, Yu L, et al. Dual- and Multi-Energy CT: Principles, Technical Approaches, and Clinical Applications. Radiology 2015;276(3): 637–53.
7. Lell MM, Kachelrieß M. Recent and Upcoming Technological Developments in Computed Tomography: High Speed, Low Dose, Deep Learning, Multienergy. Invest Radiol 2020;55(1):8–19.
8. Hsieh J, Liu E, Nett B, Tang J, Thibault J, Sahney S. A new era of image reconstruction: TrueFidelity Technical white paper on deep learning image reconstruction. 2019.
9. Noda Y, Takai Y, Asano M, et al. Comparison of image quality and pancreatic ductal adenocarcinoma conspicuity between the low-kVp and dual-energy CT reconstructed with deep-learning image reconstruction algorithm. Eur J Radiol 2022;159:110685.
10. Siegel MJ, Ramirez-Giraldo JC. Dual-Energy CT in Children: Imaging Algorithms and Clinical Applications. Radiology 2019;291(2):286–97.
11. Atwi NE, Smith DL, Flores CD, et al. Dual-energy CT in the obese: a preliminary retrospective review to evaluate quality and feasibility of the single-source dual-detector implementation. Abdom Radiol (NY) 2018. https://doi.org/10.1007/s00261-018-1774-y.
12. McNamara MM, Little MD, Alexander LF, et al. Multireader evaluation of lesion conspicuity in small pancreatic adenocarcinomas: complimentary value of iodine material density and low keV simulated monoenergetic images using multiphasic rapid kVp-switching dual energy CT. Abdominal imaging 2015;40(5):1230–40.
13. Quiney B, Harris A, McLaughlin P, et al. Dual-energy CT increases reader confidence in the detection and diagnosis of hypoattenuating pancreatic lesions. Abdom Imag 2015;40(4):859–64.
14. Mileto A, Ananthakrishnan L, Morgan DE, et al. Clinical Implementation of Dual-Energy CT for Gastrointestinal Imaging. AJR Am J Roentgenol 2020. https://doi.org/10.2214/ajr.20.25093.
15. Atwi NE, Sabottke CF, Pitre DM, et al. Follow-up Recommendation Rates Associated With Spectral Detector Dual-Energy CT of the Abdomen and Pelvis: A Retrospective Comparison to Single-Energy CT. J Am Coll Radiol : JACR 2020;17(7):940–50.

16. Tamm EP, Le O, Liu X, et al. "How to" incorporate dual-energy imaging into a high volume abdominal imaging practice. Abdom Radiol (NY) 2017;42(3):688–701.

17. Thiravit S, Brunnquell C, Cai LM, et al. Building a dual-energy CT service line in abdominal radiology. Eur Radiol 2021;31(6):4330–9.

18. Rassouli N, Etesami M, Dhanantwari A, et al. Detector-based spectral CT with a novel dual-layer technology: principles and applications. Insights into Imaging 2017;8(6):589–98.

19. Matsumoto K, Jinzaki M, Tanami Y, et al. Virtual monochromatic spectral imaging with fast kilovoltage switching: improved image quality as compared with that obtained with conventional 120-kVp CT. Radiology 2011;259(1):257–62.

20. Bamberg F, Dierks A, Nikolaou K, et al. Metal artifact reduction by dual energy computed tomography using monoenergetic extrapolation. Eur Radiol 2011;21(7):1424–9.

21. Meinel FG, Bischoff B, Zhang Q, et al. Metal artifact reduction by dual-energy computed tomography using energetic extrapolation: a systematically optimized protocol. Invest Radiol 2012;47(7):406–14.

22. Mileto A, Barina A, Marin D, et al. Virtual Monochromatic Images from Dual-Energy Multidetector CT: Variance in CT Numbers from the Same Lesion between Single-Source Projection-based and Dual-Source Image-based Implementations. Radiology. Apr 2016;279(1):269–77.

23. Mileto A, Sofue K, Marin D. Imaging the renal lesion with dual-energy multidetector CT and multi-energy applications in clinical practice: what can it truly do for you? Eur Radiol 2016. https://doi.org/10.1007/s00330-015-4180-7.

24. Shuman WP, Green DE, Busey JM, et al. Dual-energy liver CT: effect of monochromatic imaging on lesion detection, conspicuity, and contrast-to-noise ratio of hypervascular lesions on late arterial phase. AJR American journal of roentgenology. Sep 2014;203(3):601–6.

25. Voss BA, Khandelwal A, Wells ML, et al. Impact of dual-energy 50-keV virtual monoenergetic images on radiologist confidence in detection of key imaging findings of small hepatocellular carcinomas using multiphase liver CT. Acta radiologica (Stockholm, Sweden 1987) 2022;63(11):1443–52.

26. Almutairi A, Sun Z, Poovathumkadavi A, et al. Dual Energy CT Angiography of Peripheral Arterial Disease: Feasibility of Using Lower Contrast Medium Volume. PLoS One 2015;10(9):e0139275.

27. Fletcher JG, Takahashi N, Hartman R, et al. Dual-energy and dual-source CT: is there a role in the abdomen and pelvis? Radiol Clin 2009;47(1):41–57.

28. Toshav A. Economics of Dual-Energy CT: Workflow, Costs, and Benefits. Semin Ultrasound CT MR 2022;43(4):352–4.

29. Itani M, Bresnahan BW, Rice K, et al. Clinical and Payer-Based Analysis of Value of Dual-Energy Computed Tomography for Workup of Incidental Abdominal Findings. J Comput Assist Tomogr 2019;43(4):605–11.

30. Wortman JR, Shyu JY, Fulwadhva UP, et al. Impact Analysis of the Routine Use of Dual-Energy Computed Tomography for Characterization of Incidental Renal Lesions. J Comput Assist Tomogr 2019;43(2):176–82.

31. Sodickson AD, Keraliya A, Czakowski B, et al. Dual energy CT in clinical routine: how it works and how it adds value. Emerg Radiol 2021;28(1):103–17.

32. Wortman JR, Bunch PM, Fulwadhva UP, et al. Dual-Energy CT of Incidental Findings in the Abdomen: Can We Reduce the Need for Follow-Up Imaging? AJR Am J Roentgenol 2016. https://doi.org/10.2214/ajr.16.16087. W1-w11.

33. Uyeda JW, Richardson IJ, Sodickson AD. Making the invisible visible: improving conspicuity of noncalcified gallstones using dual-energy CT. Abdom Radiol (NY) 2017. https://doi.org/10.1007/s00261-017-1229-x.

34. Wortman JR, Uyeda JW, Fulwadhva UP, et al. Dual-Energy CT for Abdominal and Pelvic Trauma. Radiographics 2018;38(2):586–602.

35. Gosangi B, Mandell JC, Weaver MJ, et al. Bone Marrow Edema at Dual-Energy CT: A Game Changer in the Emergency Department. Radiographics 2020;40(3):859–74.

36. Meyer M, Nance JW Jr, Schoepf UJ, et al. Cost-effectiveness of substituting dual-energy CT for SPECT in the assessment of myocardial perfusion for the workup of coronary artery disease. Eur J Radiol 2012;81(12):3719–25.

37. Wong WD, Mohammed MF, Nicolaou S, et al. Impact of Dual-Energy CT in the Emergency Department: Increased Radiologist Confidence, Reduced Need for Follow-Up Imaging, and Projected Cost Benefit. Am J Roentgenol 2020;215(6):1528–38.

38. Patel BN, Boltyenkov AT, Martinez MG, et al. Cost-effectiveness of dual-energy CT versus multiphasic single-energy CT and MRI for characterization of incidental indeterminate renal lesions. Abdom Radiol (NY) 2020;45(6):1896–906.

39. Andersen MB, Ebbesen D, Thygesen J, et al. Impact of spectral body imaging in patients suspected for occult cancer: a prospective study of 503 patients. Eur Radiol 2020;30(10):5539–50.

Neuroradiology Applications of Dual and Multi-energy Computed Tomography

Natthawut Jarunnarumol, MD[a,b,*], Shahmir Kamalian, MD[b], Michael H. Lev, MD[b], Rajiv Gupta, MD, PhD[b]

KEYWORDS

- Dual-energy CT • Multispectral CT • Neuroimaging • Virtual monochromatic
- Material decomposition • Spectral imaging • Stroke • Head and neck imaging

KEY POINTS

- Spectral computed tomography (CT) scanners (including dual, multienergy, and photon-counting CT) have many advantages over conventional, single-energy CT (SECT) scanners; these include improved material differentiation and characterization based on spectral properties of tissue, improved image quality at same or lower radiation exposure, higher spatial and contrast resolution, and reduced contrast medium requirement due to improved image contrast.
- These advantages are leveraged using postprocessing algorithms applied to multispectral data, to create virtual monochromatic images (VMIs) and material decomposition images. VMIs simulate what the CT images would look like if a monochromatic x-ray beam at a user-selected energy level were to be used for data acquisition.
- Material decomposition leverages material-specific spectral information to differentiate between substances that have similar attenuation on SECT images. Examples include but are not limited to "virtual noncontrast," "virtual non-calcium (VN-Ca)," and, most notably for neuro applications, "hemorrhage versus iodine." VN-Ca images in particular can also be used to enhance automated and semiautomated bone subtraction image creation, which plays a major role in CT angiographic clinical practice.
- Photon-counting CT is a new, promising diagnostic tool with additional advantages over both conventional and spectral CT, including potentially marked improvements in contrast, spatial, and temporal resolution, owing to technical advances such as smaller detector pixels, lower electronic noise, and increased intrinsic spectral detector sensitivity, especially of lower energy x-ray photons.

INTRODUCTION

Computed tomography (CT) is the preferred diagnostic imaging tool for most emergency conditions. Its relative ease of use, with few contraindications, quick examination time, and cost-effectiveness compared with MR imaging, make it a go-to option in the emergency room. Recent advancements in spectral CT scanners (including dual, multienergy, and photon-counting CT) further solidify CT as the preferred diagnostic imaging technique for many emergent situations, including neurological emergencies. The superiority of spectral CT over conventional single-energy CT (SECT) is evident in several ways. For instance, it can use spectral information to differentiate between materials that

[a] Department of Diagnostic and Therapeutic Radiology, Ramathibodi Hospital, Mahidol University, Bangkok 10400, Thailand; [b] Department of Radiology, Massachusetts General Hospital, Harvard Medical School, Boston, MA 02114, USA
* Corresponding author. Department of Diagnostic and Therapeutic Radiology, Ramathibodi Hospital, Mahidol University, Bangkok 10400, Thailand.
E-mail addresses: natthawut.jar@mahidol.edu; njarunnarumol@mgh.harvard.edu

Radiol Clin N Am 61 (2023) 973–985
https://doi.org/10.1016/j.rcl.2023.05.009

exhibit the same attenuation or Hounsfield Units (HUs) on a SECT examination.

In this article, we will also demonstrate the benefits of using photon-counting detectors (PCDs) to enhance imaging quality. This includes improved spatial resolution, decreased image noise, and greater gray-white differentiation in the brain due to higher contrast resolution. These advancements are achieved using truly multispectral x-ray imaging. Furthermore, the implementation of appropriate postprocessing techniques can enhance material differentiation and tissue characterization, whereas also reducing the patient's exposure to radiation and the need for contrast media. Spectral CT provides virtual noncontrast (VNC) and bone-subtracted images, which are widely used in clinical practice. With the advent of multispectral imaging, CT holds the potential to surpass MR imaging for many clinical applications. This article will also discuss the routine clinical applications of dual, multienergy, and photon-counting CT in neuroradiology.

CLINICAL APPLICATIONS
Ischemic Stroke

Virtual NCCT from dual-energy computed tomography is equal to conventional NCCT
Imaging of ischemic stroke patients typically entails an non-contrast CT (NCCT) scan of the head followed by a CT angiographic (CTA) of the head and neck. For these patients, it may be possible to perform only the CTA portion with dual-energy CT (DECT) or multi-energy CT (MECT) and eliminate the conventional NCCT that precedes it. A VNC image may then be obtained from the DECT or MECT CTA. This not only shortens the time in the radiology department but also reduces radiation exposure. VNC-derived Alberta Stroke Program Early CT Score (ASPECTS) is equal to NCCT ASPECTS in acute ischemic stroke patients with large-vessel occlusion while offering the added benefit of a significantly reduced CT dose.[1] Similarly, A recent study published in the American Journal of Neuroradiology found that there was no significant difference in accuracy between NCCT and VNC-derived ASPECTS scores when diffusion weighted imaging (DWI) was used as the reference standard for detecting early ischemic changes[2] (**Fig. 1**).

Improved detection of infarct
DECT and MECT images allow one to retrospectively pick a virtual keV setting for visualization. By selecting an appropriate keV, the optimal stroke window can be obtained with the highest tissue contrast, making it easier to identify the infarcted area[3] (**Fig. 2**).

One can also use material discrimination to accentuate different aspects of an image. For example, a new brain edema reconstruction method has been developed using 3-material decomposition, which suppresses gray/white matter contrast while accentuating brain edema. This method improves the sensitivity and specificity of detecting acute infarctions, resulting in a more accurate ASPECT score in ischemic stroke patients within 4 hours of symptom onset compared with initial true NCCT.[4] Another study also found that noncontrast virtual monochromatic image (VMI) at 80 keV within 4.5 hours of the last seen well and at 90 keV after 4.5 hours, improved the ability to differentiate between infarcted and normal brain parenchyma compared with conventional NCCT.[3] Besides, VMI at the higher keV can reduce metallic artifacts (**Fig. 3**) and maximize the image quality compared with the conventional NCCT.[5] With higher KeV images, although the artifact is reduced, there is also a reduction of gray–white matter differentiation, the optimal point depends on the energy-level selection (**Fig. 4**).

Detection of intra-arterial thrombus
A VNC image has a different noise profile compared with NCCT because the radiation dose is split between 2 sets of images, namely, the VNC and iodine-overlay images. Therefore, the VNC images derived from DECT angiography cannot match the diagnostic accuracy of conventional NCCT images in detecting hyperdense artery signs.[6] However, in patients who have undergone mechanical thrombectomy, a recent study found that DECT can differentiate red blood cell (RBC)-rich and RBC-poor thrombi by measuring CT attenuation at a lower energy level (80 keV).[7] VNC images can also detect persistent residual clots immediately after thrombectomy. A recent study showed that arteries with residual clots have significantly higher attenuation compared with perfused contralateral arteries on VNC images.[8] This result may be important in prognosticating clinical outcomes.

Differentiating between contrast staining and hemorrhagic conversion
DECT has become a routine part of the clinical evaluation after thrombectomy. This is because it can differentiate between intraparenchymal hemorrhage secondary to reperfusion injury and iodine leakage (**Fig. 5**) caused by postischemic blood–brain barrier disruption. A DECT scan obviates MR imaging or serial CT scanning. A recent study showed that DECT with 80 and 150 kVp tube voltages is highly accurate and specific in differentiating cerebral stroke from intracerebral hemorrhage.[9] A 2020 meta-

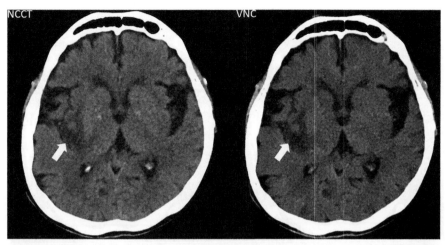

Fig. 1. A conventional NCCT (left) compared with a derived VNC image (right), for a patient with an acute stroke. There is ischemic hypodensity with loss of gray/white differentiation along the posterior aspect of the right insular cortex, the right external capsule, and the posterior limb of the right internal capsule (*arrows*), seen equally well on both NCCT and VNC images (window-level 40 HU, window-width 80 HU, for both images).

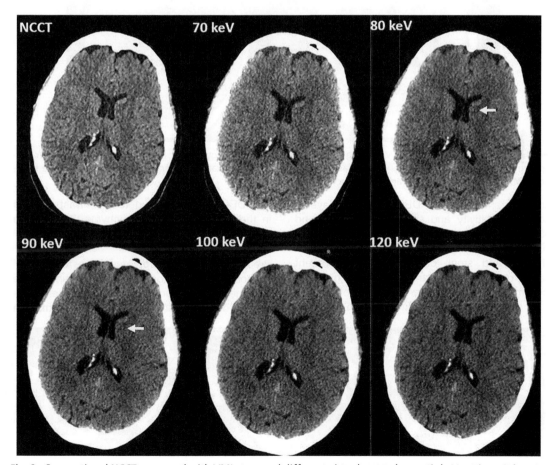

Fig. 2. Conventional NCCT compared with VMI at several different virtual monochromatic keV settings. It is noteworthy that the ischemic hypodensity at the left posterior caudate nucleus is most conspicuous (ie, optimal contrast resolution) on the 80 to 90-keV images (*arrows*; all images window-level 40 HU, window-width 50 HU).

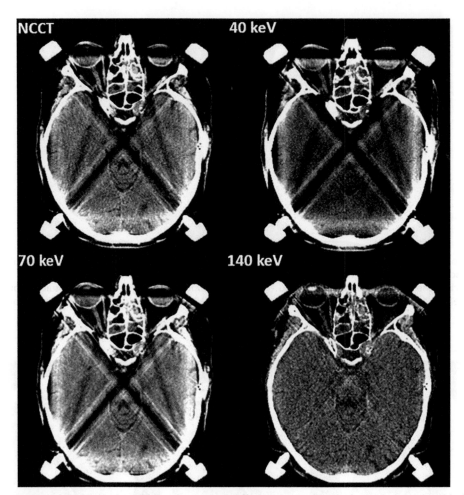

Fig. 3. Conventional NCCT versus VMI images at several different energy levels of a patient in a head-holder pre-operatively for stereotactic surgery. There as marked metallic beam-hardening artifact reduction with the high-KeV VMIs, with near complete artifact reduction at 140 virtual keV.

analysis showed that DECT has an overall pooled sensitivity and specificity of 96% and 98% for detecting intracranial hemorrhage (ICH), effectively differentiating it from contrast staining and small calcifications.[10] A recent case report of postresuscitation hypoxic/ischemic injury with an earlier history of intravenous iodine contrast administration showed

that DECT can reliably detect contrast staining in the ischemic brain parenchyma using iodine map and VNC images.[11]

Predicting risk of hemorrhagic transformation
Hemorrhagic transformation of brain tissue damaged by ischemic stroke due to intraparenchymal bleeding is a serious complication. Patients with

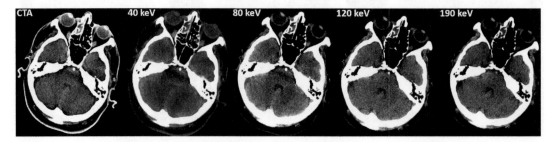

Fig. 4. Conventional NCCT versus VMI images at several different energy levels through the posterior fossa, show marked beam-hardening artifact reduction through the pons with the high-KeV VMIs. At 120 KeV, beam-hardening artifact is minimized, with clinically acceptable assessment of gray–white matter differentiation.

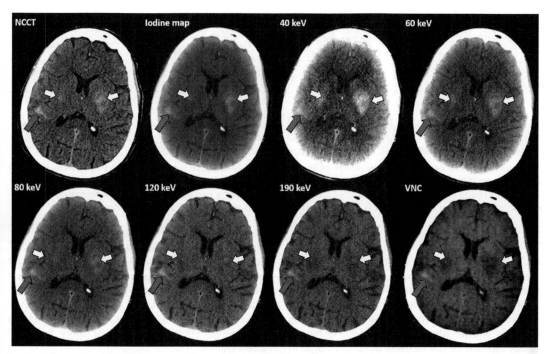

Fig. 5. Follow-up NCCT of an acute right middle cerebral artery (MCA) territory infarct following endovascular thrombectomy, compared with iodine maps, multienergy keV VMI, and VNC images. There is hyperdensity at the right posterior temporal lobe (*red arrow*), which is persistent on the iodine maps, each of the VMI energy levels, and the VNC images, which suggests hemorrhagic transformation of the right posterior temporal infarct. Other regions of hyperdensity on the NCCT and iodine map images, however, at the left greater than right basal ganglia (*white arrows*), show decreasing conspicuity on the high keV VMI and VNC images. There is near complete disappearance of the basal ganglia hyperdensity on the 120 keV, 190 keV, and VNC images, suggesting contrast staining (ie, iodine "blush") caused by blood–brain barrier breakdown in regions of severe MCA ischemia but *without* hemorrhagic conversion; hypodensity suggestive of basal ganglia infarct is best seen on the VNC-images only, without the confounding effects of iodine blush. In this example, the iodine blush is most effectively eliminated in the VNC images, however spatial and gray–white matter resolution is most effectively maintained on the 120-keV VMI images.

contrast staining after mechanical thrombectomy have a higher likelihood of experiencing unfavorable outcomes (Modified Rankin Scale [mRS] >2) and higher rates of hemorrhagic transformation. DECT after mechanical thrombectomy can predict the risk of hemorrhagic transformation. For example, studies show that higher levels of iodine extravasation (>1.35 mg/dL) detected on DECT scans after mechanical thrombectomy may indicate a higher risk for intracerebral hemorrhage development.[12] Early detection of these markers enables more aggressive treatment and close monitoring to reduce the risk of hemorrhagic transformation.

Hemorrhagic Stroke and Other Intracranial Hemorrhages

Detection of intracranial hemorrhages

DECT can improve the detection of intracranial hemorrhages. A small amount of bleeding is more easily detected on the virtual non-calcium (VN-Ca) images, especially small subdural or epidural hematomas that are adjacent to the inner table of the skull. Intraventricular hemorrhage near the calcified choroid plexus can still be seen on the VN-Ca images because the calcified portion is subtracted out in these images[13] (**Fig. 6**). Increasing the monochromatic keV level to 190 keV results in improved hematoma-brain contrast, increased spatial resolution, reduced beam-hardening artifacts, and reduced partial volume averaging on thin-section images.[14] As a result, these thin-section images have higher diagnostic value in detecting subdural hematomas, supratentorial contusions, and epidural hematomas that may not be evident on conventional CT scans. DECT also has high-diagnostic accuracy in differentiating intra-axial and extra-axial hemorrhages from iodinated contrast, without the need for repeat imaging that would expose the patient to additional radiation.[15]

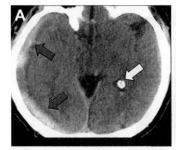 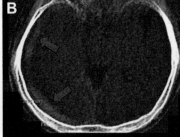 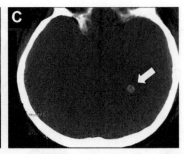

Fig. 6. Virtual monochromatic 65 keV image of the brain (*A*) reveals acute subdural hemorrhage along the right temporal convexity (*red arrows*) and calcified choroid plexus in the left lateral ventricle (*white arrow*). Acute subdural hemorrhage is hyperdense on the VN-Ca images (*B*), however is not apparent on high keV material decomposition images (*C*), although the left lateral ventricle choroid plexus calcification remains well seen.

Differentiating hemorrhage from calcification
DECT can distinguish intracranial hemorrhage from calcification by analyzing the different tissue densities at 2 different energy levels: the relative change in density is indicative of the elemental composition of each material. There are instances when it is unclear whether a faint focus of hyperdensity represents calcification or hemorrhage. In these cases, the calcium overlay and VN-Ca images derived from DECT can provide clarity. In general, DECT offers improved diagnostic accuracy compared with simulated SECT in differentiating small foci of intracranial hemorrhage from faint calcifications. Hemorrhagic foci can be identified as having a density of less than 74 HU on simulated SECT images, greater than 44 HU on VN-Ca images, and less than 7 HU on calcium images.[16,17] The overall sensitivity and specificity of DECT in differentiating intracerebral hemorrhage from contrast staining or small calcifications are 96% and 98%, respectively.[10]

Spot sign
The "spot sign" is a focus on a contrast-containing blood pool visible on an arterial or delayed phase CTA. It is an indicator of active bleeding at the time of the scan because it shows intravenous contrast extravasating into the brain parenchyma. The spot sign is a powerful predictor of hematoma expansion. DECT can improve the detection of spot sign (**Fig. 7**). On iodine overlay maps, the presence of iodinated contrast material on arterial phase and/or delayed images signals active extravasation.[13] Although the true spot sign is most specific for primary intracranial hemorrhage, there are several spot sign mimics that account for 31% of intracranial hemorrhages, including vascular (microAVM, aneurysm, and Moya Moya) or nonvascular causes (tumors and choroid plexus calcification).[18] According to a recent study, the use of DECT to detect the iodine concentration

within the entire hematoma and the focal brightest spot within the hematoma has proven to be more effective in predicting hematoma expansion compared with the conventional spot sign.[19] Therefore, the use of DECT can enhance the identification of patients who require more aggressive treatments, such as surgical or other forms of interventions.

Detection of contrast enhancement in hemorrhage or calcified lesions
DECT has the ability to differentiate between various tissues based on their density and composition and can also identify contrast enhancements in hemorrhagic or calcified lesions. Unlike SECT, it is not challenging for DECT to identify contrast enhancement in hemorrhagic or calcified lesions using iodine overlay maps. In diagnosing intracranial hemorrhages of uncertain origin, the fusion images created by DECT using iodine overlay and VNC images can accurately distinguish between a hemorrhagic tumor and pure intracranial hemorrhage.[20] As such, DECT greatly improves the accuracy of diagnoses made by radiologists. This, in turn, helps guide clinicians in determining the best treatment plan for their patients.

Computed tomography Arteriography and Venography

Improved contrast-to-noise ratio and differentiation of low-contrast tissues
The contrast-to-noise ratio (CNR) measures the visibility of 2 tissues with similar attenuation relative to each other, compared with the surrounding image noise. DECT improves CNR by using 2 x-ray beams with different energy levels and thereby enhancing the differences in the attenuation of various tissue types based on their composition. DECT can make it easier to identify small or subtle lesions or structures that may be difficult to detect on a conventional SECT scan. For example, in a

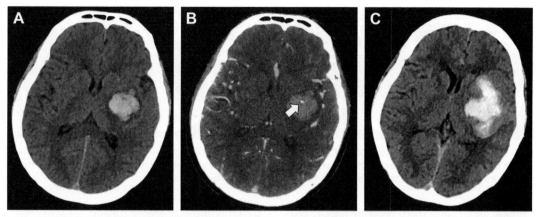

Fig. 7. Conventional NCCT image (*A*) reveals an acute intraparenchymal hematoma centered in the left basal ganglia, with mild peripheral hypodense vasogenic edema. The DECT iodine overlay map (*B*) demonstrates a spot sign (*arrow*), corresponding to a focus of active contrast extravasation, within the hematoma. The presence of a spot-sign is highly predictive of hematoma expansion. Follow-up 24-hour NCCT (*C*) confirms increased size of the left basal ganglia hematoma with an increased mass effect, resulting in the effacement of the left lateral ventricle and a minimal rightward midline shift.

study using an 80-kVp beam, there was a significant improvement in arterial enhancement with a sharper appearance of cerebral arteries and heightened diagnostic image quality. Additionally, the radiation dose was reduced by 22.2% compared with the standard 120-kVp beam.[21]

Using virtual monochromatic images (VMIs), one can use different keV levels to enhance gray/white differentiation in the brain. A study by Pomerantz and colleagues[5] showed that a 65 to 70-keV level provides the best contrast for visualizing the cortical ribbon and the deep gray nuclei as compared with the adjacent gray matter.

Reducing the dosage of contrast media in imaging studies

DECT has the added benefit of reducing the amount of contrast material required for a scan. One can retrospectively increase the conspicuity of iodinated contrast by selecting a VMI energy level to one that is closer to the K-edge of iodine (33.4 keV). As can be seen in **Fig. 8**, the brightness of iodine increases when the virtual photon energy is decreased. The improved CNR also allows for a reduction in the contrast dose. This is especially important for patients who are prone to contrast-induced nephropathy. The use of low-kVp images with optimized noise and advanced reconstruction techniques results in a reduction in iodine dose.[22,23] This not only reduces the risk of side effects associated with the contrast material but also makes the procedure more cost-effective.

Bone removal

In many regions such as the head, neck, and spine, bones can obscure clear visualization of

structures of interest (**Fig. 9**), especially contrast-enhanced structures such as blood vessels. DECT enables the separation of bone from other tissues, leading to improved clarity and visibility of the structures of interest. DECT-based bone subtraction in head and neck imaging has been found to be effective with a lower radiation dose compared with conventional SECT techniques.[24] DECT-based bone subtraction enhances efficiency in interpretation as radiologists can make maximum intensity projection (MIP) images of a 3D stack of axial images, allowing for a more global analysis of the structures of interest such as blood vessels. A study found that DECT angiography for stroke patients improved vessel delineation, reducing the reading time from 4.60 minutes to 3.49 minutes ($P < .001$), with no decrease in diagnostic accuracy compared with standard CT angiography.[25]

Improved detection of small aneurysms

Detection of small aneurysms can be challenging with traditional CT imaging because they may blend in with the surrounding tissue. Small aneurysms are especially difficult to identify on conventional CTA near the skull base. CTA with dual-energy bone removal has demonstrated high-diagnostic accuracy in detecting intracranial aneurysms, particularly small ones (<3 mm) at the skull base CTA.[26] Improved detection and more confident diagnosis may facilitate appropriate triage including follow-up, surgical clipping, or endovascular coiling.

Evaluation of carotid artery stenosis

DECT can improve the assessment of carotid artery stenosis, a condition that increases the risk

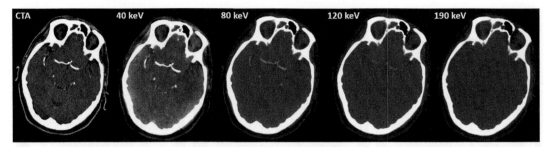

Fig. 8. CTA source image, obtained using dual source spectral CT scanning, through the circle-of-Willis. VMIs at multiple different keV energy levels show maximal contrast conspicuity at the lowest keV images that are closest to the "k-edge" of iodine (33.4 keV) at which the photoelectric effect is optimal.

of stroke. DECT, and more recently MECT, provides a detailed and accurate map of the carotid artery, enabling precise assessment of the degree of stenosis that is not confounded by atherosclerotic calcifications. The main challenge in the evaluation of carotid artery stenosis is the presence of heavily calcified plaque, which may be difficult to differentiate from the iodinated contrast in the lumen. Automated plaque removal available with DECT, which can differentiate calcified plaque from iodinated contrast, may be used as an adjunct to standard reconstructions to effectively evaluate high-grade stenosis.[27]

Determining vulnerable carotid plaques

DECT provides valuable insight into the characteristics and composition of carotid artery stenosis including the location, shape, size, and different constituents of the plaque. It can also detect the presence of calcification, thrombus, ulceration, subintimal intravasation, or other abnormalities. All these characteristics of atherosclerotic plaque are important in determining the vulnerability of the plaque. Research has shown that factors such as a thin fibrous cap, a large lipid-rich core, intraplaque hemorrhage, calcified nodule, and vasa vasorum enhancement can increase the risk

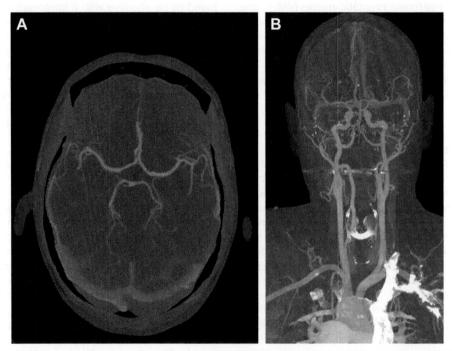

Fig. 9. An axial MIP head CTA image through the circle-of-Willis, with automated bone removal that leverages the spectral source image dataset (*A*). Similar bone removal is shown in the arch-to-vertex MIP reconstruction of the head and neck CTA performed in this patient with transient-ischemic-attack symptoms (*B*). Efficient, accurate bone removal, augmented by spectral CTA datasets, is of value in reducing the need for complex image postprocessing by dedicated "3D-lab" technologists or by radiologists during image interpretation, which can help speed lesion detection in both the arterial and venous head and neck vasculature.

of future strokes.[28] Additionally, the use of effective atomic number (Z value) maps generated by gemstone spectral imaging can further differentiate between vulnerable and stable carotid plaques.[29] In fact, early evidence suggests that carotid plaque characterization using DECT may be able to predict imminent ischemic stroke in the next 30 days.[30,31]

Head and Neck Imaging

Detecting early abscess formation
Early detection of abscesses can be challenging because they often lack distinct borders and blend into the surrounding tissue. DECT improves visualization of enhancing tissues, increases tissue contrast, and reduces bone and artifact interference. These features can facilitate accurate diagnosis. DECT also improves visualization of the absence of iodine in the central part of an abscess, thereby making it easier to identify the abscess and assess the severity of surrounding soft tissue infection.[13] Although large abscesses declare themselves, both clinically as well as on imaging, DECT makes it easier to detect small abscesses that may not be noticeable on a SECT scan.

Evaluation of nonmalignant neck lesions
The diagnosis of nonmalignant neck lesions, such as cysts, thyroid nodules, lymph nodes, and salivary gland tumors, can be improved with the use of DECT. DECT not only offers the same diagnostic capabilities as conventional CT in assessing the location, size, and shape of the lesion but also provides additional information on the composition of the lesion. The absence of iodine on the iodine maps and the lack of obvious enhancement on VMIs can further confirm the benignity of most neck lesions.[32]

Differentiation of tumor recurrence from posttreatment changes
Differentiating between tumor recurrence and posttreatment changes can be challenging for patients who have undergone cancer treatment such as radical neck dissection, lymph node exploration, chemotherapy, and radiation. Conventional imaging methods may be limited in distinguishing posttreatment changes from tumor recurrence, DECT may provide a more detailed assessment of tissue changes. Typically, tumor recurrence will exhibit a similar density and enhancement pattern as the primary tumor. Posttreatment changes, such as fibrosis and granulation tissue, may display distinct density and enhancement patterns. By using low-keV VMIs and analyzing the tissue composition with iodine maps, DECT can enhance tissue contrast and differentiate between the density and enhancement patterns of tumor recurrence and posttreatment changes such as fibrosis.[33,34]

Tumor invasion versus nonossified thyroid cartilage
On conventional CT imaging, it may be challenging to differentiate between the nonossified thyroid cartilage and an adjacent tumor due to their similar appearance. However, by utilizing a DECT-derived iodine map and calcium suppression images, the density and enhancement characteristics of the 2 can be contrasted, enabling differentiation between cartilage invasion by squamous cell carcinoma and nonossified thyroid cartilage.[35,36]

Cervical nodal metastases
The evaluation of cervical nodal metastases can be improved using DECT. Similar to conventional imaging, DECT provides detailed images of the cervical lymph nodes and accurately assesses their size, shape, and location. In addition, DECT can differentiate benign from malignant lymph nodes by analyzing their density, enhancement pattern, and presence of calcifications, providing a more comprehensive assessment. Accurate staging of head and neck cancer may be achieved by analyzing iodine concentration on iodine maps in addition to HU assessment, with or without ultrasonography, to diagnose cervical lymph node metastases.[37–39]

Spine Imaging

Metallic artifact reduction
Metallic artifacts can severely affect the quality of images, causing blurring and distorting the structures of interest. By using high-keV VMIs to reduce these artifacts, the visualization of the interface between metal and bone in spinal fixation is improved. Such high-keV imaging provides a more accurate assessment of periprosthetic lucencies and hardware loosening.[40] DECT provides a simple method for metal artifact reduction (MAR) that is available on demand. If desired, one can also push the high-keV images to the Picture Archiving and Communication System (PACS) for archival.

Bone marrow edema and other marrow replacing lesions
Bone marrow edema is characterized by inflammation and increased water content in the bone marrow. Using material decomposition, it is possible to suppress the calcium in the bone marrow in the so-called VN-Ca images. In a VN-Ca image, the marrow effectively consists of marrow fat and any other non-calcium materials.

As a result, VN-Ca images accentuate bone marrow edema in vertebral compression fractures, a feature that can help to differentiate acute vertebral compression fractures from chronic vertebral compression fractures.[41,42] Additionally, VN-Ca images can be used to detect bone marrow replacement in multiple myeloma, even when there are no obvious osteolytic lesions present on conventional CT scans.[43] This makes it easier to identify metastatic lesions in the bone marrow that may not be visible on SECT scans. Additionally, virtual monochromatic very-low keV images can be adjunct to maximize enhancement to search for enhancing spinal tumor or epidural collections for whom MR imaging may be contraindicated (Fig. 10).

Utilizing computed tomography myelogram
DECT can be used for CT myelography to assess the spinal cord and surrounding structures. The injection of contrast material into the spinal canal helps to highlight the spinal cord and certain abnormalities, such as herniated discs and tumors. Several case reports have demonstrated that DECT myelography can enhance iodinated contrast attenuation and differentiate between calcified osteophytes and extradural contrast, thus improving the diagnosis of cerebrospinal fluid leaks.[44,45]

PHOTON-COUNTING COMPUTED TOMOGRAPHY

The recent introduction of the advanced photon-counting CT holds great promise as a diagnostic tool. The main advantage of photon-counting CT over conventional and other spectral CT imaging is its specialized detector that counts and bins individual x-ray photons instead of the traditional method of measuring the total amount of energy that is incident on a detector element. Unlike PCDs, traditional energy-integrating detectors lose information about the energy of the incoming x-ray photons. PCD enables more accurate measurement of the energy of incoming x-rays, resulting in improved accuracy and higher resolution images.[46–48] This can be particularly useful in detecting small tumors or abnormalities that may not be visible on traditional CT scans.

Photon-counting CT also offers the advantage of smaller detector sizes and lower electronic noise, resulting in ultrahigh-resolution scans. This contributes to improved image quality with reduced radiation dose compared with conventional and other spectral CT imaging. In addition, optimal image contrast can be achieved with photon-counting CT with equal contribution of low-energy spectra for image reconstruction, leading to increased iodine contrast and lower iodine dose requirements. Brain scans with photon-counting CT have been shown to have higher gray–white matter contrast with a decrease in beam-hardening and streak artifacts in the posterior fossa.[49–51] The reduction of metal artifacts in neurovascular coils and spinal hardware can be achieved and further optimized by the use of photon-counting CT in combination with MAR techniques, as supported by several studies.[51,52] Similarly, the quality of head and neck CTA is improved with photon-counting CT compared with energy integrating detector CT, making it easier to diagnose conditions such as CNS vasculitis, particularly small vessel

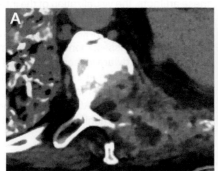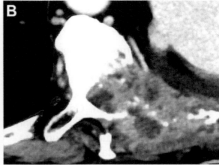

Fig. 10. Virtual monochromatic very-low keV images through a lower thoracic vertebral body, with (*A*) and without (*B*) colorized iodine overlay, shows lytic destructive changes in the left pedicle, lamina, transverse process, and rib, from an aggressive soft tissue lesion with necrotic components. With conventional contrast-enhanced CT, assessment for possible involvement within the spinal canal is typically suboptimal, due to marked beam-hardening effects from circumferential surrounding bone and poor CNR. In patients for whom MR imaging is not possible or contraindicated, however, spectral CT can help maximize iodine conspicuity, improving accuracy for the evaluation of the degree and extent of abnormal enhancing phlegmon or collections within the spinal canal.

vasculitis, and tiny aneurysms.[53] Additionally, this technique offers improved spatial resolution with dose reduction for sinus and temporal bone imaging.[54,55] Imaging of vessel walls with photon-counting CT has the potential to become a clinically useful clinical tool, owing to its faster scanning, higher spatial resolution, and higher temporal resolution, compared with current conventional and other spectral CT imaging. In conclusion, with its many potential advantages over conventional and spectral CT, photon-counting CT is likely to become a routine part of the clinical standard of care in the future.

CLINICS CARE POINTS

- Dual and multi-spectral CT may be used in routine clinical care for differentiating hemorrhage from iodinated contrast or calcifications, optimizing contrast-to-noise ratio for improved gray-white differentiation, artifact suppression, and multiple other applications.
- Advent to newer photon-counting CT scanners has enabled ultra-high spatial resolution and multi-spectral imaging in every CT scan.

ACKNOWLEDGMENTS

This research was supported in part by NIH 5R01CA212382-05 (PI: Yoshida, Hiroyuki), NIH 5R01EB024343-04 (PI: Bonmassar, Giorgio), and NIH 1R03EB032038-01 (PI: Gupta, Rajiv).

DISCLOSURE

- N. Jarunnarumol and S. Kamalian have no commercial or financial conflicts of interest to disclose that are relevant to this article.
- M. Lev would like to disclose the following interests that are not relevant to the current article.
  - Consultant: GE Healthcare, Seagen/Roche-Genentech/Takeda Pharm,
  - Grant support: GE Healthcare, Co-investigator on NIH Grants with Dr Larry Wald & Dr Giorgio Bonmassar.
- R. (Raj) Gupta would like to declare the following interests that are not relevant to the current article:
  - Idorsia, Inc, Consulting/Advising and member of Image Review Committee.
  - Mosaic Research Management, Consulting/Advising
  - Braintale Inc., Scientific Advisory Board.

- Mary Hitchcock Memorial Hospital, Expert testimony.
- Siemens Medical Solutions, USA: Speaker honorarium.
- Samsung: Research Grant.
- University of Wisconsin: CT Protocols Advisory Board
- The Risk Management Foundation of the Harvard Medical Institutions Incorporated (RMF): Legal consulting
- "Spectral precision imaging for early diagnosis of colorectal lesions with CT colonography," NIH, 5R01CA212382-05, (PI: Yoshida, Hiroyuki)
- "Dense array image-compatible EEG for enhanced neonatal care–Administrative Supplement," NIH-National Institutes of Health, 5R01EB024343-04, (PI: Bonmassar, Giorgio)
- "A Simulation Framework for X-Ray Phase-Contrast Imaging," (NIH-National Institutes of Health, 1R03EB032038–01, PI: Gupta, Rajiv).

REFERENCES

1. van den Broek M, Byrne D, Lyndon D, et al. ASPECTS estimation using dual-energy CTA-derived virtual non-contrast in large vessel occlusion acute ischemic stroke: a dose reduction opportunity for patients undergoing repeat CT? Neuroradiology 2022;64(3):483–91.
2. Kauw F, Ding VY, Dankbaar JW, et al. Detection of early ischemic changes with virtual noncontrast dual-energy CT in Acute ischemic stroke: a noninferiority analysis. AJNR Am J Neuroradiol 2022;43(9):1259–64.
3. van Ommen F, Dankbaar JW, Zhu G, et al. Virtual monochromatic dual-energy CT reconstructions improve detection of cerebral infarct in patients with suspicion of stroke. Neuroradiology 2021;63(1):41–9.
4. Mohammed MF, Marais O, Min A, et al. Unenhanced dual-energy computed tomography: visualization of brain edema. Invest Radiol 2018;53(2):63–9.
5. Pomerantz SR, Kamalian S, Zhang D, et al. Virtual monochromatic reconstruction of dual-energy unenhanced head CT at 65-75 keV maximizes image quality compared with conventional polychromatic CT. Radiology 2013;266(1):318–25.
6. Winklhofer S, Vittoria De Martini I, Nern C, et al. Dual-energy computed tomography in stroke imaging: technical and clinical considerations of virtual non-contrast images for detection of the hyperdense artery sign. J Comput Assist Tomogr 2017;41(6):843–8.

7. Panyaping T, Udomkaewkanjana N, Keandoungchun J. Utility of dual-energy CT in differentiating clot in acute ischemic stroke. NeuroRadiol J 2022. https://doi.org/10.1177/19714009221147234. 19714009221147234.

8. Mangesius S, Janjic T, Steiger R, et al. Dual-energy computed tomography in acute ischemic stroke: state-of-the-art. Eur Radiol 2021;31(6):4138–47.

9. Grkovski R, Acu L, Ahmadli U, et al. A novel dual-energy CT method for detection and differentiation of intracerebral hemorrhage from contrast extravasation in stroke patients after endovascular thrombectomy : feasibility and first results. Clin Neuroradiol 2022. https://doi.org/10.1007/s00062-022-01198-3.

10. Choi Y, Shin NY, Jang J, et al. Dual-energy CT for differentiating acute intracranial hemorrhage from contrast staining or calcification: a meta-analysis. Neuroradiology 2020;62(12):1617–26.

11. Nayab A, Wijdicks EF, Luetmer PH, et al. Value of dual energy CT in post resuscitation coma. Differentiating contrast retention and ischemic brain parenchyma. Radiol Case Rep 2022;17(10):3722–6.

12. Bonatti M, Lombardo F, Zamboni GA, et al. Iodine extravasation quantification on dual-energy CT of the brain performed after mechanical thrombectomy for acute ischemic stroke can predict hemorrhagic complications. AJNR Am J Neuroradiol 2018;39(3):441–7.

13. Potter CA, Sodickson AD. Dual-energy CT in emergency neuroimaging: added value and novel applications. Radiographics 2016;36(7):2186–98.

14. Bodanapally UK, Archer-Arroyo KL, Dreizin D, et al. Dual-energy computed tomography imaging of head: virtual high-energy monochromatic (190 keV) images are more reliable than standard 120 kV images for detecting traumatic intracranial hemorrhages. J Neurotrauma 2019;36(8):1375–81.

15. Phan CM, Yoo AJ, Hirsch JA, et al. Differentiation of hemorrhage from iodinated contrast in different intracranial compartments using dual-energy head CT. AJNR Am J Neuroradiol 2012;33(6):1088–94.

16. Wiggins WF, Potter CA, Sodickson AD. Dual-energy CT to differentiate small foci of intracranial hemorrhage from calcium. Radiology 2020;294(1):129–38.

17. Kotsenas AL. Using dual-energy CT to identify small foci of hemorrhage in the emergency setting. Radiology 2020;294(1):139–40.

18. Gazzola S, Aviv RI, Gladstone DJ, et al. Vascular and nonvascular mimics of the CT angiography "spot sign" in patients with secondary intracerebral hemorrhage. Stroke 2008;39(4):1177–83.

19. Tan CO, Lam S, Kuppens D, et al. Spot and diffuse signs: quantitative markers of intracranial hematoma expansion at dual-energy CT. Radiology 2019;290(1):179–86.

20. Kim SJ, Lim HK, Lee HY, et al. Dual-energy CT in the evaluation of intracerebral hemorrhage of unknown origin: differentiation between tumor bleeding and pure hemorrhage. AJNR Am J Neuroradiol 2012;33(5):865–72.

21. Cho ES, Chung TS, Oh DK, et al. Cerebral computed tomography angiography using a low tube voltage (80 kVp) and a moderate concentration of iodine contrast material: a quantitative and qualitative comparison with conventional computed tomography angiography. Invest Radiol 2012;47(2):142–7.

22. Parakh A, Macri F, Sahani D. Dual-energy computed tomography: dose reduction, series reduction, and contrast load reduction in dual-energy computed tomography. Radiol Clin North Am 2018;56(4):601–24.

23. Cecco CND. New contrast injection strategies for low kV and keV imaging. Appl Radiol 2018;47(1):7–11.

24. Deng K, Liu C, Ma R, et al. Clinical evaluation of dual-energy bone removal in CT angiography of the head and neck: comparison with conventional bone-subtraction CT angiography. Clin Radiol 2009;64(5):534–41.

25. Morhard D, Fink C, Becker C, et al. Value of automatic bone subtraction in cranial CT angiography: comparison of bone-subtracted vs. standard CT angiography in 100 patients. Eur Radiol 2008;18(5):974–82.

26. Zhang LJ, Wu SY, Niu JB, et al. Dual-energy CT angiography in the evaluation of intracranial aneurysms: image quality, radiation dose, and comparison with 3D rotational digital subtraction angiography. AJR Am J Roentgenol 2010;194(1):23–30.

27. Thomas C, Korn A, Ketelsen D, et al. Automatic lumen segmentation in calcified plaques: dual-energy CT versus standard reconstructions in comparison with digital subtraction angiography. AJR Am J Roentgenol 2010;194(6):1590–5.

28. Kamalian S, Lev MH, Pomerantz SR. Dual-energy computed tomography angiography of the head and neck and related applications. Neuroimaging Clin N Am 2017;27(3):429–43.

29. Shinohara Y, Sakamoto M, Kuya K, et al. Assessment of carotid plaque composition using fast-kV switching dual-energy CT with gemstone detector: comparison with extracorporeal and virtual histology-intravascular ultrasound. Neuroradiology 2015;57(9):889–95.

30. Yuenyongsinchai K, Tan C, Vranic J, et al. Carotid plaque characterization using dual-energy computed tomography: predicting imminent ipsilateral ischemic stroke in 30 days. Stroke: Vascular and Interventional Neurology 2022;2. https://doi.org/10.1161/SVIN.121.000313.

31. Choi E, Byun E, Kwon SU, et al. Carotid plaque composition assessed by CT predicts subsequent cardiovascular events among subjects with carotid stenosis. AJNR Am J Neuroradiol 2021;42(12):2199–206.

32. Perez-Lara A, Forghani R. Dual-energy computed tomography of the neck: a pictorial review of normal anatomy, variants, and pathologic entities using different energy reconstructions and material decomposition maps. Neuroimaging Clin N Am 2017;27(3):499–522.

33. Yamauchi H, Buehler M, Goodsitt MM, et al. Dual-energy CT-Based differentiation of benign posttreatment changes from primary or recurrent malignancy of the head and neck: comparison of spectral hounsfield units at 40 and 70 keV and iodine concentration. AJR Am J Roentgenol 2016; 206(3):580–7.

34. Lam S, Gupta R, Levental M, et al. Optimal virtual monochromatic images for evaluation of normal tissues and head and neck cancer using dual-energy CT. AJNR Am J Neuroradiol 2015;36(8): 1518–24.

35. Kuno H, Onaya H, Iwata R, et al. Evaluation of cartilage invasion by laryngeal and hypopharyngeal squamous cell carcinoma with dual-energy CT. Radiology 2012;265(2):488–96.

36. Forghani R, Levental M, Gupta R, et al. Different spectral hounsfield unit curve and high-energy virtual monochromatic image characteristics of squamous cell carcinoma compared with nonossified thyroid cartilage. AJNR Am J Neuroradiol 2015; 36(6):1194–200.

37. Luo YH, Mei XL, Liu QR, et al. Diagnosing cervical lymph node metastasis in oral squamous cell carcinoma based on third-generation dual-source, dual-energy computed tomography. Eur Radiol 2023; 33(1):162–71.

38. Yoon J, Choi Y, Jang J, et al. Preoperative assessment of cervical lymph node metastases in patients with papillary thyroid carcinoma: Incremental diagnostic value of dual-energy CT combined with ultrasound. PLoS One 2021;16(12):e0261233.

39. Li L, Cheng SN, Zhao YF, et al. Diagnostic accuracy of single-source dual-energy computed tomography and ultrasonography for detection of lateral cervical lymph node metastases of papillary thyroid carcinoma. J Thorac Dis 2019;11(12):5032–41.

40. Liao E, Srinivasan A. Applications of dual-energy computed tomography for artifact reduction in the head, neck, and spine. Neuroimaging Clin N Am 2017;27(3):489–97.

41. Wang C-K. Bone marrow edema in vertebral compression fractures: detection with dual-energy CT. Radiology 2013;269. Number 2—November 2013.

42. Bierry G, Venkatasamy A, Kremer S, et al. Dual-energy CT in vertebral compression fractures: performance of visual and quantitative analysis for bone marrow edema demonstration with comparison to MRI. Skeletal Radiol 2014;43(4):485–92.

43. Thomas C, Schabel C, Krauss B, et al. Dual-energy CT: virtual calcium subtraction for assessment of bone marrow involvement of the spine in multiple myeloma. AJR Am J Roentgenol 2015;204(3): W324–31.

44. Houk JL, Marin DM, Malinzak MD, et al. Dual energy CT for the identification of CSF-Venous Fistulas and CSF leaks in spontaneous intracranial hypotension: Report of four cases. Radiol Case Rep 2022;17(5): 1824–9.

45. Iyama Y, Nakaura T, Iyama A, et al. The usefulness of dual-layer spectral computed tomography for myelography: a case report and review of the literature. Case Rep Orthop 2018;2018:1468929.

46. Esquivel A, Ferrero A, Mileto A, et al. Photon-counting detector CT: key points radiologists should know. Korean J Radiol 2022;23(9):854–65.

47. Nakamura Y, Higaki T, Kondo S, et al. An introduction to photon-counting detector CT (PCD CT) for radiologists. Jpn J Radiol 2022. https://doi.org/10.1007/s11604-022-01350-6.

48. Tortora M, Gemini L, D'Iglio I, et al. Spectral photon-counting computed tomography: a review on technical principles and clinical applications. J Imaging 2022;8(4). https://doi.org/10.3390/jimaging8040112.

49. Pourmorteza A, Symons R, Reich DS, et al. Photon-counting CT of the brain: in vivo human results and image-quality assessment. AJNR Am J Neuroradiol 2017;38(12):2257–63.

50. Michael AE, Boriesosdick J, Schoenbeck D, et al. Image-quality assessment of polyenergetic and virtual monoenergetic reconstructions of unenhanced CT scans of the head: initial experiences with the first photon-counting CT approved for clinical use. Diagnostics 2022;12(2). https://doi.org/10.3390/diagnostics12020265.

51. Leng S, Bruesewitz M, Tao S, et al. Photon-counting detector CT: System design and clinical applications of an emerging technology Radiographics 2019; 39(3):729–43.

52. Schmitt N, Wucherpfennig L, Rotkopf LT, et al. Metal artifacts and artifact reduction of neurovascular coils in photon-counting detector CT versus energy-integrating detector CT - in vitro comparison of a standard brain imaging protocol. Eur Radiol 2022. https://doi.org/10.1007/s00330-022-09073-y.

53. Symons R, Reich DS, Bagheri M, et al. Photon-counting computed tomography for vascular imaging of the head and neck: first in vivo human results. Invest Radiol 2018;53(3):135–42.

54. Grunz JP, Petritsch B, Luetkens KS, et al. Ultra-low-dose photon-counting CT imaging of the paranasal sinus with tin prefiltration: how low can we go? Invest Radiol 2022;57(11):728–33.

55. Rajendran K, Voss BA, Zhou W, et al. Dose reduction for sinus and temporal bone imaging using photon-counting detector CT with an additional tin filter. Invest Radiol 2020;55(2):91–100.

Dual-Energy Computed Tomography Applications in Lung Cancer

Zachary J. Hartley-Blossom, MD, MBA[a,b], Subba R. Digumarthy, MD[a,b],*

KEYWORDS

- Dual-energy CT • Lung cancer • Thoracic imaging • Clinical application • Treatment response
- Iodine concentration • Iodine maps

KEY POINTS

- Dual-energy computed tomography (DECT) is an evolving tool in the evaluation of lung cancer, including differentiating benign from malignant pulmonary nodules.
- Monitoring treatment response with DECT offers additional information over single energy CT including evaluation of metastatic mediastinal lymph nodes and primary tumor.
- Iodine quantification is a surrogate for tumor vascularity and viability and important in determining prognostic features, such as tumor necrosis and hypoxia.
- DECT also helps in assessment of response after systemic and locoregional therapy, such as thermal ablation and radiation.

INTRODUCTION

Although prostate and breast cancer remain the most prevalent cancers in men and women, respectively, lung cancer accounts for more deaths in men than prostate and colorectal cancers combined and in women more than breast and colorectal cancers combined.[1,2] Although clinical treatment options and imaging technology have expanded over recent decades, utilization of these technological advances has lagged in clinical practice. As a result, PET/computed tomography (PET/CT) and standard CT remains the workhorse in diagnosing, staging, and surveillance of lung cancer.[3]

Recent advancements in CT technology have allowed for near-simultaneous imaging and acquisition at two different energy levels (in kilovoltage or kV), which provide the information for derived dual-energy CT (DECT) images. Applications of DECT in various body parts have been previously reported, including within the thorax.[4–8] This article examines the intrathoracic applications for DECT, focusing on lung cancer.

PHYSICS AND TECHNOLOGY OF DUAL-ENERGY COMPUTED TOMOGRAPHY

The details of the physics and applied technology of DECT are extensively discussed elsewhere within this collection of articles; we will briefly discuss the salient features. DECT operates under the principle that imaging data acquired with high (120–150 kV) and low energy (80–100 kV) can distinguish between materials of high different atomic numbers.[9] The vastly different atomic numbers in calcium, iodine, and soft tissue (water) allow for material decompensation maps by subtracting calcium from water and iodine, iodine from calcium and water, or water from calcium and calcium iodine. This subtraction allows for creating of virtual non-contrast images (using the subtraction of iodine)[10] or images that accentuate enhancement characteristics (using the subtraction of water).[11] In thoracic imaging, these are referred to as pulmonary blood volume images and allow for evaluation of enhancement characteristics of lung tissue and in better detection and assessment of pulmonary emboli.[12,13]

[a] Division of Thoracic Imaging and Intervention, Massachusetts General Hospital, Boston, MA, USA; [b] Harvard Medical School, Boston, MA, USA
* Corresponding author. 55 Fruit Street, Founders 202 Boston, MA, 02114.
E-mail address: sdigumarthy@mgh.harvard.edu

Radiol Clin N Am 61 (2023) 987–994
https://doi.org/10.1016/j.rcl.2023.06.001

Differing techniques can acquire imaging data from two different energy levels. First, scanners can simultaneously use two independent x-ray sources operating at different kV over the same anatomic region with a compromised field of view. Second, a single x-ray source can rapidly acquire two independent sequential acquisitions at different kV; however, with some misregistration artifacts due to the time lag between the two acquisitions and patient movement.[14,15] Third, a gold and tin filter splits an x-ray beam at the source into low- and high-energy photons, which are then detected by a single detector and used to create the required DECT images. Finally, the exiting x-ray beam from the patient is detected by two layers of detectors to separate the low- and high-energy photons to generate the DECT images subsequently. Regardless of the technique, additional information can be extracted from the resultant data set.

IMAGE DATA SETS
Virtual Monoenergetic Images

Regardless of the acquisition method of DECT data, all vendors allow users to reconstruct virtual monoenergetic images at a single spectral energy between 40 and 200 keV (kilo electron volt). Lower keV images have higher image noise and contrast because they are close to the K-edge of the iodine. Conversely, the higher keV images have lower contrast and less noise (Fig. 1). Therefore, it is possible on some scanners to combine the high contrast of lower keV with the lower noise of higher keV to generate lower keV to generate Mono + images with lower noise.

At our institution, most chest DECT scans are reconstructed at 40 keV (Siemens) or 60 keV (GE Healthcare); these are auto-generated either on the scanner user interface or using postprocessing server-based DECT application. However, users can select any keV level on the DECT postprocessing server-based application (such as GE AW server Siemens Syngo.via).

Similar to DECT, data from energy-integrating detectors in recently commercialized photon-counting detector (PCD) CT scanners (Siemens Naeotom Alpha) also allow the reconstruction of monoenergetic images between 40 and 190 keV.[16] In addition, these scanners set detector energy thresholds for spectral acquisitions, such as in rigid thresholds of 20 and 60 keV for 120 kV acquisition and 20 and 70 keV for 140 kV.

Iodine Quantification

DECT and PCD-CT scanners allow users to measure contrast enhancement-related Hounsfield units (HU) values and iodine quantity in the selected region of interest (ROI) or volume of interest(VOI) (Fig. 2). Iodine density refers to iodine concentration (displayed as mg/mL or mg/cm³) within the ROI. Normalized iodine concentration or density refers to how iodine density within an ROI/VOI is normalized against another ROI/VOI in a tissue or blood vessel to reduce the patient variability related to contrast concentration or iodine delivery rate. Another variable is a relative enhancement (in percentage) which refers to the ratio of the iodine enhancement in the ROI relative to the iodine enhancement in the normalized ROI. Finally, the iodine-related attenuation (HU) measures the HU of the iodine enhancement in the ROI. Although HU is measured on a digital imaging and communications in medicine (DICOM) image workstation or picture archiving and communication system (PACS), a dedicated, vendor-specific DECT image processing software/workstation is generally essential for measuring iodine density or concentration. It is helpful to draw ROI in other regions such as non-enhancing chest wall musculature and within the lumen of vessels for comparison.

DUAL-ENERGY COMPUTED TOMOGRAPHY APPLICATIONS IN THORACIC ONCOLOGY
Evaluation of the Solitary Pulmonary Nodule

Single-energy CT is very sensitive in detecting pulmonary nodules but has low specificity to differentiate benign and malignant nodules. Therefore,

Mono+ 40 keV   Mono+ 60 keV   Mono+ 80 keV   Mono+ 100 keV   Mono+ 140 keV

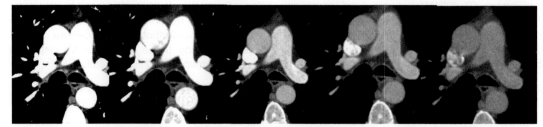

Fig. 1. Effect of keV on image contrast and noise. High contrast and high noise in pulmonary arteries and thoracic aorta at low keV transitions to low contrast and low noise at higher keV. The high contrast makes noise less perceptible in vasculature after IV contrast.

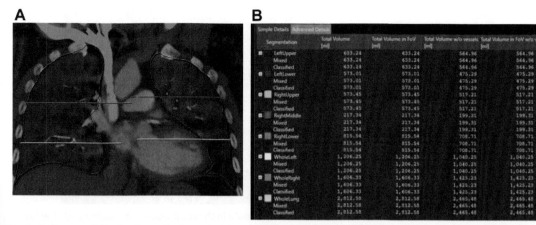

Fig. 2. Pulmonary blood volume (iodine map) images. (*A*) The iodine distribution estimated in the lung zones is a surrogate for perfusion. ROI can also be drawn in localized lung tumors and mediastinal nodes. (*B*) The accompanying displays the blood volume in the upper, mid, and lower zones in both lungs.

results in numerous follow-up examinations and invasive procedures to determine the composition of an indeterminate nodule. These diagnostic steps can cause undue stress and anxiety for the patient and add to health care costs. DECT can differentiate benign from malignant nodules at a single scan to alleviate some of these unintended downstream effects.

Lung nodule characterization is a common indication for PET/CT, and this indication was among the first to receive reimbursement from the Centers for Medicare and Medicaid Services. However, evaluating solitary pulmonary nodules by DECT predates PET/CT by nearly a decade. Higashi and colleagues[17] generated DECT images for 20 solitary pulmonary nodule (SPNs) and concluded that calcium-equivalent density images improved the detection of subtle calcifications in benign nodules. Since then, several studies examined the application of DECT for solitary pulmonary nodules. A study by Chae and colleagues[18] compared the absolute HU and degree of enhancement of 49 SPNs on virtual non-contrast DECT images compared with enhanced images. There was a significant difference between the absolute HU of benign and malignant nodules on the virtual non-contrast images and the degree of enhancement compared with the contrast-enhanced images (**Fig. 3**). In a study by Lee and colleagues[19] benign nodules demonstrated lower CT attenuation value, iodine-related value, and iodine concentration (see **Fig. 3**). However, it is essential to understand the limitations of evaluating pulmonary nodules. For example, a phantom study showed that DECT could detect calcium and iodine in artificial nodules over 16 mm, but in smaller nodules, clear differentiation was not achieved.[20] The same study, however, demonstrated contrast enhancement within

ground glass nodules, later found to be adenocarcinomas, but not within pulmonary hemorrhage or infectious/inflammatory opacities (**Fig. 4**).

Lung Cancer

Relationships between iodine measurements by DECT and subsequent histopathologic correlation of lung cancers have also been described (**Fig. 5**). For example, in a study of 60 patients, the correlation between iodine volume and subsequent tumor differentiation on pathologic specimens was examined.[21] The study was performed with a dual-phase DECT protocol, with the early phase acquired using automatic bolus tracking and a subsequent scan after a 90-second delay. The results for HU measurements in the delayed phase were as follows: 59.6 HU $\pm$ 18.6 in grade 1 tumors; 46.5 HU $\pm$ 11.3 in grade 2 tumors; 34.3 HU $\pm$ 15 in grade 3 tumors; and 28.8 HU $\pm$ 6.4 in grade 4 tumors. These differences were significant with increased contrast washout for higher grade tumors.

In a recent study by Tian and colleagues,[22] DECT was used to correlate levels of marker of cell division and mitosis (Ki-67) in patients with non-small cell lung cancer (NSCLC) and more specifically, solid lung adenocarcinoma. Expression levels of Ki-67 were separated into high-level expression (>30%), mid-level expression (10%–30%), and low-level expression (<10%). In this study, iodine concentration, among several other parameters, was higher in the high-level group than in the middle- or low-level groups ($P < .05$). The iodine concentration performed better in distinguishing the high-level and low-level groups but was less clear with the middle-level group. This offers a potential noninvasive way to monitor

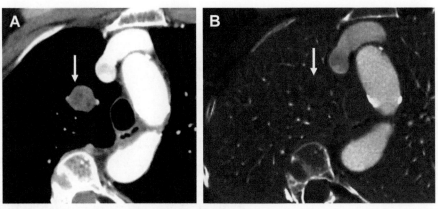

Fig. 3. Hamartoma. (*A*) CT image demonstrates low-density nodule in the right upper lobe (*arrow*). (*B*) The iodine concentration was low with a value of 0.3 mg/cc (similar to chest wall musculature 0.5 mg/cc).

the proliferation and treatment response in solid NSCLC, particularly given the prognostic implication of varying levels of Ki-67 expression.[23]

Jia and colleagues[24] used serologic markers and imaging characteristics to differentiate histologic subtypes of lung cancer. Although no specific imaging differences were detected among the attenuation characteristics between histologic subtypes, there was a difference in iodine concentration and the slope of the spectral curve between various subtypes, which became more profound with the addition of serum tumor markers. Although only applicable to a small subset of patients, this offers insights into potential applications in the future.

Evaluation of Mediastinal Lymph Nodes

Accurate delineation of lymph node involvement is crucial for staging lung cancer and choosing treatment algorithms. Unfortunately, the accuracy is still low for all the benefits of PET/CT, and nodal sampling is considered the gold standard.[25] Therefore, invasive tissue sampling is routine practice to rule out metastatic disease.

The iodine concentration and normalized iodine concentration from DECT could be used to differentiate benign from metastatic lymph nodes in NSCLC (**Fig. 6**). A study by Li and colleagues[26] was able to differentiate between benign and metastatic lymph nodes with a sensitivity of 80%; specificity of 70%; positive predictive value of 70%, and negative predictive value of 76%, and achieved 73% accuracy using a threshold of 29.32 $\mu g/cm^3$ for iodine concentration. Within this study, no difference was detected based on the histologic subtype of lung cancer.

A recent study from Nagano and colleagues[27] corroborates these findings. In this study, 57 patients had preoperative DECT and PET/CT and subsequent surgical dissection and pathologic analysis of 117 lymph nodes. The sensitivity, specificity, and accuracy of metastatic nodes were 15.2%, 98.8%, and 75.2% for the presence of necrosis; 54.5%, 85.7%, and 76.9% for short-axis diameter greater than 8.5 mm and 87.9%, 58.3%, and 66.7% for electron density of $3.48 \times 1023/cm^3$ or less, respectively. Further evaluation of pairs of these features demonstrated that the combination of electron density and short-axis diameter was better than either feature alone ($P < .05$) (sensitivity 54.5%, specificity 94.0%, and accuracy 82.9%), as was the combination of

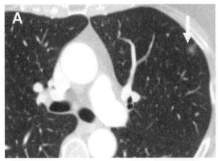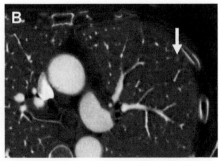

Fig. 4. Adenocarcinoma. (*A*) CT image demonstrates part-solid nodule in the left upper lobe (*arrow*). (*B*) The iodine concentration was 1.8 mg/cc.

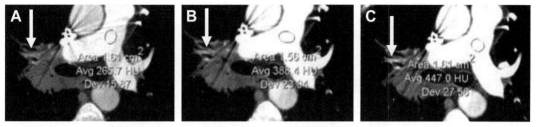

Fig. 5. High-grade adenocarcinoma with intra-tumoral vascularity. CT images at 120 KV (*A*), 65 keV (*B*), and 60 keV (*C*) demonstrate increased conspicuity of intra-tumoral vessels and increased CT HU values at lower mono-energetic images (*arrows*). There was high iodine concentration of 3 mg/cc in iodine maps (not shown here). Also notice the high contrast density in the pulmonary artery at low monoenergetic images.

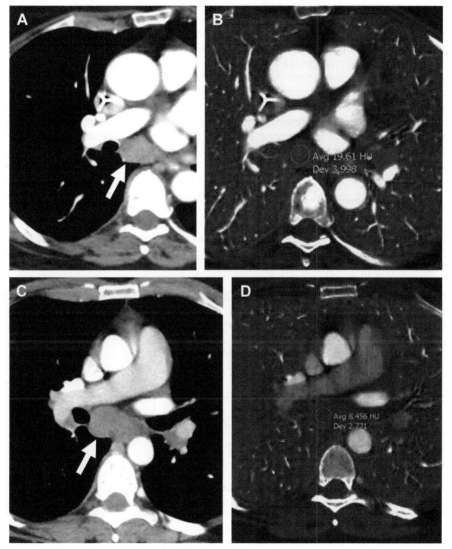

Fig. 6. Metastatic and benign mediastinal lymph nodes. Metastatic subcarinal lymph nodes in mediastinal window (*A*) and iodine images (*B*) demonstrate high CT enhancement and iodine concentration (2 mg/cc) compared with lymph nodes in sarcoidosis in mediastinal (*C*) and iodine images (*D*) with a low iodine concentration of 0.8 mg/cc.

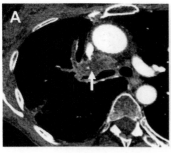
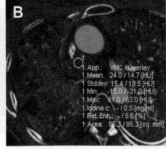
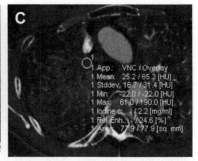

Fig. 7. Mediastinal nodes treated with chemoradiation. (*A*) CT demonstrates necrotic right paratracheal lymphadenopathy. Iodine map demonstrates low central iodine concentration of 0.5 mg/mL (*B*) and high peripheral iodine concentration of 2.2 mg/mL suggestive of residual viable tumor (*C*) in apparently necrotic nodes.

electron density and positive fluorodeoxyglucose (FDG) activity (sensitivity 60.6%, specificity 90.5%, and accuracy 82.9%).

An additional study from Ogawa and colleagues[28] demonstrated that patients undergoing a single-phase DECT scan could replace a dual-phase single-energy CT to evaluate both mediastinal structures, including vessels and lymph nodes, and enhancement in pulmonary lesions. In addition, using a single phase DECT scan allows for decreased radiation (depending on technique) than a dual-phase single-energy study and additional lesion characterization.

Evaluating Lesion Characteristics and Treatment Response

To this point, assessing metabolic activity and associated treatment response have been a primary differentiator when comparing the utility of single-energy CT versus PET/CT. DECT can add incremental value over single-energy CT. Several studies examined the use of DECT to assess treatment response after different treatments. A study by Baxa and colleagues[29] found that iodine concentration values in metastatic lymph nodes remained elevated in non-responding lymph nodes and decreased in responding lymph nodes (**Fig. 7**).[7] A study by Liu and colleagues[30] examined the utility of DECT in patients after undergoing radiofrequency ablation (RFA) for primary lung cancer and demonstrated that the iodine concentration of the lesions significantly decreased after treatment (**Fig. 8**). Whereas, increasing iodine concentration on follow-up examinations can predict early recurrence in tumors terates with RFA.[31]

A recent dual-phase DECT study found a correlation between peripheral and central iodine

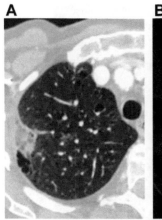
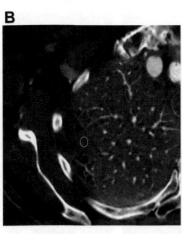
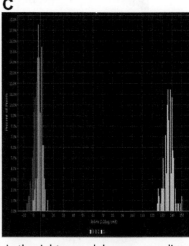

Fig. 8. Lung cancer treated with thermal ablation. (*A*) Peripheral opacity in the right upper lobe corresponding to treatment zone that resembles a pulmonary infarct. (*B*) Iodine map demonstrates no iodine concentration. Region of interests was drawn in the shoulder musculature (*red ellipse*), ablated cancer (*pink ellipse*) and in the right brachiocephalic artery (*yellow ellipse*). The iodine concentration is displayed as a graph (*C*). The nonenhancing musculature and the ablated tumor have iodine concentration of less than 0.3 mg/cc and the contrast opacified blood in the right brachiocephalic artery has reached a concentration over 12 mg/cc.

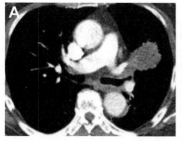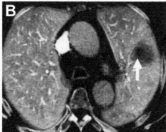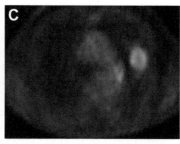

Fig. 9. Tumor necrosis and hypoxia. (*A*) CT demonstrates homogeneous density mass in the central left upper lobe. (*B*). Iodine images demonstrate low central iodine concentration of 0.5 mg/mL (*arrow*) suggesting necrosis and intra-tumoral hypoxia and possible poor response to radiation therapy. (*C*) 18F FDG PET shows increased uptake in the tumor above the level of mediastinal blood pool.

concentration and tumor hypoxia on pathology. It offers a new noninvasive approach to evaluating tumor characteristics and predicting response to therapy,[32] as tumor hypoxia is associated with poor response to radiation therapy (**Fig. 9**). This degree of detail is not possible given the spatial resolution of PET and is a unique capability of DECT. PET/CT remains the gold standard for assessing metabolic activity and is used after lung-distorting treatment, such as external beam radiation therapy and ablation. However, DECT offers an exciting alternative to PET that does not require patient preparation or long scan times and can be used for radiation treatment planning.[33]

SUMMARY

DECT demonstrates added value in the imaging of patients with thoracic malignancies particularly lung cancer from diagnosis through treatment response and treatment planning in radiation therapy. In addition, the clinical application of DECT can provide additional information about tumor growth and biology to optimize dose modulation to the areas of greatest concern in radiation therapy. More extensive prospective studies comparing DECT with PET/CT and in the future photon-counting CT can validate the clinical application of DECT and increase utilization.

CLINICS CARE POINTS

- Dual-energy computed tomography (DECT) can be single-source or dual-source scanner with one or two x-ray tubes. The image data sets can be predetermined and sent directly to the PACS to improve efficiency. If needed the desired image data sets can also be generated by radiologists.

- The applications of DECT in lung cancer are mostly derived by measuring iodine-related enhancement, iodine concentration, and generating iodine maps. These features help to differentiate benign and malignant nodules and low and high grades of lung cancer.

- Assessment of iodine values in lymph nodes helps to improve prediction of metastasis and determining residual disease after treatment.

- Detection of hypoxia and necrosis in the primary tumor may have prognostic value and helps in guiding the treatment plan, particularly for radiation therapy. The success of thermal ablation of lung cancers can also be predicted by residual iodine concentration and iodine-related enhancement.

DISCLOSURES

Dr S.R. Digumarthy provides independent image analysis for hospital-contracted clinical research trials programs for Merck, Pfizer, Bristol Myers Squibb, Novartis, Roche, Polaris, Cascadian, Abbvie, Gradalis, Bayer, Zai laboratories, Biengen, Resonance, Analise. Research grants from Lunit Inc, Korea, GE, United States, Qure AI, Vuno Inc and honorarium from Siemens.

REFERENCES

1. Cancer facts & figures 2022. Available at: Cancer.org. Available at: https://www.cancer.org/research/cancer-facts-statistics/all-cancer-facts-figures/cancer-facts-figures-2022.html Accessed May 2023.
2. USCS data visualizations - CDC. Centers for Disease Control and Prevention. Available at: https://gis.cdc.gov/Cancer/USCS/#/AtAGlance/. Accessed May 2023.
3. NCCN Imaging Appropriate Use Criteria™. Available at: https://www.nccn.org/professionals/imaging/content/. Accessed May 2023.

4. Hamid S, Nasir MU, So A, et al. Clinical Applications of Dual-Energy CT. Korean J Radiol 2021;22(6):970–82.

5. Sanghavi PS, Jankharia BG. Applications of dual energy CT in clinical practice: A pictorial essay. Indian J Radiol Imaging 2019;29(3):289–98.

6. Khan AU, Khanduri S, Tarin Z, et al. Dual-Energy Computed Tomography Lung in patients of Pulmonary Tuberculosis. J Clin Imaging Sci 2020;10:39.

7. Canellas R, Digumarthy SR, Otrakji A, et al. Applications of DECT in Thoracic Oncology: Evidence So Far. Clin Oncol 2016;1:1148.

8. D'Angelo T, Albrecht MH, Caudo D, et al. Virtual noncalcium dual-energy CT: clinical applications. Eur Radiol Exp 2021;5(1):38.

9. Liu X, Yu L, Primak AN, et al. Quantitative imaging of element composition and mass fraction using dual-energy CT: three-material decomposition. Med Phys 2009;36:1602–9.

10. Toepker M, Moritz T, Krauss B, et al. Virtual noncontrast in second-generation, dual-energy computed tomography: reliability of attenuation values. Eur J Radiol 2012;81:e398–405.

11. Sakamoto A, Sakamoto I, Nagayama H, et al. Quantification of lung perfusion blood volume with dual-energy CT: assessment of the severity of acute pulmonary thromboembolism. AJR Am J Roentgenol 2014;203:287–91.

12. Hong YJ, Shim J, Lee SM, et al. Dual-Energy CT for Pulmonary Embolism: Current and Evolving Clinical Applications. Korean J Radiol 2021 Sep;22(9):1555–68.

13. Digumarthy SR, Singh R, Rastogi S, et al. Low contrast volume dual-energy CT of the chest: Quantitative and qualitative assessment. Clin Imaging 2021 Jan;69:305–10.

14. Mangold S, Gatidis S, Luz O, et al. Single-source dual-energy computed tomography: use of monoenergetic extrapolation for a reduction of metal artifacts. Invest Radiol 2014;49:788–93.

15. Ginat DT, Gupta R. Advances in computed tomography imaging technology. Annu Rev Biomed Eng 2014;16:431–53.

16. Willemink MJ, Persson M, Pourmorteza A, et al. Photon-counting CT: Technical Principles and Clinical Prospects. Radiology 2018 Nov;289(2):293–312.

17. Higashi Y, Nakamura H, Matsumoto T, et al. Dual-energy computed tomographic diagnosis of pulmonary nodules. J Thorac Imaging 1994;9:31–4.

18. Chae EJ, Song JW, Seo JB, et al. Clinical utility of dual-energy CT in the evaluation of solitary pulmonary nodules: initial experience. Radiology 2008; 249:671–81.

19. Lee SH, Hur J, Kim YJ, et al. Additional value of dual-energy CT to differentiate between benign and malignant mediastinal tumors: an initial experience. Eur J Radiol 2013 Nov;82(11):2043–9.

20. Kawai T, Shibamoto Y, Hara M, et al. Can dual-energy CT evaluate contrast enhancement of ground-glass attenuation? Phantom and preliminary clinical studies. Acad Radiol 2011;18:682–9.

21. Iwano S, Ito R, Umakoshi H, et al. Evaluation of lung cancer by enhanced dual-energy CT: association between three-dimensional iodine concentration and tumour differentiation. Br J Radiol 2015;88: 20150224.

22. Tian S, Jianguo X, Tian W, et al. Application of dual-energy computed tomography in preoperative evaluation of Ki-67 expression levels in solid non-small cell lung cancer. Medicine (Baltim) 2022;101(31): e29444.

23. Chirieac LR. Ki-67 expression in pulmonary tumors. Transl Lung Cancer Res 2016 Oct;5(5):547–51.

24. Jia Y, Xiao X, Sun Q, et al. CT spectral parameters and serum tumor markers to differentiate histological types of cancer histology. Clin Radiol 2018;73:1033–40.

25. Kligerman S, Digumarthy S. Staging of non-small cell lung cancer using integrated PET/CT. AJR Am J Roentgenol 2009 Nov;193(5):1203–11.

26. Li GJ, Gao J, Wang GL, et al. Correlation between vascular endothelial growth factor and quantitative dual-energy spectral CT in non-small-cell lung cancer. Clin Radiol 2016;71:363–8.

27. Nagano H, Takumi K, Nakajo M, et al. Dual-Energy CT-Derived Electron Density for Diagnosing Metastatic Mediastinal Lymph Nodes in Non-Small Cell Lung Cancer: Comparison with Conventional CT and FDG PET/CT Findings. AJR Am J Roentgenol 2022 Jan;218(1):66–74.

28. Ogawa M, Hara M, Imafuji A, et al. Dual-energy CT can evaluate both hilar and mediastinal lymph nodes and lesion vascularity with a single scan at 60 seconds after contrast medium injection. Acad Radiol 2012;19:1003–10.

29. Baxa J, Vondráková A, Matoušková T, et al. Dual-phase dual-energy CT in patients with lung cancer: assessment of the additional value of iodine quantification in lymph node therapy response. Eur Radiol 2014;24:1981–8.

30. Liu L, Zhi X, Liu B, et al. Utilizing gemstone spectral CT imaging to evaluate the therapeutic efficacy of radiofrequency ablation in lung cancer. Radiol Med 2016 Apr;121(4):261–7.

31. Izaaryene J, Vidal V, Bartoli JM, et al. Role of dual-energy computed tomography in detecting early recurrences of lung tumours treated with radiofrequency ablation. Int J Hyperthermia 2017 Sep; 33(6):653–8.

32. Dewaguet J, Copin MC, Duhamel A, et al. Dual-Energy CT Perfusion of Invasive Tumor Front in Non-Small Cell Lung Cancers. Radiology 2022 Feb; 302(2):448–56.

33. Zhu J, Penfold SN. Dosimetric comparison of stopping power calibration with dual-energy CT and single-energy CT in proton therapy treatment planning. Med Phys 2016 Jun;43(6):2845–54.

Dual-Energy Computed Tomography in Cardiac Imaging

Benjamin Böttcher, MD[a,b], Emese Zsarnoczay, MD[c,d],
Akos Varga-Szemes, MD, PhD[c], Uwe Joseph Schoepf, MD[c],
Felix G. Meinel, MD[b], Marly van Assen, MSc, PhD[a],
Carlo N. De Cecco, MD, PhD[e,*]

KEYWORDS

- Dual-energy computed tomography • Cardiovascular imaging • Coronary plaque imaging
- Myocardial perfusion imaging • Myocardial tissue characterization • Photon counting

KEY POINTS

- Dual-energy computed tomography (CT) imaging provides virtual monoenergetic images with improved image quality and contrast attenuation allowing significant reduction of contrast volume.
- Dual-energy CT-derived virtual non-contrast images enable coronary artery calcium scoring from contrast-enhanced scans.
- Dual-energy CT offers material decomposition for advanced coronary plaque analysis.
- Dual-energy CT-based myocardial perfusion imaging adds incremental value over cardiac CT angiography for assessment of coronary artery disease.
- Dual-energy CT imaging enables noninvasive myocardial fibrosis evaluation.

INTRODUCTION

Cardiovascular diseases (CVDs) are the leading cause for hospitalization and death worldwide.[1,2] Noninvasive imaging plays a major role in treatment and prognosis of CVD. Computed tomography (CT) provides anatomical and functional information and is implemented in various guidelines.[3–6] Various techniques such as coronary artery calcium (CAC) scoring, cardiac CT angiography (CCTA), CT-derived fractional flow reserve (CT-FFR), and myocardial perfusion imaging (MPI) enable numerous facets of CVD. Especially the high

negative predictive value of CCTA allows CT to act as a gatekeeper for invasive treatment techniques, such as invasive coronary angiography or transcatheter aortic valve implantation.[5]

Cardiac CT imaging is performed mainly using single-energy CT (SECT) acquisition where images are acquired on a single predefined energy level. Thus, recommended energy levels represent a compromise between low-energy acquisition settings providing high soft tissue contrast but susceptible for metal, beam-hardening and blooming artifacts, and high-energy acquisitions with opposite characteristics.[7] New generation

[a] Division of Cardiothoracic Imaging, Department of Radiology and Imaging Sciences, Emory University Hospital, 1364 Clifton Road NE, Suite D112, Atlanta, GA 30322, USA; [b] Institute of Diagnostic and Interventional Radiology, Pediatric Radiology and Neuroradiology, University Medical Centre Rostock, Ernst-Heydemann-Strasse 6, 18057 Rostock, Germany; [c] Division of Cardiovascular Imaging, Department of Radiology and Radiological Science, Medical University of South Carolina, Clinical Science Building, 96 Jonathan Lucas Street, Suite 210, MSC 323 Charleston, SC 29425, USA; [d] MTA-SE Cardiovascular Imaging Research Group, Medical Imaging Center, Semmelweis University, Üllői út 26, 1085 Budapest, Hungary; [e] Division of Cardiothoracic Imaging and Imaging Informatics, Department of Radiology and Imaging Sciences, Emory University Hospital, Emory Healthcare, Inc. 1365 Clifton Road NE, Suite - AT503, Atlanta, GA 30322, USA
* Corresponding author. Department of Radiology and Imaging Sciences Emory University Hospital, Emory Healthcare, Inc., 1365 Clifton Road NE, Suite - AT503, Atlanta, GA 30322.
E-mail address: carlo.dececco@emory.edu

Radiol Clin N Am 61 (2023) 995–1009
https://doi.org/10.1016/j.rcl.2023.05.004

CT scanners allow image acquisitions with two energy spectra—dual-energy CT (DECT) or spectral CT, respectively. DECT imaging allows multiple new image reconstruction options which have an incremental value in optimizing image quality and quantifying materials such as iodine.[8]

DECT technique has reached clinical practice for a limited number of applications; however, DECT imaging is still it its development stage.[9–11] Although DECT shows potential for improving diagnostic imaging of CVD, plenty of challenges remain before DECT can be implemented in standard care on a large scale.[12] This review aims to outline current cardiac applications of DECT, summarizing recent literature and discussing their findings.

DUAL-ENERGY COMPUTED TOMOGRAPHY TECHNIQUES FOR CARDIAC IMAGING

Cardiac CT imaging is challenging because of complex anatomical structures, such as coronary arteries in addition to cardiac and respiratory motion. Dual-energy imaging refers to acquisition and processing of CT data using two different energies. Different DECT systems are available, including dual-source DECT (Siemens Healthineers), single-source rapid kV-switching DECT (GE Healthcare), and dual-layer DECT (Philips Medical Systems), which differ in image acquisition and processing methodology but provide similar image reconstructions.[13] DECT provides several key features which can enhance cardiac imaging, as summarized in **Table 1**. First, using two energy levels allows the reconstruction of virtual monoenergetic images (VMIs). These images combine data of both high- and low-energy CT acquisition using characteristics of each energy level to simulate single-energy acquisitions at multiple keV levels.[7] Suggested optimum energy level for cardiac evaluation is 70 keV for traditional VMI algorithms[14] and 40 keV for noise-optimized VMI algorithms.[15] Lower energy reconstruction can be used to improve contrast attenuation, whereas higher kV reconstruction can be used to reduce artifacts, for example, in stent imaging.

The second feature provided by DECT is material decomposition. DECT enables material identification using the unique attenuation profiles of different materials, identified by using both energy levels.[16] Thus, material-specific signals can be suppressed or increased during image reconstruction. Most relevant reconstruction techniques for cardiovascular imaging are virtual non-contrast (VNC) and calcium subtraction images. VNC images remove iodine signals from contrast-enhanced DECT scans allowing coronary calcium score assessment without need for additional non-contrast CT scan.[10] Calcium subtraction images remove calcium from contrast-enhanced DECT images, improving vessel depiction and lumen visualization in coronary arteries, for example.[17] In addition, material decompensation allows for the quantification of material concentrations, such as iodine, which can be used to quantify myocardial perfusion.[8] See **Fig. 1** for an overview of DECT key features.

EFFECTS OF DUAL-ENERGY COMPUTED TOMOGRAPHY ON RADIATION DOSE, ENHANCEMENT, AND ARTIFACT REDUCTION

Sufficient contrast attenuation and detailed visualization of fine anatomical structures is needed to meet diagnostic requirements. Impaired image quality caused by motion artifacts and metal artifacts from cardiac support devices represent unique challenges for cardiac imaging.

DECT imaging improves diagnostic interpretation of the cardiovascular system while using similar radiation doses as SECT acquisitions. Studies on different approaches for DECT such as dual-source, dual–layer, and rapid kV-switching show that radiation dose is similar or can even be reduced across all available DECT scanner technologies while increasing image quality.[18–20] However, most of these studies are performed using 120 kV SECT scans as reference. The current trend is to image at lower kV levels to decrease radiation dose where possible, however, DECT has the disadvantage of need for high-energy acquisition.

The volume of contrast agent used during image acquisition is critical to ensure sufficient attenuation within target structures. Impaired renal function is not uncommon in cardiac patients, and therefore, the volume of contrast agents needs to be minimized. DECT VMI allows for greater than 50% contrast volume reduction in dual-energy CCTA providing similar image interpretability and diagnostic accuracy as single-energy protocols with standard contrast dose.[21–24] Similar results were found for pre-TAVR DECT angiography.[25] An example of increasing contrast attenuation with decreasing VMI energy level is visualized in **Fig. 2**.

The increasing prevalence of cardiac devices (such as ICDs and pacemakers), valve protheses, and coronary stents increase the prevalence of artifacts causing impaired image quality and reduced diagnostic performance. DECT VMI at high energy levels significantly decreases blooming artifacts and improves stent lumen visualization.[26,27] However, higher energy levels provide lower contrast attenuation and contrast-to-noise ratio (CNR) hampering in-stent restenosis

Table 1
Overview of dual-energy computed tomography techniques for advanced cardiac imaging

DECT Technique	Characteristics	Advantages Over SECT	Qualitative Versus Quantitative Analysis	PCD-CT Improvements
Virtual monoenergetic images (VMIs)	Simulated single-energy images ranging from 40–140 keV Optimal energy level for cardiac imaging 70 keV or noise-optimized 40 keV Optimal energy level for stent imaging 80 keV	Improved image quality Significant reduction of contrast volume possible Improved stent imaging	Qualitative + semiquantitative	Electronic noise filtering reduces image noise and increases CNR Advanced spatial resolution Extended energy spectrum
Material decomposition	Attenuation-based using unique attenuation profiles of materials or based on calculation of electron density (ρ_e) and effective atomic number (Z_{eff})	Improved diagnostic accuracy for plaque characterization. Quantitative assessment of plaque components	Qualitative + quantitative	k-edge imaging using spectral singularities of materials allows advanced material decomposition
Virtual non-contrast (VNC) images	Material decomposition-based suppression of contrast attenuation	Provides unenhanced images without need for true non-contrast scan	Qualitative	Advanced virtual non-contrast Virtual non-iodine images Quantification of calcium mass
Calcium subtraction images	Material decomposition-based suppression of calcium attenuation	Improved vessel und lumen depiction in heavily calcified coronary arteries	Qualitative	Advanced material separation
Iodine distribution maps	Material decomposition-based amplification of iodine attenuation	Direct visualization of iodine distribution as indirect surrogate of myocardial perfusion and detection of late iodine distribution to calculate extracellular volume fraction	Qualitative + quantitative	Advanced material separation and spatial resolution

Abbreviations: DECT, dual-energy computed tomography; PCD-CT, photon-counting computed tomography; SECT, single-energy computed tomography.

| Image acquisition | Image reconstruction | Cardiac imaging Task |

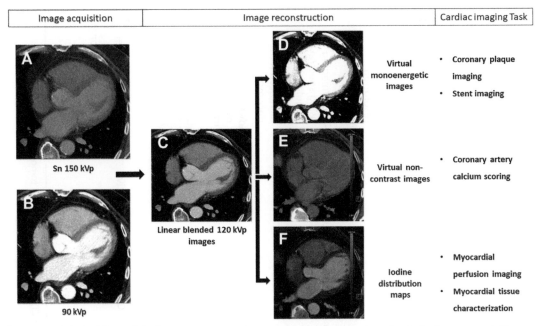

Fig. 1. Imaging workflow of dual-energy computed tomography for cardiac imaging tasks. Image acquisition was performed with a dual-source dual-energy CT system at Sn150 kVp (*A*) and 90 kVp (*B*). Image reconstruction provides (*C*) linear blended images simulating conventional single-energy images acquired at 120 kVp. (*D*) Virtual monoenergetic images suitable for advanced coronary plaque and stent imaging. (*E*) Virtual non-contrast images enabling coronary artery calcium scoring from contrast-enhanced scans. (*F*) Iodine distribution maps providing myocardial perfusion and myocardial tissue assessment.

evaluation. VMI at lower energy levels improves contrast enhancement but increases artifacts and cannot be recommended for stent imaging.[28] Studies have showed that DECT VMI at 80 keV is optimal for coronary stent imaging, combining sufficient enhancement with significant reduction of beam hardening and blooming artifacts.[29] The evaluation of in-stent restenosis using dual-source and dual-layer DECT showed no significant differences indicating improved stent imaging.[30]

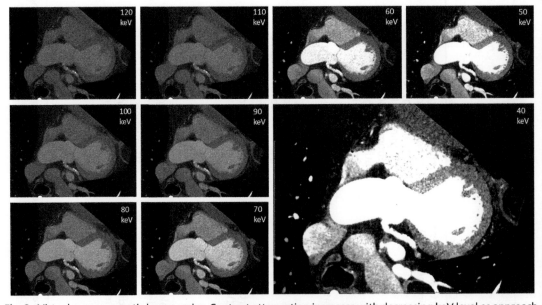

Fig. 2. Virtual monoenergetic image series. Contrast attenuation increases with decreasing keV level as approaching the k-edge of iodine at 33.2 keV. Also note the increase of image noise with decreasing energy level.

CORONARY ARTERY ASSESSMENT
Coronary Artery Calcium Scoring

CAC quantification based on the Agatston score[31] on CT is used to assess calcium burden in patients with suspected coronary artery disease (CAD).[4,6] DECT offers the possibility of VNC reconstructions. An example is visualized in **Fig. 3**. This enables CAC scoring on contrast-enhanced acquisitions, allowing complete coronary artery assessment in a single acquisition offering radiation dose reduction[32] and decreasing scanning times and costs.

Efficient iodine removal in VNC images is critical for accurate CAC scoring since remaining iodine attenuation or falsely removed calcifications mistaken as iodine could cause inaccurate scoring. VNC reconstructions have shown to provide excellent iodine removal efficiency and reliability.[33–35] However, iodine removal quality is notably impacted by radiation dose, size, and density of calcified stenoses[36] and should therefore be interpreted with caution.

DECT-derived CAC scores, volumes, and mass highly correlate with measurements from true non-contrast (TNC) SECT data sets on per-patient and per-vessel level[32–35,37] as well as on per-stenosis level.[36] However, DECT tends to underestimate small and low-density calcified plaques, whereas large and high-density plaques are overestimated.[36]

DECT CCTA-derived VNC images can rule-out coronary calcifications with high accuracy and false-positive results predominantly related to imaging artifacts.[32–35] Excellent correlation is also reported for CAC scoring in VNC images obtained from contrast-enhanced non-gated chest DECT.[38,39]

However, occasionally false-negative results are shown, most likely caused by cardiac motion artifacts.[39] DECT systematically underestimates absolute CAC compared with TNC SECT with more noticeable deviation in non-gated chest DECT,[32–39] possibly caused by reduced blooming and beam hardening artifacts in VNC images. Advanced reconstruction algorithms such as contrast material extraction processing and new contrast agents can reduce mean deviation of DECT-derived CAC scoring.[40] Scanner adjusted

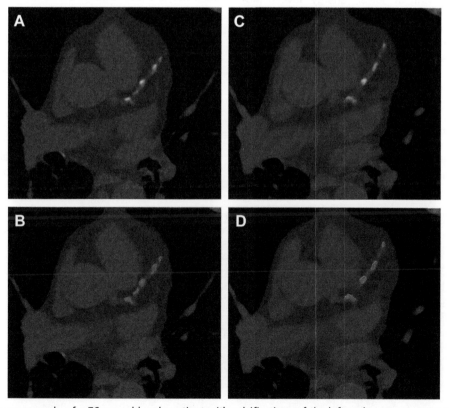

Fig. 3. Image example of a 76-year-old male patient with calcifications of the left main coronary artery (LM) and left anterior descending artery (LAD). True non-contrast image (A, B) and virtual non-contrast (C, D) reconstructions at the same slice positions with color overlay of CAC scoring (CACS). Total true non-contrast CACS = 624.6 and total virtual non-contrast CACS = 636.3.These spectral images were acquired using a PCD-CT system. However, images acquired with EID-CT systems in dual-energy mode have similar ability to create virtual non-contrast images.

Agatston scores and regression models can be used to correct underestimation of absolute values enabling direct comparison with TNC SECT-derived CAC values.

Overall, CAC scoring using DECT VNC images is feasible, showing high correlation to state-of-the-art TNC SECT scores. However, DECT VNC shows a systemic underestimation of absolute CAC values, requiring the use of adjusted Agatston scores or correction algorithms for correct interpretation.

Coronary Artery Plaque Analysis

Detection, quantification, and characterization of coronary artery plaques are a key task for cardiac CT imaging. DECT provides very high sensitivity for detection of calcified plaques, non-inferior to SECT.[41] However, blooming artifacts and partial volume effects greatly limit SECT-derived plaque quantification.[42] DECT VMI can improve accuracy of stenosis quantification, offering the highest accuracy in 90 keV VMI for calcified and partly calcified plaques and 140 keV VMI for non-calcified plaques.[43] VMI at lower energy levels (40–70 keV) provides higher CNR improving delineation between contrast enhancement and plaques but suffer from negative effects of calcium blooming similarly to SECT images.[14]

Calcium subtraction images, as visualized in **Fig. 4**, significantly reduce blooming artifacts improving image quality and diagnostic accuracy in patients with high calcium burden.[44,45] Calcium subtraction images showed improved lumen depiction with increased diagnostic confidence of radiologists while providing similar image quality as SECT acquisitions.[17]

Plaque composition is critical for cardiac risk assessment as several features are associated with increased risk for major adverse cardiac events.[46–48] DECT-derived plaque characterization can be performed with attenuation-based (or hounsfield-unit-[HU]-based) methods and calculation of electron density (ρ_e) and effective atomic number (Z_{eff}).

Attenuation-based DECT material composition uses changing attenuation values of elements in different energy spectra. Calcium shows a significant change of attenuation over the x-ray energy spectrum, whereas soft tissue components remain similar. DECT material decomposition increases diagnostic accuracy of plaque characterization compared with SECT.[49,50] Machine learning approaches have been used for combined assessment of multiple DECT reconstructions further improving discrimination between lipid and fibrous plaques.[51] However, attenuation-based material decomposition remains challenging for plaque characterization due to overlapping HU values for soft tissue components.

Electron density (ρ_e) and effective atomic number (Z_{eff}) can be obtained from DECT data using numerical algorithms. Subsequent comparison of calculated values with theoretical known ρ_e and Z_{eff} values allows identification and quantification of tissue components. DECT-derived Z_{eff} can detect different components of coronary artery plaques.[52] DECT enables quantitative analysis of lipid, fibrous, and calcium components in non-calcified plaques,[53] which allows the detection of vulnerable plaques in ex vivo coronary artery samples.[54] Computational simulations suggest quantification of coronary plaque components such water, lipid, calcium, and protein contents are also possible.[55]

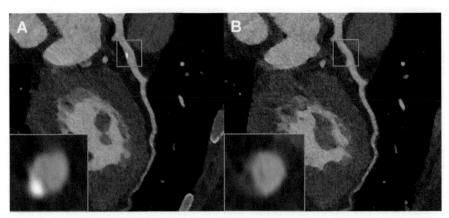

Fig. 4. Image example of a 56-year-old man with a calcification in the left anterior descending artery (LAD). Coronary CT angiography (*A*) shows a mild stenosis in the LAD. By using a calcium removal algorithm (*B*), calcium attenuation can be suppressed resulting in improved lumen depiction. This specific case used a PCD-CT for image acquisition. However, similar calcium subtraction algorithms are available for dual-energy EID-CT.

Very few studies are performed on the clinical application and accuracy of DECT-based plaque characterization. Studies have showed higher diagnostic performance and sensitivity for Z_{eff} measurements compared with attenuation-based material decomposition in non-calcified plaques.[56] Recent research on the identification of culprit lesions suggests that both attenuation-based and Z_{eff}-based analysis improve sensitivity and diagnostic accuracy in combination with conventional CT plaque characteristics.[57]

In summary, DECT plaque characterization can provide detailed analysis of calcified plaques and plaque stability. Non-calcified plaque classification remains challenging but new methods including calculation of ρ_e and Z_{eff} from DECT data showed promising results in preclinical studies. Although initial results are promising, large trials in a clinical setting are missing.

MYOCARDIAL PERFUSION IMAGING

MPI provides functional assessment of CAD. Myocardial perfusion can be performed by using static and dynamic MPI acquisitions, whereas infarcted areas can be detected by using late iodine enhancement imaging similarly to late gadolinium enhancement with MR imaging.[58]

Using VMI, hypo-attenuation in areas with perfusion defects can be identified visually and semi-quantitatively. Attenuation-based DECT VMI for MPI offers superior image quality with high robustness against beam-hardening artifacts resulting in better diagnostic accuracy compared with SECT.[59] VMI at low energy levels provides higher sensitivity for iodine enhancing differences between normal myocardium and perfusion defects and is therefore preferable for MPI providing better diagnostic accuracy.[60] Overall, VMI reconstructions of stress–rest DECT MPI showed reliably high accuracy for detection of perfusion defects using SPECT as reference.[59–61] Combined evaluation of CCTA and stress–rest DECT MPI from VMI shows superior diagnostic performance over CCTA alone.[61] The individual analysis of rest acquisitions found similar attenuation values for normal myocardium and ischemic defects.[60] It is therefore likely that reversible perfusion defects are missed using rest-only imaging, indicating a higher diagnostic benefit of using stress acquisitions.

Quantitative iodine distribution maps can be reconstructed from DECT data sets, these iodine maps can subsequently be interpreted visually or quantitatively, see Fig. 5, for an example. Visual assessment of iodine maps showed high accuracy when compared with MR imaging,[62–64] SPECT,[65]

and PET[66] MPI. Significant improvements of diagnostic performance for detection of hemodynamically relevant CAD by adding iodine maps to CCTA assessment are demonstrated for stress-only,[63] stress–rest,[67,68] and rest-only[66] DECT protocols. In addition, combined CCTA/stress–rest DECT MPI showed non-inferior results when compared with CCTA/SPECT[68] while omitting the need for second imaging modality.

Highest improvement in accuracy of CCTA/stress–rest DECT MPI over CCTA assessment alone is in patients with coronary stents.[68] DECT MPI is capable to overcome the limitation of impaired image quality caused by stents by detecting these in-stent restenosis through detection of the resulting myocardial perfusion defects.

Investigations on usage of rest and stress acquisitions indicate that CCTA combined with rest-only has inferior diagnostic performance compared with a CCTA stress-only combination.[62,65] Rest-only protocols especially fall short in detecting reversible defects which are apparent only under stress. The comparison of stress-only versus stress–rest protocols showed no difference in diagnostic performance,[65] indicating that the stress acquisition is the most important one for perfusion purposes.

Beyond visual analysis, iodine concentrations can be obtained from DECT iodine distribution maps for quantitative analysis. Various phantom-based studies have shown high accuracy of iodine quantification across a wide spectrum of DECT scanner technologies,[69–71] with decreasing accuracy with increasing patient size.[69] Accuracy improved with increasing energy separation used during image acquisition.[70] Myocardial iodine concentrations derived from DECT strongly correlated with myocardial blood flow values from dynamic CT perfusion images and could correctly determine perfusion defects in a porcine model with invasive FFR as reference standard.[72] Iodine concentration thresholds were determined using MR imaging stress–rest perfusion as reference standard and in stress-only[73] and stress–rest[74] DECT settings in small sample size studies. Threshold iodine concentration of 2.5 mg/mL at rest[74] and 2.1 mg/mL at stress[73,74] showed optimal discrimination between normal myocardium and perfusion defects; however, further investigation of these thresholds is needed. The differentiation between ischemia and infarction is challenging due to overlapping concentration values particularly in stress DECT MPI and reduced quantification accuracy at lower iodine concentrations.[70] Thresholds for differentiation between ischemia and infarction are only described in one small study for rest DECT acquisitions (1.0 mg/mL).[74] A recent

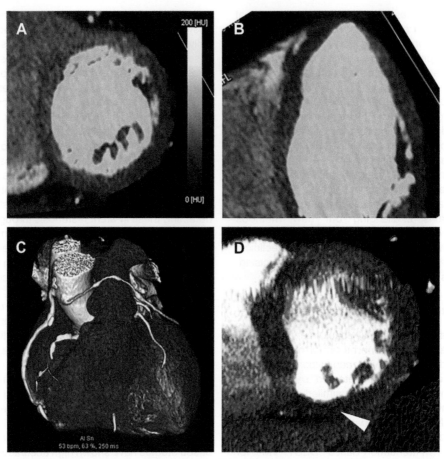

Fig. 5. Dual-energy computed tomography iodine distribution maps acquired in different individuals at rest (*A* and *B*) and stress (*D*).Case 1, top row: Iodine maps in (*A*) short axis view and (*B*) long axis view with homogeneous iodine distribution indicating normal myocardial perfusion at rest. Case 2, bottom row: Dual-energy-based 3D reconstruction (*C*) and iodine distribution map (*D*) of a patient with multiple coronary artery bypass grafts. (*C*) 3D reconstruction of computed tomography images visualizing coronary arteries and bypass grafts. (*D*) Iodine distribution map indicates an inferior wall transmural defect (see *arrowhead*) consistent with chronic myocardial infarct in the right coronary artery territory.

investigation on different contrast injection protocols found significant variations of absolute iodine concentration values.[75] Iodine quantification and its use to detect myocardial perfusion defects need further investigation and standardization to be clinically applicable. However, the quantitative assessment of iodine distribution maps showed superior diagnostic performance compared with visual analysis.[76] The combined use of available DECT techniques suggests optimal perfusion assessment.[77]

It can be concluded that DECT MPI is feasible and showed good accuracy in detecting myocardial perfusion defects. Stress and stress–rest DECT acquisitions add the most value over anatomical evaluation alone with superior diagnostic capabilities over rest-only protocols. Although quantitative analysis shows potential in

small studies, further research is needed to prove clinical value.

MYOCARDIAL TISSUE CHARACTERIZATION

Myocardial fibrosis is a major cause of impaired myocardial contractility and reduced cardiac function. Fibrotic remodeling can be induced after acute myocardial injury such as myocarditis or myocardial infarction as well as by chronic cardiac overload and infiltrative diseases such as amyloidosis and Fabry disease.[78,79] Appropriate treatment can interrupt or reverse certain fibrotic changes.[80] Thus, myocardial tissue characterization is beneficial to guide clinical management and treatment in various cardiac diseases.[81]

The gold standard for myocardial fibrosis detection is endomyocardial biopsy. However, major tradeoffs are periprocedural complications and sampling errors. The latter can cause false-negative results and is not capable of determining the extent of fibrosis.[82]

Extracellular volume (ECV) refers to the proportion of extracellular compartment in myocardial tissue, and ECV values correlate with the collagen volume fraction as reported for various cardiac pathologies.[83–87] The assessment of ECV is commonly performed with cardiac MR imaging.[81] However, late iodine enhancement imaging using CT has emerged as an alternative solution with high correlation to both MR imaging and histology.[88–91] To calculate ECV values, CT attenuation pre- and post-contrast administration within myocardium and blood pool as well as the hematocrit level needs to be determined. SECT requires two separate CT acquisitions (ie, non-contrast and late iodine enhancement images) to discriminate the change of CT attenuation.[88,89] DECT provides VNC images omitting the need for a separate TNC scan.[92] In addition, changes in CT attenuation can be derived from DECT iodine maps by measuring the iodine distribution equilibrium in the myocardium and blood pool.[91] Because iodine concentration pre-contrast administration is zero, this approach only requires a post-contract acquisition. An example is visualized in **Fig. 6**. Previous investigations showed high correlation between SECT- and DECT-derived ECV indicating potential reduction of radiation dose, scanning time, and mis-registration by DECT.[88,89,91,92] In comparison to SECT, DECT was reported to provide more accurate and reliable measurements especially at higher heart rates for diagnosis of myocardial fibrosis.[93] Further, segmental comparison between ECV measurements from DECT and MR imaging showed strong correlation.[94]

The evaluation of diffuse myocardial fibrosis in multiple cardiac pathologies using DECT demonstrated good agreement compared with cardiac MR imaging and excellent interobserver agreement.[91] A recent study suggests a threshold ECV value of greater than 29.5% to discriminate cardiomyopathic from healthy myocardium.[95] DECT-derived ECV showed reliable detection of diffuse myocardial fibrosis in patients with heart failure with the same inverse association with ejection fraction and cardiac output as MR imaging-derived ECV.[96] However, the same study found slightly overestimated ECV by DECT compared with MR imaging. This might be explained by lower soft tissue contrast resolution of CT and needs to be considered when measuring ECV with DECT.

Aortic stenosis can cause cardiac remodeling, myocardial hypertrophy, and consequently myocardial fibrosis.[97] The early detection of myocardial fibrosis and risk stratification are critical in patients with aortic stenosis, as increasing fibrosis is associated with progressing heart failure.[98] DECT-based ECV values are reported as independent predictors of all-cause mortality and hospitalization for heart failure in patients with severe aortic stenosis.[99]

Acute myocarditis causes edema, hyperemia, and myocyte necrosis/fibrosis,[100] and diagnosis is challenging. The significant increase of DECT-derived myocardial ECV (>31.6%) was demonstrated in patients with verified acute myocarditis.[101] Further, DECT ECV is suggested as early predictor of major adverse events in patients with acute myocarditis with a proposed cutoff of $\geq$39.5%.[102]

Myocardial tissue characterization using DECT ECV is shown to be feasible with reliable accuracy and predictive value for patient outcome and risk stratification. However, existing studies were conducted only in small patient cohorts, and further research especially on potential systemic ECV overestimation is needed.

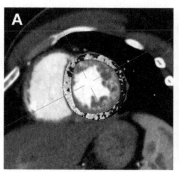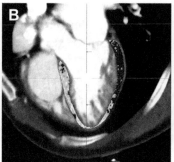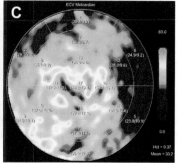

Fig. 6. Representative case of septal involvement in arrhythmogenic right ventricular dysplasia in a 30-year-old female patient. Basal short axis (*A*) and long axis (*B*) Dual energy (DE)-based CT-ECV images are shown. (*C*) Representative CT-ECV polar map based on the 17-segment American Heart Association (AHA) model. (Note that the inner and outer 25% of the myocardial wall are excluded to avoid artifacts.)

FUTURE PERSPECTIVE: PHOTON-COUNTING COMPUTED TOMOGRAPHY: CARDIAC APPLICATIONS

Photon-counting detectors (PCDs) use semiconductors to convert individual x-ray photons directly into electronic signals whereas conventional SECT and DECT use energy-integrating detectors (EIDs). PCD-CT enables discrimination of single incident photons and their assignment to certain energy bins, resulting in improved spectral resolution.[103] Recent research on clinical PCD-CT demonstrated promising results including decreased electronic noise, improved CNR, high spatial resolution, and potential reduction of required iodine contrast volumes.[104–107] PCD-CT provides all multienergy reconstructions also available from DECT but without a decrease in temporal resolution.

Comparing objective image quality of PCD-CT to EID-CT systems, improved CNR was demonstrated in low-energy VMIs under 60 keV in a thorax phantom.[108] Therefore, PCDs are expected to enhance image quality in patients as well, especially with increasing Body-Mass-Index (BMI), leading to reduced radiation doses and improved detection of coronary artery disease.

CAC scoring is an established noninvasive imaging-based screening tool which is predicted to be further optimized using PCD-CT. High spatial resolution provided by PCD-CT systems might result in less calcium blooming and more precise CAC scores.[109] PCD-CT provides improved VNC (two-material separation) and virtual non-iodine (multi-material separation) images compared with dual-energy EID-CT. Moreover, PCD material decomposition enables quantification of the physical mass of calcium promising more reproducible CAC measurements independent of acquisition and reconstruction parameters of the scanner. VMIs and differing iterative reconstruction levels can affect CAC scores, and PCD-related adjustments of these parameters might improve CAC quantification accuracy.[109]

The risk of iodine contrast is well-known,[110] and therefore, the reduction of iodine contrast use for cardiovascular CT is a long-desired goal. One successful strategy to decrease contrast media volume is using VMI reconstructions at lower keV levels. Similar or higher vessel sharpness, CNR, and attenuation were reported for a dynamic phantom using PCD-CT with VMI reconstructions at 40, 50, and 55 keV at 75% and 40 keV at 50% contrast volume.[104] However, it is important to keep in mind that postprocessed VMIs at low energy levels lead to higher image noise levels.

Coronary CT angiography with conventional EID-CT systems tends to overestimate coronary artery stenosis especially in the presence of high coronary calcification burden due to blooming artifacts.[42,111] However, dual-energy based postprocessing algorithms potentially solve this issue in the near future. VMI affects the accuracy of coronary artery stenosis quantification, increasing calcium blooming artifacts at lower energy levels while increasing keV levels reduce calcium blooming; however, iodinated contrast attenuation also decreases. A calcium removal algorithm—based on spectrally resolved multi-threshold PCD-CT data—can improve image interpretability by decreasing calcium blooming and measuring the stenosis degree closer to its real size as described in a phantom study.[112]

In summary, current literature suggests that PCD-CT has the potential to provide new pathways in cardiovascular imaging toward more precise diagnostics, but further clinical investigations are needed to validate present results and translate them into clinical routine.

SUMMARY

DECT offers a variety of reconstruction techniques for improved cardiac imaging. VMIs decrease artifacts improving coronary plaque and stent visualization. Further, contrast attenuation is increased allowing significant reduction of contrast dose. VNC reconstructions enable CAC scoring from contrast-enhanced scans. DECT provides advanced plaque imaging with detailed analysis of plaque components, indicating plaque stability. ECV assessment using DECT offers noninvasive detection of myocardial fibrosis.

CLINICS CARE POINTS

- Dual-energy computed tomography (CT)-derived virtual monoenergetic images showed best results for cardiac evaluation at 70 keV or noise-optimized 40 keV energy levels. Coronary stents are best visualized using 80 keV images.

- Virtual monoenergetic images improve contrast attenuation allowing for up to 50% reduction of contrast volume use.

- Virtual non-contrast reconstructions enable coronary artery calcium scoring without the need for true non-contrast scans but showed systemic underestimation of absolute calcium scoring values requiring the use of adjusted scores or correction algorithms for correct interpretation.

- Dual-energy CT-derived plaque characterization can provide detailed analysis of plaque components and plaque stability but is not yet validated for clinical settings.
- Dual-energy CT-based myocardial perfusion using stress and stress–rest protocols add incremental value over cardiac CT angiography evaluation alone and showed superior diagnostic capabilities over rest-only protocols.
- Myocardial tissue characterization by dual-energy CT is feasible but existing studies suggest potential systemic overestimation of extracellular volume fraction.

DISCLOSURE

Dr C.N. De Cecco receives institutional research support and/or personal fees from Bayer and Siemens. Dr M. van Assen receives research funding from Siemens Healthineers, Germany. Dr F.G. Meinel has received research funding from GE Healthcare and speaker honoraria from GE Healthcare, United Kingdom, Circle Cardiovascular Imaging and Bayer Vital. Dr A. Varga-Szemes receives institutional research support and/or personal fees from Bayer, Elucid Bioimaging and Siemens. Dr U.J. Schoepf receives institutional research support and/or personal fees from Bayer, Germany, Bracco, Elucid Bioimaging, Guerbet, United States, HeartFlow, Inc, Keya Medical, and Siemens. All other authors have no disclosures.

REFERENCES

1. Timmis A, Vardas P, Townsend N, et al. European Society of Cardiology: cardiovascular disease statistics 2021. Eur Heart J 2022;43(8):716–99.

2. Tsao CW, Aday AW, Almarzooq ZI, et al. Heart Disease and Stroke Statistics-2022 Update: A Report From the American Heart Association. Circulation 2022;145(8):e153–639.

3. Collet JP, Thiele H, Barbato E, et al. 2020 ESC Guidelines for the management of acute coronary syndromes in patients presenting without persistent ST-segment elevation. Eur Heart J 2021; 42(14):1289–367.

4. Knuuti J, Wijns W, Saraste A, et al. 2019 ESC Guidelines for the diagnosis and management of chronic coronary syndromes. Eur Heart J 2020; 41(3):407–77.

5. Vahanian A, Beyersdorf F, Praz F, et al. 2021 ESC/ EACTS Guidelines for the management of valvular heart disease. Eur Heart J 2022;43(7):561–632.

6. Writing Committee M, Gulati M, Levy PD, et al. 2021 AHA/ACC/ASE/CHEST/SAEM/SCCT/SCMR Guideline for the Evaluation and Diagnosis of Chest Pain: A Report of the American College of Cardiology/American Heart Association Joint Committee on Clinical Practice Guidelines. J Cardiovasc Comput Tomogr 2022;16(1):54–122.

7. Albrecht MH, Vogl TJ, Martin SS, et al. Review of Clinical Applications for Virtual Monoenergetic Dual-Energy CT. Radiology 2019;293(2):260–71.

8. Albrecht MH, De Cecco CN, Schoepf UJ, et al. Dual-energy CT of the heart current and future status. Eur J Radiol 2018;105:110–8.

9. De Cecco CN, Schoepf UJ, Steinbach L, et al. White Paper of the Society of Computed Body Tomography and Magnetic Resonance on Dual-Energy CT, Part 3: Vascular, Cardiac, Pulmonary, and Musculoskeletal Applications. J Comput Assist Tomogr 2017;41(1):1–7.

10. De Santis D, Eid M, De Cecco CN, et al. Dual-Energy Computed Tomography in Cardiothoracic Vascular Imaging. Radiol Clin North Am 2018;56(4):521–34.

11. Lempel M, Frishman WH. Cardiac Applications of Dual-Energy Computed Tomography. Cardiol Rev 2019;27(4):208–10.

12. Kay FU. Dual-energy CT and coronary imaging. Cardiovasc Diagn Ther 2020;10(4):1090–107.

13. Megibow AJ, Kambadakone A, Ananthakrishnan L. Dual-Energy Computed Tomography: Image Acquisition, Processing, and Workflow. Radiol Clin North Am 2018;56(4):507–20.

14. Symons R, Choi Y, Cork TE, et al. Optimized energy of spectral coronary CT angiography for coronary plaque detection and quantification. J Cardiovasc Comput Tomogr 2018;12(2):108–14.

15. Arendt CT, Czwikla R, Lenga L, et al. Improved coronary artery contrast enhancement using noise-optimised virtual monoenergetic imaging from dual-source dual-energy computed tomography. Eur J Radiol 2020;122:108666.

16. Patino M, Prochowski A, Agrawal MD, et al. Material Separation Using Dual-Energy CT: Current and Emerging Applications. Radiographics 2016; 36(4):1087–105.

17. De Santis D, Jin KN, Schoepf UJ, et al. Heavily Calcified Coronary Arteries: Advanced Calcium Subtraction Improves Luminal Visualization and Diagnostic Confidence in Dual-Energy Coronary Computed Tomography Angiography. Invest Radiol 2018;53(2):103–9.

18. Lenga L, Leithner D, Peterke JL, et al. Comparison of Radiation Dose and Image Quality of Contrast-Enhanced Dual-Source CT of the Chest: Single-Versus Dual-Energy and Second-Versus Third-Generation Technology. AJR Am J Roentgenol 2019;212(4):741–7.

19. van Ommen F, de Jong H, Dankbaar JW, et al. Dose of CT protocols acquired in clinical routine using a dual-layer detector CT scanner: A preliminary report. Eur J Radiol 2019;112:65–71.

20. Papadakis AE, Perisinakis K, Damilakis J. The effect of heart rate, vessel angulation and acquisition protocol on the estimation accuracy of calcified artery stenosis in dual energy cardiac CT: A phantom study. Phys Med 2020;70:208–15.

21. Carrascosa P, Leipsic JA, Capunay C, et al. Monochromatic image reconstruction by dual energy imaging allows half iodine load computed tomography coronary angiography. Eur J Radiol 2015;84(10):1915–20.

22. Raju R, Thompson AG, Lee K, et al. Reduced iodine load with CT coronary angiography using dual-energy imaging: a prospective randomized trial compared with standard coronary CT angiography. J Cardiovasc Comput Tomogr 2014;8(4):282–8.

23. Yi Y, Zhao X-M, Wu R-Z, et al. Low Dose and Low Contrast Medium Coronary CT Angiography Using Dual-Layer Spectral Detector CT. Int Heart J 2019;60(3):608–17.

24. Rotzinger DC, Si-Mohamed SA, Yerly J, et al. Reduced-iodine-dose dual-energy coronary CT angiography: qualitative and quantitative comparison between virtual monochromatic and polychromatic CT images. Eur Radiol 2021;31(9):7132–42.

25. Dubourg B, Caudron J, Lestrat JP, et al. Single-source dual-energy CT angiography with reduced iodine load in patients referred for aortoiliofemoral evaluation before transcatheter aortic valve implantation: impact on image quality and radiation dose. Eur Radiol 2014;24(11):2659–68.

26. Hickethier T, Baessler B, Kroeger JR, et al. Monoenergetic reconstructions for imaging of coronary artery stents using spectral detector CT: In-vitro experience and comparison to conventional images. J Cardiovasc Comput Tomogr 2017;11(1):33–9.

27. Mangold S, Cannao PM, Schoepf UJ, et al. Impact of an advanced image-based monoenergetic reconstruction algorithm on coronary stent visualization using third generation dual-source dual-energy CT: a phantom study. Eur Radiol 2016;26(6):1871–8.

28. Stehli J, Fuchs TA, Singer A, et al. First experience with single-source, dual-energy CCTA for monochromatic stent imaging. Eur Heart J Cardiovasc Imaging 2015;16(5):507–12.

29. Liu Q, Wang Y, Qi H, et al. Exploring the best monochromatic energy level in dual energy spectral imaging for coronary stents after percutaneous coronary intervention. Sci Rep 2021;11(1):17576.

30. Hickethier T, Wenning J, Bratke G, et al. Evaluation of soft-plaque stenoses in coronary artery stents using conventional and monoenergetic images: first in-vitro experience and comparison of two different dual-energy techniques. Quant Imaging Med Surg 2020;10(3):612–23.

31. Agatston AS, Janowitz WR, Hildner FJ, et al. Quantification of coronary artery calcium using ultrafast computed tomography. J Am Coll Cardiol 1990;15(4):827–32.

32. Yamada Y, Jinzaki M, Okamura T, et al. Feasibility of coronary artery calcium scoring on virtual unenhanced images derived from single-source fast kVp-switching dual-energy coronary CT angiography. J Cardiovasc Comput Tomogr 2014;8(5):391–400.

33. Fuchs TA, Stehli J, Dougoud S, et al. Coronary artery calcium quantification from contrast enhanced CT using gemstone spectral imaging and material decomposition. Int J Cardiovasc Imaging 2014;30(7):1399–405.

34. Nadjiri J, Kaissis G, Meurer F, et al. Accuracy of Calcium Scoring calculated from contrast-enhanced Coronary Computed Tomography Angiography using a dual-layer spectral CT: A comparison of Calcium Scoring from real and virtual non-contrast data. PLoS One 2018;13(12):e0208588.

35. Schwarz F, Nance JW, Ruzsics B, et al. Quantification of Coronary Artery Calcium on the Basis of Dual-Energy CCTA. Radiology 2012;264(3). https://doi.org/10.1148/radiol.12112455/-/DC1.

36. Li Q, Berman BP, Hagio T, et al. Coronary artery calcium quantification using contrast-enhanced dual-energy computed tomography scans in comparison with unenhanced single-energy scans. Phys Med Biol 2018;63(17):175006.

37. Kumar V, Min JK, He X, et al. Computation of Calcium Score With Dual-Energy Compted Tomography: A Phantom Study. J Comput Assist Tomogr 2017;41(1):156–8.

38. Lee SY, Kim TH, Han K, et al. Feasibility of Coronary Artery Calcium Scoring on Dual-Energy Chest Computed Tomography: A Prospective Comparison with Electrocardiogram-Gated Calcium Score Computed Tomography. J Clin Med 2021;10(4). https://doi.org/10.3390/jcm10040653.

39. Song I, Yi JG, Park JH, et al. Virtual Non-Contrast CT Using Dual-Energy Spectral CT: Feasibility of Coronary Artery Calcium Scoring. Korean J Radiol 2016;17(3):321–9.

40. Lambert JW, Sun Y, Ordovas KG, et al. Improved Calcium Scoring at Dual-Energy Computed Tomography Angiography Using a High-Z Contrast Element and Novel Material Separation Technique. J Comput Assist Tomogr 2018;42(3):459–66.

41. Henzler T, Porubsky S, Kayed H, et al. Attenuation-based characterization of coronary atherosclerotic plaque: comparison of dual source and dual energy CT with single-source CT and histopathology. Eur J Radiol 2011;80(1):54–9.

42. Vavere AL, Arbab-Zadeh A, Rochitte CE, et al. Coronary artery stenoses: accuracy of 64-detector row CT angiography in segments with mild, moderate,

or severe calcification–a subanalysis of the CORE-64 trial. Radiology 2011;261(1):100–8.

43. Stehli J, Clerc OF, Fuchs TA, et al. Impact of monochromatic coronary computed tomography angiography from single-source dual-energy CT on coronary stenosis quantification. J Cardiovasc Comput Tomogr 2016;10(2):135–40.

44. Andreini D, Pontone G, Mushtaq S, et al. Diagnostic Accuracy of Rapid Kilovolt Peak-Switching Dual-Energy CT Coronary Angiography in Patients With a High Calcium Score. JACC Cardiovasc Imaging 2015;8(6):746–8.

45. Yunaga H, Ohta Y, Kaetsu Y, et al. Diagnostic performance of calcification-suppressed coronary CT angiography using rapid kilovolt-switching dual-energy CT. Eur Radiol 2017;27(7):2794–801.

46. Narula J, Nakano M, Virmani R, et al. Histopathologic characteristics of atherosclerotic coronary disease and implications of the findings for the invasive and noninvasive detection of vulnerable plaques. J Am Coll Cardiol 2013;61(10):1041–51.

47. Williams MC, Moss AJ, Dweck M, et al. Coronary Artery Plaque Characteristics Associated With Adverse Outcomes in the SCOT-HEART Study. J Am Coll Cardiol 2019;73(3):291–301.

48. Jinnouchi H, Sato Y, Sakamoto A, et al. Calcium deposition within coronary atherosclerotic lesion: Implications for plaque stability. Atherosclerosis 2020;306:85–95.

49. Gianni U, Tantawy S, Amoa F, et al. Dual-energy Coronary Computed Tomography Angiography Is Superior To Single Energy Computed Tomography For Evaluation Of Necrotic Core In Sudden Cardiac Death. Journal of Cardiovascular Computed Tomography 2020;14(3):S77–8.

50. Obaid DR, Calvert PA, Gopalan D, et al. Dual-energy computed tomography imaging to determine atherosclerotic plaque composition: a prospective study with tissue validation. J Cardiovasc Comput Tomogr 2014;8(3):230–7.

51. Yamak D, Panse P, Pavlicek W, et al. Non-calcified coronary atherosclerotic plaque characterization by dual energy computed tomography. IEEE J Biomed Health Inform 2014;18(3):939–45.

52. Matsui K, Machida H, Mitsuhashi T, et al. Analysis of coronary arterial calcification components with coronary CT angiography using single-source dual-energy CT with fast tube voltage switching. Int J Cardiovasc Imaging 2015;31(3):639–47.

53. Haghighi RR, Chatterjee S, Tabin M, et al. DECT evaluation of noncalcified coronary artery plaque. Med Phys 2015;42(10):5945–54.

54. Mandal SR, Bharati A, Haghighi RR, et al. Non-invasive characterization of coronary artery atherosclerotic plaque using dual energy CT: Explanation in ex-vivo samples. Phys Med 2018;45:52–8.

55. Ding H, Wang C, Malkasian S, et al. Characterization of arterial plaque composition with dual energy computed tomography: a simulation study. Int J Cardiovasc Imaging 2021;37(1):331–41.

56. Nakajima S, Ito H, Mitsuhashi T, et al. Clinical application of effective atomic number for classifying non-calcified coronary plaques by dual-energy computed tomography. Atherosclerosis 2017;261:138–43.

57. Sheta HM, Moller S, Heinsen LJ, et al. Characteristics of culprit lesion in patients with non-ST-elevation myocardial infarction and improvement of diagnostic utility using dual energy cardiac CT. Int J Cardiovasc Imaging 2021;37(5):1781–8.

58. Assen MV, Vonder M, Pelgrim GJ, et al. Computed tomography for myocardial characterization in ischemic heart disease: a state-of-the-art review. Eur Radiol Exp 2020;4(1):36.

59. Carrascosa PM, Cury RC, Deviggiano A, et al. Comparison of myocardial perfusion evaluation with single versus dual-energy CT and effect of beam-hardening artifacts. Acad Radiol 2015;22(5):591–9.

60. Carrascosa P, Deviggiano A, de Zan M, et al. Improved Discrimination of Myocardial Perfusion Defects at Low Energy Levels Using Virtual Monochromatic Imaging. J Comput Assist Tomogr 2017;41(4):661–7.

61. Carrascosa PM, Deviggiano A, Capunay C, et al. Incremental value of myocardial perfusion over coronary angiography by spectral computed tomography in patients with intermediate to high likelihood of coronary artery disease. Eur J Radiol 2015;84(4):637–42.

62. Ko SM, Park JH, Hwang HK, et al. Direct comparison of stress- and rest-dual-energy computed tomography for detection of myocardial perfusion defect. Int J Cardiovasc Imaging 2014;30(Suppl 1):41–53.

63. Ko SM, Song MG, Chee HK, et al. Diagnostic performance of dual-energy CT stress myocardial perfusion imaging: direct comparison with cardiovascular MRI. AJR Am J Roentgenol 2014;203(6):W605–13.

64. Pelgrim GJ, Dorrius M, Xie X, et al. The dream of a one-stop-shop: Meta-analysis on myocardial perfusion CT. Eur J Radiol 2015;84(12):2411–20.

65. Meinel FG, De Cecco CN, Schoepf UJ, et al. First-arterial-pass dual-energy CT for assessment of myocardial blood supply: do we need rest, stress, and delayed acquisition? Comparison with SPECT. Radiology 2014;270(3):708–16.

66. Li W, Yu F, Liu M, et al. Clinical value of resting cardiac dual-energy CT in patients suspected of coronary artery disease. BMC Med Imaging 2022;22(1):32.

67. De Cecco CN, Harris BS, Schoepf UJ, et al. Incremental value of pharmacological stress cardiac

dual-energy CT over coronary CT angiography alone for the assessment of coronary artery disease in a high-risk population. AJR Am J Roentgenol 2014;203(1):W70–7.

68. Chung HW, Ko SM, Hwang HK, et al. Diagnostic Performance of Coronary CT Angiography, Stress Dual-Energy CT Perfusion, and Stress Perfusion Single-Photon Emission Computed Tomography for Coronary Artery Disease: Comparison with Combined Invasive Coronary Angiography and Stress Perfusion Cardiac MRI. Korean J Radiol 2017;18(3):476–86.

69. Koonce JD, Vliegenthart R, Schoepf UJ, et al. Accuracy of dual-energy computed tomography for the measurement of iodine concentration using cardiac CT protocols: validation in a phantom model. Eur Radiol 2014;24(2):512–8.

70. Pelgrim GJ, van Hamersvelt RW, Willemink MJ, et al. Accuracy of iodine quantification using dual energy CT in latest generation dual source and dual layer CT. Eur Radiol 2017;27(9):3904–12.

71. Jacobsen MC, Schellingerhout D, Wood CA, et al. Intermanufacturer Comparison of Dual-Energy CT Iodine Quantification and Monochromatic Attenuation: A Phantom Study. Radiology 2018;287(1):224–34.

72. Poulter R, Wood DA, Starovoytov A, et al. Quantified dual energy computed tomography perfusion imaging using myocardial iodine concentration: Validation using CT derived myocardial blood flow and invasive fractional flow reserve in a porcine model. J Cardiovasc Comput Tomogr 2019;13(2):86–91.

73. Delgado Sanchez-Gracian C, Oca Pernas R, Trinidad Lopez C, et al. Quantitative myocardial perfusion with stress dual-energy CT: iodine concentration differences between normal and ischemic or necrotic myocardium. Initial experience. Eur Radiol 2016;26(9):3199–207.

74. van Assen M, Lavra F, Schoepf UJ, et al. Iodine quantification based on rest/stress perfusion dual energy CT to differentiate ischemic, infarcted and normal myocardium. Eur J Radiol 2019;112:136–43.

75. Boccalini S, Si-Mohamed S, Matzuzzi M, et al. Effect of contrast material injection protocol on first-pass myocardial perfusion assessed by dual-energy dual-layer computed tomography. Quant Imaging Med Surg 2022;12(7):3903–16.

76. Nakahara T, Toyama T, Jinzaki M, et al. Quantitative Analysis of Iodine Image of Dual-energy Computed Tomography at Rest: Comparison With 99mTc-Tetrofosmin Stress-rest Single-photon Emission Computed Tomography Myocardial Perfusion Imaging as the Reference Standard. J Thorac Imaging 2018;33(2):97–104.

77. Mochizuki J, Nakaura T, Yoshida N, et al. Spectral imaging with dual-layer spectral detector computed tomography for the detection of perfusion defects in acute coronary syndrome. Heart Ves 2022;37(7):1115–24.

78. Hosch W, Kristen AV, Libicher M, et al. Late enhancement in cardiac amyloidosis: correlation of MRI enhancement pattern with histopathological findings. Amyloid 2008;15(3):196–204.

79. Moon JC, Sachdev B, Elkington AG, et al. Gadolinium enhanced cardiovascular magnetic resonance in Anderson-Fabry disease. Evidence for a disease specific abnormality of the myocardial interstitium. Eur Heart J 2003;24(23):2151–5.

80. López B, Querejeta R, González A, et al. Effects of loop diuretics on myocardial fibrosis and collagen type I turnover in chronic heart failure. J Am Coll Cardiol 2004;43(11):2028–35.

81. Messroghli DR, Moon JC, Ferreira VM, et al. Clinical recommendations for cardiovascular magnetic resonance mapping of T1, T2, T2* and extracellular volume: A consensus statement by the Society for Cardiovascular Magnetic Resonance (SCMR) endorsed by the European Association for Cardiovascular Imaging (EACVI). J Cardiovasc Magn Reson 2017;19(1):75.

82. Mewton N, Liu CY, Croisille P, et al. Assessment of myocardial fibrosis with cardiovascular magnetic resonance. J Am Coll Cardiol 2011;57(8):891–903.

83. Scully PR, Bastarrika G, Moon JC, et al. Myocardial Extracellular Volume Quantification by Cardiovascular Magnetic Resonance and Computed Tomography. Curr Cardiol Rep 2018;20(3):15.

84. Pucci A, Aimo A, Musetti V, et al. Amyloid Deposits and Fibrosis on Left Ventricular Endomyocardial Biopsy Correlate With Extracellular Volume in Cardiac Amyloidosis. J Am Heart Assoc 2021;10(20):e020358.

85. Everett RJ, Treibel TA, Fukui M, et al. Extracellular Myocardial Volume in Patients With Aortic Stenosis. J Am Coll Cardiol 2020;75(3):304–16.

86. Whittaker P, Boughner DR, Kloner RA. Analysis of healing after myocardial infarction using polarized light microscopy. Am J Pathol 1989;134(4):879–93.

87. Díez J, Querejeta R, López B, et al. Losartan-dependent regression of myocardial fibrosis is associated with reduction of left ventricular chamber stiffness in hypertensive patients. Circulation 2002;105(21):2512–7.

88. Nacif MS, Kawel N, Lee JJ, et al. Interstitial myocardial fibrosis assessed as extracellular volume fraction with low-radiation-dose cardiac CT. Radiology 2012;264(3):876–83.

89. Bandula S, White SK, Flett AS, et al. Measurement of myocardial extracellular volume fraction by using equilibrium contrast-enhanced CT: validation against histologic findings. Radiology 2013;269(2):396–403.

90. Jablonowski R, Wilson MW, Do L, et al. Multidetector CT measurement of myocardial extracellular

volume in acute patchy and contiguous infarction: validation with microscopic measurement. Radiology 2015;274(2):370–8.

91. Lee HJ, Im DJ, Youn JC, et al. Myocardial Extracellular Volume Fraction with Dual-Energy Equilibrium Contrast-enhanced Cardiac CT in Nonischemic Cardiomyopathy: A Prospective Comparison with Cardiac MR Imaging. Radiology 2016;280(1):49–57.

92. van Assen M, De Cecco CN, Sahbaee P, et al. Feasibility of extracellular volume quantification using dual-energy CT. Journal of Cardiovascular Computed Tomography 2019;13(1):81–4.

93. Emoto T, Oda S, Kidoh M, et al. Myocardial Extracellular Volume Quantification Using Cardiac Computed Tomography: A Comparison of the Dual-energy Iodine Method and the Standard Subtraction Method. Acad Radiol 2021;28(5):e119–26.

94. Ohta Y, Kishimoto J, Kitao S, et al. Investigation of myocardial extracellular volume fraction in heart failure patients using iodine map with rapid-kV switching dual-energy CT: Segmental comparison with MRI T1 mapping. Journal of Cardiovascular Computed Tomography 2020;14(4):349–55.

95. Abadia AF, van Assen M, Martin SS, et al. Myocardial extracellular volume fraction to differentiate healthy from cardiomyopathic myocardium using dual-source dual-energy CT. J Cardiovasc Comput Tomogr 2020;14(2):162–7.

96. Wang R, Liu X, Schoepf UJ, et al. Extracellular volume quantitation using dual-energy CT in patients with heart failure: Comparison with 3T cardiac MR. Int J Cardiol 2018;268:236–40.

97. Dweck MR, Boon NA, Newby DE. Calcific aortic stenosis: a disease of the valve and the myocardium. J Am Coll Cardiol 2012;60(19):1854–63.

98. Park SJ, Cho SW, Kim SM, et al. Assessment of Myocardial Fibrosis Using Multimodality Imaging in Severe Aortic Stenosis: Comparison With Histologic Fibrosis. JACC Cardiovasc Imaging 2019;12(1):109–19.

99. Suzuki M, Toba T, Izawa Y, et al. Prognostic Impact of Myocardial Extracellular Volume Fraction Assessment Using Dual-Energy Computed Tomography in Patients Treated With Aortic Valve Replacement for Severe Aortic Stenosis. J Am Heart Assoc 2021;10(18):e020655.

100. Friedrich MG, Sechtem U, Schulz-Menger J, et al. Cardiovascular Magnetic Resonance in Myocarditis: A JACC White Paper. J Am Coll Cardiol 2009;53(17):1475–87.

101. Si-Mohamed SA, Restier LM, Branchu A, et al. Diagnostic Performance of Extracellular Volume Quantified by Dual-Layer Dual-Energy CT for Detection of Acute Myocarditis. J Clin Med 2021;10(15). https://doi.org/10.3390/jcm10153286.

102. Si-Mohamed SA, Congi A, Ziegler A, et al. Early Prediction of Cardiac Complications in Acute Myocarditis by Means of Extracellular Volume Quantification With the Use of Dual-Energy Computed Tomography. JACC (J Am Coll Cardiol): Cardiovascular Imaging 2021;14(10):2041–2.

103. Leng S, Bruesewitz M, Tao S, et al. Photon-counting Detector CT: System Design and Clinical Applications of an Emerging Technology. Radiographics 2019;39(3):729–43.

104. Emrich T, O'Doherty J, Schoepf UJ, et al. Reduced Iodinated Contrast Media Administration in Coronary CT Angiography on a Clinical Photon-Counting Detector CT System: A Phantom Study Using a Dynamic Circulation Model. Invest Radiol 2022;58(2). https://doi.org/10.1097/rli.0000000000000911.

105. Sandstedt M, Marsh J Jr, Rajendran K, et al. Improved coronary calcification quantification using photon-counting-detector CT: an ex vivo study in cadaveric specimens. Eur Radiol 2021;31(9):6621–30.

106. Euler A, Higashigaito K, Mergen V, et al. High-Pitch Photon-Counting Detector Computed Tomography Angiography of the Aorta: Intraindividual Comparison to Energy-Integrating Detector Computed Tomography at Equal Radiation Dose. Invest Radiol 2022;57(2):115–21.

107. Boccalini S, Si-Mohamed SA, Lacombe H, et al. First In-Human Results of Computed Tomography Angiography for Coronary Stent Assessment With a Spectral Photon Counting Computed Tomography. Invest Radiol 2022;57(4):212–21.

108. Booij R, van der Werf NR, Dijkshoorn ML, et al. Assessment of Iodine Contrast-To-Noise Ratio in Virtual Monoenergetic Images Reconstructed from Dual-Source Energy-Integrating CT and Photon-Counting CT Data. Diagnostics 2022;12(6):1467.

109. Eberhard M, Mergen V, Higashigaito K, et al. Coronary Calcium Scoring with First Generation Dual-Source Photon-Counting CT-First Evidence from Phantom and In-Vivo Scans. Diagnostics 2021;11(9). https://doi.org/10.3390/diagnostics11091708.

110. van der Molen AJ, Reimer P, Dekkers IA, et al. Post-contrast acute kidney injury – Part 1: Definition, clinical features, incidence, role of contrast medium and risk factors. Eur Radiol 2018;28(7):2845–55.

111. Zhang S, Levin DC, Halpern EJ, et al. Accuracy of MDCT in assessing the degree of stenosis caused by calcified coronary artery plaques. AJR Am J Roentgenol 2008;191(6):1676–83.

112. Allmendinger T, Nowak T, Flohr T, et al. Photon-Counting Detector CT-Based Vascular Calcium Removal Algorithm: Assessment Using a Cardiac Motion Phantom. Invest Radiol 2022;57(6):399–405.

Vascular Applications of Dual-Energy Computed Tomography

Prabhakar S. Rajiah, MBBS, MD, FRCR[a],*,
Avinash Kambadakone, MD, DNB, FRCR, FSABI, FSAR[b],
Lakshmi Ananthakrishnan, MD[c], Patrick Sutphin, MD[b],
Sanjeeva P. Kalva, MD[b]

KEYWORDS

• Vascular • Spectral • Dual-energy • Multi-energy • Computed tomography

KEY POINTS

- Low-energy virtual monoenergetic images boost iodine attenuation which can salvage suboptimal enhanced studies or perform low-contrast material dose studies
- High energy VMIs reduce artifacts from metal, calcium blooming and beam hardening.3. Iodine maps and virtual non contrast images are useful in lesion characterization

INTRODUCTION

Dual-energy computed tomography (CT) (DECT) or multi-energy CT (MECT) imaging provides the attenuation characteristics of tissues at different x-ray energies based on image acquisition and reconstruction at multiple energy levels.[1] This allows differentiation and quantification of tissues and materials with different atomic numbers that may otherwise have similar attenuation values on conventional single-energy computed tomography (CT). DECT is the more commonly used term as the primary technique involves using incident x-ray beams of two different energies. The term spectral CT encompasses all the different methods, including those techniques that use only a single x-ray beam. Source-based MECT technologies include dual-source, rapid kV-switching, and sequential/dual-spin and twin-beam CT, whereas detector-based technologies include dual-layer detector and photon-counting detector (PCD) CT[2–4] (Table 1). MECT generates additional material decomposition (MD) images such as iodine maps, virtual non-contrast (VNC), and effective atomic number-based images

(Fig. 1, Table 2). Virtual monoenergetic images (VMIs) that mimic a single-energy x-ray beam can be generated between 35 and 200 keV (Fig. 2).[5,6] The tissue attenuation values at different VMI energy levels can be plotted for characterization. In this article, the authors review and illustrate the applications of MECT in vascular imaging (Table 3).

INCREASED SIGNAL OF IODINATED CONTRAST MATERIAL

Photoelectric attenuation of iodine increases at x-ray energies that are closer to k-edge of iodine, 33 keV. Hence, if 70 keV is used as a surrogate for 120 kVp, the attenuation values (HU) of iodinated contrast material progressively increases as VMI energy levels decrease below 70 keV (see Fig. 2). This boost in the HU of iodine in low-energy VMIs (<70 keV) can be useful in vascular imaging in several ways. First, suboptimal contrast-enhanced studies, either due to patient or technical factors, can be salvaged using low-energy VMIs with maintained diagnostic accuracy (Fig. 3).[7,8] This saves the need for a repeat

[a] Department of Radiology, Mayo Clinic, 200 1st Street Southwest, Rochester, MN 55905, USA; [b] Department of Radiology, Massachusetts General Hospital, Boston, MA, USA; [c] Department of Radiology, UT Southwestern Medical Center, Dallas, TX, USA
* Corresponding author.
E-mail address: radpr73@gmail.com

Radiol Clin N Am 61 (2023) 1011–1029
https://doi.org/10.1016/j.rcl.2023.05.005

Table 1
Key features of commercially available multi-energy computed tomography technologies

Technology	Vendor	Decomposition	Advantages	Disadvantages
Dual source	Siemens	Image	Independent adjustment of tube voltage and tube current Good spectral separation, augmented by filters	Prospective selection of DE mode over single energy or high-pitch helical mode required. Smaller FOV for one tube Imperfect spatial/temporal registration Cross-scatter
Rapid kVp switching	GE Canon	Projection	Near synchronous acquisition No cross-scatter Full FOV	Prospective selection of DE mode required Cannot modulate voltage and tube current independently Mixing of spectral data due to same filter Slower gantry time and temporal resolution
Dual spin • Sequential • Helical	GE, Canon Siemens	Projection Image	Optimized filters No cross-scatter Dose reduction techniques available	Prospective selection of DE mode required Motion and different contrast phase for two acquisitions
Twin beam	Siemens	Image	Conventional CT scanner can be converted using a filter No FOV issues No cross-scatter Dose reduction techniques available	Prospective selection of DE mode required Suboptimal spectral separation Powerful x-ray tube required Limited maximum volume coverage speed Absorption of x-ray flux by filtration
Dual-layer detector	Philips	Projection	Prospective DE selection not needed Perfect spatiotemporal alignment No FOV limitation No cross-scatter No gantry time limitation Dose reduction techniques available	Same filter for high and low energies limits spectral separation Limited choice of tube potential to 120 or 140 kVp Earlier generation had smaller z-axis coverage of 4 cm
Photon-counting detector	Siemens	Projection	Prospective DE selection not needed Improved spatial registration and temporal resolution than dual source. Multi-energy binning K-edge imaging High spatial resolution	Higher amount of available data Limited choice of tube potential to 120 or 140 kVp

(continued on next page)

Table 1 (*continued*)				
Technology	**Vendor**	**Decomposition**	**Advantages**	**Disadvantages**
			Higher radiation dose efficiency Lower noise and artifacts Combined modes: multi-energy with high-pitch helical or high resolution	

CT (with associated increased in iodinated contrast material load and radiation exposure) or pursuing an alternative imaging study[9,10] and avoids patient anxiety. Second, this principle can be used to perform contrast-enhanced CTs at a lower iodinated contrast material dose, especially in patients with severe renal dysfunction. Several studies on MECT imaging with low-dose intravenous contrast material in different vascular beds have demonstrated maintained or improved image quality at low-energy VMIs.[11–14] Iodinated contrast material load reduction of 70%, contrast material volume as low as 25 mL and iodine dose as low as 15 g have been reported.[11–14] The optimal VMI level that allows high image contrast as well as low noise depends on the scanner, reconstruction algorithm, injection protocols, body habitus, metal instrumentation/prosthesis and the vascular bed. Most of the early studies concluded that 50 to 60 keV was the optimal energy level,[10,12] with further lower energy images limited by increased image noise. Most vendors, however, now offer noise-optimized algorithms, as a result of which 40 to 50 keV has been shown to have the highest image quality with visualization of tiny arterial branches (**Fig. 4**).[1,3,15–18]

Third, low-energy VMI also generates angiographic quality images from routine CT scans that are not optimized for vascular imaging.[10] For example, 40-keV VMI has been shown to be capable of diagnosing incidental PE even on portal venous CT scans in oncologic patients.[19] Nontarget arterial beds which typically do not get opacified to the same extent as the target vasculature can also be evaluated. For example, although a conventional CT pulmonary angiogram demonstrates suboptimal opacification of the thoracic aorta, this vessel can be evaluated using low-energy VMI.[20] Low-energy VMI generated from venous phase images (aka virtual arterial phase reconstructions) has been shown to be effective in the evaluation of abdominal aorta post-endovascular aneurysm repair.[21]

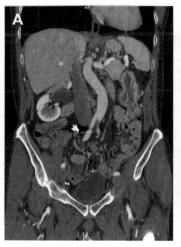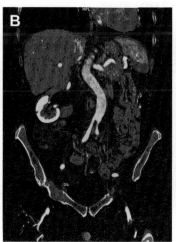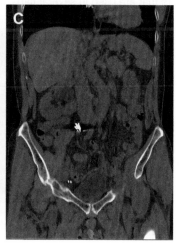

Fig. 1. Images obtained from a dual-source MECT scanner. (*A*) Mixed type of image obtained by 50-50 blending of low-energy (90 kVp) and high-energy (150 kVp) images. (*B*) Iodine map with the pixels color coded based on their iodine content. (*C*) Virtual non-contrast (VNC) images obtained by removing signal of iodine from pixels.

Table 2
Images derived from a multi-energy computed tomography scanner that are used in vascular imaging

Image Type	Basis Materials	Image Generation Technique
Routine diagnostic		Linear blending of low- and high-energy images in dual-source CT Combination of data from low- and high-energy detectors in dual-layer CT Using all incident photons incident on the detector >20 keV energy (T3D)
Virtual monoenergetic images	Iodine/water; photoelectric/compton	Linear combination of basis images allows creation of virtual images at various monoenergetic levels from 35 to 200 keV
Iodine maps (iodine-only)	Iodine, water	2 or 3 material decomposition
Virtual non-contrast (water-only)	Iodine, water	2 or 3 material decomposition
Calcium/bone separation	Calcium, iodine, soft tissue/blood	Virtual separation line between iodine and bone Morphological basis or material decomposition
Effective atomic number-weighted		Material decomposition

Improved Visualization of Anatomy and Lesions

MECT images can improve visualization of vascular anatomy and some lesions. Visualization of small vessels, such as spinal arteries, the artery of Adamkiewicz, intercostal arteries, and bronchial arteries can be improved using low-energy VMI due to increased attenuation of iodinated contrast material.[11,22] This is particularly useful in small perforators that are used in several flaps, including fibular perforator arteries and deep inferior epigastric arteries. Visualization of veins, including varicose veins can be improved in indirect CT venography by using low-energy VMI and iodine/water MD images.[8] Low-energy VMIs also improve the detection of endoleaks[23] (**Fig. 5**) and leaks in the perigraft space of surgical grafts.[24–27] The detection of endoleaks is possible even in a routine CT (*rather than a CTA*) with the use of low-energy VMI.[27] Iodine maps also improve the detection of endoleaks (see **Fig. 5**C). Low-energy VMI and iodine

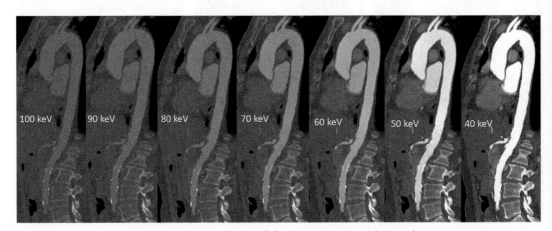

Fig. 2. Virtual monoenergetic images: Sagittal view of the thoracic aorta with virtual monoenergetic reconstructions at different energy levels from 100 to 40 keV. Note that the contrast material signal in the aorta progressively increases with decreasing energy levels, with the highest contrast material signal seen at 40 keV.

Table 3
Applications of multi-energy computed tomography in vascular imaging

Application	Use	Type of Image
Improving iodine signal from the lumen	Salvage suboptimal study	Low-energy VMI
	Low dose of contrast material	Low-energy VMI
	CTA quality from routine CT images	Low-energy VMI
Improved visualization	Improved visualization of lesions	Low-energy VMI
		Iodine maps
	Improved visualization of small vessels	Low-energy VMI
Decreased artifacts	Decreasing beam hardening, calcium blooming, metallic artifacts	High-energy VMI
Improved 3D reconstructions	Improved 3D reconstructions of CT arteriograms	Bone subtracted images
Separation of calcium	Improved visualization of lumen, decreased calcium blooming	Calcium separated images
Saving radiation doses	Decreasing phases of multiphasic CTAs	Virtual non-contrast
		Low-energy VMI
	Characterization of incidental lesions	Iodine map
		Virtual non-contrast
		Effective atomic number
	Salvaging suboptimal enhanced studies and avoiding repeat CTs	Low-energy VMI

maps can also improve the conspicuity of gastrointestinal bleeds (**Fig. 6**) and bleeds in the abdomen/pelvis.[28] In addition, low-energy VMI and iodine maps help in diagnosis of bowel ischemia by increasing the contrast between normal bowel and non-enhancing ischemic bowel.[29,30]

LESION CHARACTERIZATION

MECT can characterize several lesions, including those which are incidental. For example, a high-attenuation lesion on a post-contrast CT or CT Angiography (CTA) of a patient with bleeding could be either due to active extravasation of contrast material, hematoma, or calcification. Distinguishing these entities is important, because active bleeding may require further intervention. In the absence of a true non-contrast (TNC) acquisition, VNC image and iodine map can help to distinguish these entities (**Fig. 7**) as well as ingested material such as pills (**Fig. 8**). Hematoma and calcification, but not the actively extravasating contrast material, demonstrates hyperattenuation on VNC images. On the contrary, hematoma and calcification show no iodine content on the iodine map, whereas active contrast extravasation does (**Fig. 9**). Iodine maps also help in evaluating an underlying enhancing lesion as a source of GI bleeding.[31]

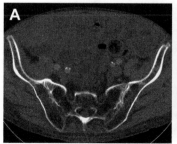 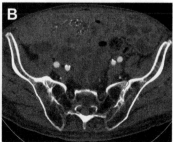 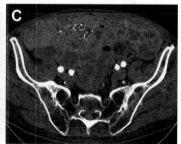

Fig. 3. Salvage of suboptimal vascular study with low-energy VMI. (*A*) Conventional mixed image shows suboptimal opacification of arteries in the pelvis due to poor contrast. (*B*) The 50-keV VMI in the same patient shows that the signal of contrast is increased due to the energy being closer to the k-edge of iodine. This obviates the need for administering another dose of contrast. (*C*) The 40-keV VMI in the same patient shows further increase of the vascular signal.

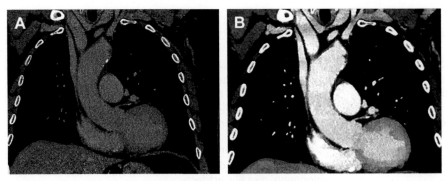

Fig. 4. Low-contrast study with low-energy VMI. (*A*) Conventional CT image in a patient who had only 30 mL of intravenous contrast material due to renal dysfunction shows that the signal in the vascular structures is not adequate for optimal evaluation. (*B*)The 40-keV VMI at the same level shows significantly increased contrast material signal.

In later stages of bowel ischemia with intramural hemorrhage, iodine map and VNC can distinguish hemorrhage from similarly appearing contrast enhancement in post-contrast CT/CTA, with the former indicating bowel ischemia. Similarly, high attenuation within the mural thrombus of an aneurysm on a contrast CT can either represent fresh bleed (*which indicates impending rupture*), calcification, or active contrast extravasation. Calcium appears dark on iodine/calcium MD images and bright on calcium/iodine MD images, whereas contrast material appears bright on iodine/calcium MD images and dark on calcium/iodine MD images. Fresh hematoma may appear bright on

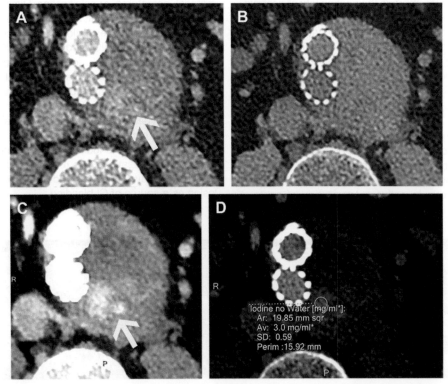

Fig. 5. Detection of endoleaks using dual energy CT. Dual-layer detector delayed phase acquisition for detection of an endoleak (*arrow*) (*A*), with VNC (*B*), 40 keV VMI (*C*), and iodine-no-water (*D*) reconstructions created from the delayed phase. The VNC is an appropriate surrogate for a true unenhanced acquisition for endoleak identification. Endoleak is more conspicuous on the 40-keV VMI reconstruction and is confirmed and quantified on the iodine-no-water reconstruction.

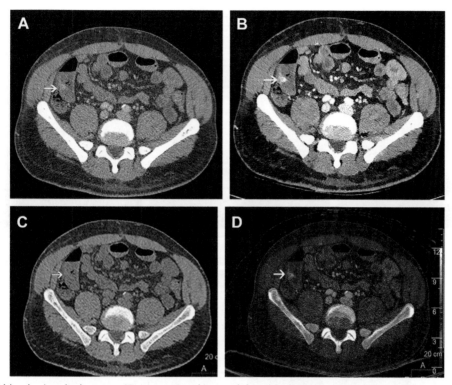

Fig. 6. GI bleed using dual-energy CT: conventional image (*A*) and 40-keV VMI reconstruction (*B*) in a patient with hematochezia. There is a faint contrast blush in the cecum (*arrow*) on conventional images, but this is subtle and could easily be overlooked. This is more conspicuous on the 50-keV VMI reconstruction (*arrow*), where it follows the expected behavior of iodine. VNC (*C*) does not show high attenuation and iodine map (*D*) shows iodine uptake, confirming that this is active contrast extravasation.

iodine/calcium MD images, but it is also bright on blood/calcium MD images and low on calcium/blood MD images.[32–34]

Iodine maps can also be used to distinguish bland thrombus from tumor thrombus or artifacts. A bland thrombus shows no significant iodine content, whereas a tumor thrombus has significant iodine content (**Fig. 10**). In some areas such as the left atrial appendage, hypoattenuation can be seen either due to thrombus or artifact from mixing of contrast material. The threshold for normal versus abnormal iodine is variable depending on the clinical indication, scanner, and acquisition parameters. For example, using the rapid kVp-switching technology, an iodine concentration cutoff 1.74 mg/mL was used to distinguish thrombus from artifact in the left atrial appendage.[35]

There has been some success in characterizing atherosclerotic plaque with an MECT particularly in the identification of lipid, which indicates a high-risk plaque that is prone for rupture and leads to acute events. A fat/water MD map can identify fat within a plaque. A spectral attenuation plot may also be used, because fat characteristically shows lower attenuation values at lower energies, which is the reverse of iodine.[36] Similarly, in Zeff images, lipid-rich plaque shows the attenuation of fat.[36]

MECT can be used to characterize incidentally encountered lesions in vascular imaging such as renal and adrenal masses. A combination of VNC and iodine map can characterize hyperattenuating lesion on post-contrast CT studies. A hemorrhagic/complicated cyst is hyperattenuating in VNC without iodine content, whereas an enhancing renal tumor is not hyperattenuating in VNC but shows iodine content in iodine map. An adrenal nodule with an attenuation of less than 10 HU on VNC image is more likely a lipid-rich adenoma than a metastasis.[37] However, an important pitfall is that lesion enhancement cannot be excluded on a VNC obtained from early arterial phase image before contrast has reached the organ parenchyma. Incidentally encountered hyperattenuation such as in mediastinum could be either calcification, surgical material, or contrast extravasation. Iodine maps and VNC can help in distinguishing these using the above-highlighted principles.

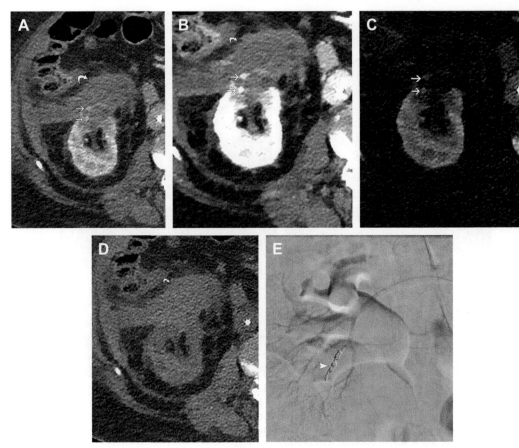

Fig. 7. Active bleed in dual-energy CT. Patient is status post recent partial nephrectomy and presented to the emergency department with pain. Single portal venous phase CT (*A*) (not a CTA) showed hemorrhage in the surgical bed (*curved arrow*) with two rounded high-attenuation foci (*straight arrows*). Those areas demonstrated the expected behavior of iodinated contrast on all series, becoming higher in attenuation on 50 keV reconstructions (*B*), showing iodine signal on the iodine map (*C*) and disappearing on the virtual unenhanced image (*D*). In addition to characterizing the high-attenuation foci, dual-energy CT also saved the need for an additional CTA which is not ideal in this patient post recent nephron sparing surgery. The patient was taken straight to angiography and embolization (*arrow*) (*E*).

ARTIFACT REDUCTION

MECT provides an additional option for decreasing some of the artifacts that are encountered in vascular imaging. Beam-hardening artifact is secondary to the disproportionate absorption of low-energy photons from a polyenergetic x-ray beam by a high-attenuation object, leading to a greater proportion of high-energy photons at the detector. This results in streaks and dark bands surrounding hyperattenuating objects such as orthopedic hardware, embolization coils, and dense contrast material in veins, which limits the evaluation of the adjacent tissues and obscures important findings.[36,38] High-energy VMI (>70 keV) are effective in reducing beam-hardening artifacts,[39,40] due to their inherent monoenergetic nature. Beam hardening progressively decreases at

higher energies above 70 keV, with the least artifacts observed at 200 keV. Because image contrast also decreases at higher energy levels, 100 to 130 keV has been shown to be the optimal energy that decreases artifact while maintaining vascular and soft tissue contrast. A study on beam hardening from dense contrast material in the axillary and subclavian veins showed lower artifacts at energy levels $\geq$ 90 keV, with the best diagnostic assessment achieved at 130 keV.[41]

Artifacts from metallic prosthesis and devices are due to beam hardening and photon starvation. Photon starvation occurs due to complete absorption of the x-ray photons by the devices with resultant zero-transmission projections.[42] Using high-energy VMI, the metallic artifacts can be reduced with improved assessment of adjacent structures.[43] The optimal energy level to decrease

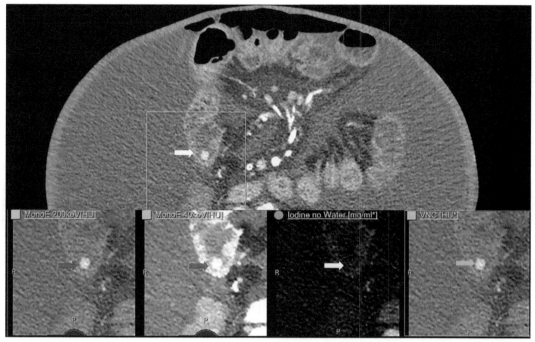

Fig. 8. Characterization of GI contents. Conventional image on the top shows a rounded focus of high attenuation (*arrow*) in the lumen of the small bowel in this cirrhotic patient. Use of dual-energy reconstructions for problem-solving demonstrates that this lesion disappears on the iodine map (*yellow arrow*), persists on the VNC reconstruction (*blue arrow*), and does not significantly change on the low- and high-keV VMI (*red arrows*), confirming that it is not an active GI bleed, but ingested material.

these artifacts depends on the device and anatomy, with ranges from 95 to 150 keV.[42,44] The reduction of metallic artifact by MECT depends on the atomic number and size of the metallic device. Embolization coils placed in aneurysms or bleeding vessels obscure evaluation of the parent vessel due to extensive artifacts. Iodine maps can reduce artifacts from metals with high atomic number (eg, *platinum-based embolization coils*)[45] (**Fig. 11**). An additional option is to subtract the low- and high-energy images, for example, 70 and 140 keV images. Coils with high attenuation in both these images will be subtracted, whereas the vessels stay bright due to the higher attenuation at low energy images.[36] Iodine-specific imaging can also reduce artifact related to adjacent

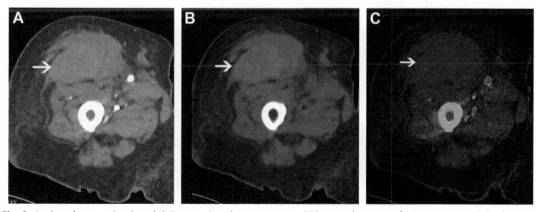

Fig. 9. Lesion characterization. (*A*) Conventional post-contrast CT image shows a soft tissue mass with high attenuation in the right thigh (*arrow*). (*B*) VNC reconstruction at the same level shows the persistence of high attenuation (*arrow*) indicating that this is hematoma and not contrast material extravasation. (*C*) Iodine map shows the absence of iodine in the lesion (*arrow*), confirming no contrast material extravasation.

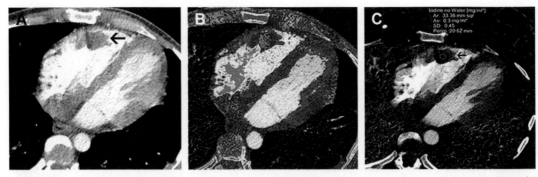

Fig. 10. Lesion characterization. (*A*) Conventional axial CT image demonstrates a right ventricular mass (*arrow*) in a patient with prior right-sided central venous catheter. (*B*) Corresponding iodine overlay image demonstrates no significant iodine within this mass (*arrow*). (*C*). Iodine map demonstrates the lack of iodine uptake associated with this mass (*arrow*). Findings are consistent with right ventricular bland thrombus.

tantalum powder in ethylene vinyl liquid embolic material allowing for detection of persistent endoleak.[46]

Blooming is another artifact in CTA, caused by a combination of partial volume averaging and beam hardening. It is commonly seen in dense calcific plaques, which appears larger than its actual size, resulting in overestimation of luminal stenosis and inaccurate diagnosis. High-energy VMI can reduce calcium blooming.[47] Similar blooming artifacts can be seen with stents, limiting intraluminal evaluation of stent patency. High-energy VMI can be used to decrease blooming from stents,[48] but they will also reduce the intraluminal signal from the contrast material.[36] A combination of 72-keV VMI and 50% iterative construction algorithm was shown to have better image quality than conventional CTA.[49] VMI at 130 keV improved visualization of stents less than 3 mm in diameter in coronary arteries[50] (**Fig. 12**). Iodine map can also reduce calcium blooming without loss of contrast signal,[36] but no overall improvement in evaluation of stent has been shown.[51] Metal artifact reduction

algorithms can be combined with VMIs to reduce artifacts from stents, metal, and clips, especially from dense metals such as cobalt alloy.[52] The advent of PCD CT provides additional options for improving visualization of stents due to its high spatial resolution.[4]

Improved reconstructions and calcium separation

CTA of peripheral arteries requires high-quality 3D reconstructions including maximum intensity projection (MIP) and volume renderings. Bone and calcium are also present in these reconstructions due to their high atomic number. In a conventional single-energy CT, the bone can be removed by subtracting pre- from post-contrast images, but this involves two acquisitions and misregistration artifacts. An attenuation threshold-based algorithm is more commonly used, which is labor-intensive, and prone to several pitfalls, including removal of signal of vessels adjacent to the bone, which may result in overestimation of

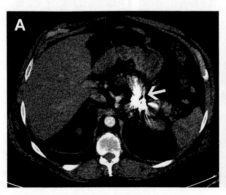
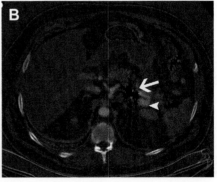

Fig. 11. Decreased artifact of embolization coil using iodine map (*A*). Axial CT scan in a 42-year-old man with proximal splenic artery embolization from rupture of prior splenic artery aneurysm shows extensive artifacts from the coil (*arrow*). (*B*) The artifacts are significantly decreased in iodine map image (*arrow*) allowing superior visualization of distal splenic artery (*arrowhead*).

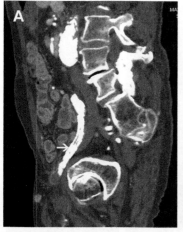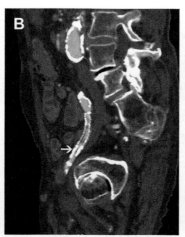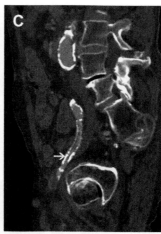

Fig. 12. Decreased blooming artifact using VMI. (*A*) Sagittal multiplanar reconstruction (MPR) conventional CT image at the level of pelvis shows extensive stent-related blooming artifact in the common iliac artery (*arrow*). (*B*) The 80-keV VMI at the same level shows decreased blooming artifact. (*C*)The 100-keV VMI at the same level shows further improvement in blooming and superior evaluation of the lumen.

luminal stenosis. MECT can achieve a more robust bone subtraction. Using MD, pixels attributed to bone are assigned a highly negative attenuation (eg, −1024 HU) and displayed as dark on the CT images. On MIP or three-dimension (3D) volume rendering (VR), bone is completely subtracted, generating high-quality MIPs or volume renderings of the vasculature containing iodinated contrast material (**Fig. 13**). The dual-energy bone subtraction technique has been shown to be fast, robust, and associated with fewer pitfalls and higher diagnostic performance compared to single-energy technique in several vascular beds.[53–55] This technique is successful in proximal and large arteries and bypass grafts but limited in smaller arteries. Occasionally, the algorithm can erroneously subtract the calcium as well and in large patients may not subtract bone in the areas excluded from the MECT field of view (FOV) in dual source dual energy CT (*ds*DECT). In the thorax, conventional techniques require multiple clip planes in addition to thresholding, whereas dual-energy techniques are faster and do not erode intercostal arteries.[22]

On 3D reconstructions, the presence of calcium limits the evaluation of luminal stenosis and results in overestimation of luminal stenosis. Subtracting calcium from the vessel wall helps in accurate quantification of luminal stenosis and generation of accurate 3D reconstructions. Following dual-energy bone subtraction as discussed above, calcium plaques can be subtracted in a *ds*DECT technique by using morphological criteria for plaques (**Fig. 14**). This provides an excellent MIP luminogram which provides a good overview of vascular anatomy. Similar to MECT bone separation, this technique also works better in proximal vessels[53] and is suboptimal below the level of the thigh.[56–58] Occasionally, there may be overremoval of calcific plaques, which can result in overestimation of stenosis.

Improved calcium separation and higher diagnostic accuracy can be achieved by using novel dedicated calcium subtraction material algorithms, which uses calcium as a primary basis material.[59,60] Because the arterial calcification is made of calcium hydroxyapatite, iodine/calcium or iodine/hydroxyapatite MD images can also improve delineation of vessels.[61] This calcium subtraction is another option to reduce calcium blooming artifact discussed in the previous section. Zeff images have shown that Zeff of arterial calcium is equivalent of calcium oxalate monohydrate.[62] Hence, iodine/calcium monohydrate oxalate material decomposition image (MDI) can also subtract calcium effectively.[36,62]

DECREASED RADIATION DOSE

MECT provides an option for reducing the radiation dose of CTA, particularly in multiphasic CTA studies. For example, CTA to evaluate for endoleaks after endovascular aortic aneurysm repair (EVAR) is typically performed at three phases, namely non-contrast, arterial, and delayed. The non-contrast phase is acquired to characterize high-attenuation areas (*such as calcium and endoleak*) seen within the aneurysmal sac in postcontrast CT. Because the attenuation numbers on the VNC images are almost like that of TNC

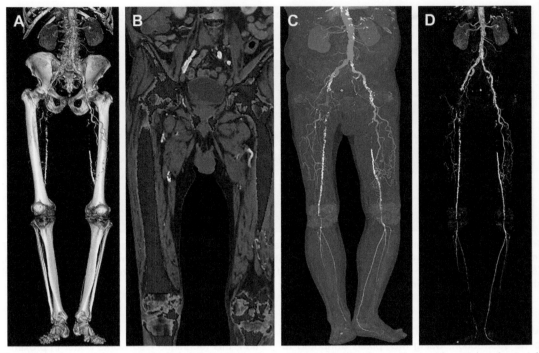

Fig. 13. Dual-energy bone subtraction. (*A*) Coronal volume-rendered image in a patient with peripheral arterial disease shows the vascular anatomy which is largely obscured by bones. (*B*) Using dual-energy material decomposition, bones can be identified and color coded. (*C*) MIP images of the peripheral arteries obtained after subtraction of bones using dual-energy material separation. (*D*) Three-dimensional volume rendered images of peripheral arteries with subtraction of bones by dual-energy material separation.

images, VNC images can be used to distinguish calcification from endoleak (**Fig. 15**). However, occasionally, there may be artifactual high attenuation on VNC images, especially if the VNC images are derived from an arterial phase acquisition with dense contrast material. In addition, calcium is sometimes subtracted on VNC images, which may lead to confusion. Iodine maps can further improve the sensitivity and specificity of endoleak detection, with the presence of iodine in a hyperattenuating area indicating an endoleak. Hence, the TNC acquisition can be safely eliminated in multiphasic CTA studies providing significant radiation dose savings.

Several studies have shown comparable sensitivity and specificity for detection of endoleaks after thoracoabdominal aneurysm repair when using a VNC/or an iodine map in lieu of a TNC acquisition.[25,26,63–65] Further radiation dose savings can be achieved by a single DECT delayed phase acquisition, decreasing the number of scans from 3 to 1.[21,64,66,67] Buffa and colleagues found 100% agreement in endoleak identification when interpreting the triphasic examination compared with the delayed phase alone with its associated VNC reconstruction.[66] The low-keV VMI generated from a single delayed venous phase acquisition

can simulate a "virtual arterial phase" with similar CNR and SNR.[21] With single-phase DECT studies, it is more appropriate to use the venous rather than the arterial phase, because arterial phase images may miss small, slow-filling endoleaks and there may be higher attenuation on VNC images derived from arterial phase images.[63,68]

Another similar protocol is the multiphasic acquisition for GI bleeding, with non-contrast, arterial, and venous phases.[69] The unenhanced phase is used to distinguish high-attenuating areas on post-contrast CT to distinguish active bleeding and preexisting ingested contents or medications. Using VNC/iodine map instead of TNC provides similar diagnostic performance (accuracy: 95% vs 92%; area under curve [AUC]: 0.95 vs 0.94; positive predictive value: 98.8% in both) and higher negative predictive value (82% VNC vs 74% TNC) with decrease in radiation dose.[70–72] VNC images from an indirect CT venography can show an acute clot.[36] VNC images can accurately quantify calcium from contrast material enhanced CT saving the need for another non-contrast acquisition.[73] The characterization of incidental lesions described in the section above also reduces the cumulative radiation dose by avoiding a follow-up dedicated CT scan.

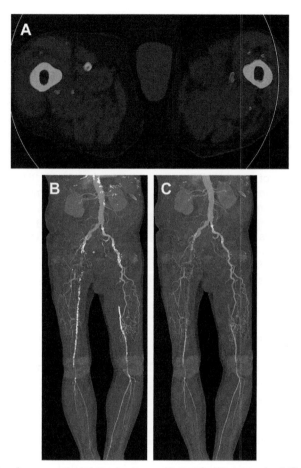

Fig. 14. Calcium separation from vessels. (*A*) Dual-energy color-coded images of calcified plaque (*orange color*) separated from contrast-filled lumen (*blue color*). (*B*) MIP with removal of bone. (*C*) MIP with removal of bone and calcium plaques. This gives an estimate of the severity of luminal stenosis.

EVALUATION OF ORGAN PERFUSION

The iodine map provides quantification of iodine, and thus is an effective surrogate for tissue perfusion, and is most used in the lungs and heart. In the lungs, it is used to evaluate the hemodynamic impact of a pulmonary embolism (PE). This is performed either using a traditional iodine overlay image or a pulmonary blood volume map, which color codes perfusion in areas with attenuation between −900 and −600 HU (ie, *lung tissue*).[1] In acute PE, wedge-shaped perfusion defects are

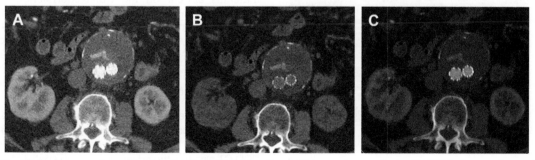

Fig. 15. Dual energy in endoleak detection. (*A*) Conventional CT image in a patient with EVAR shows a focus of high attenuation in the excluded aneurysmal sac. (*B*) Virtual non-contrast image shows the presence of high-attenuation material, which confirms this is calcification and not endoleak. The use of VNC instead of a true non-contrast image provides significant radiation dose savings. (*C*) Iodine map also shows the absence of iodine in the high attenuation, confirming this is calcium.

seen in a segmental and subsegmental distribution (**Fig. 16**). This is used either for diagnosing acute PE or to improve the detection of small subsegmental emboli which may be erroneously missed on a regular CTA or to provide hemodynamic information which is essential for prognosis.[74] Wedge-shaped, mottled, mosaic, or heterogeneous perfusion defects can also be seen in chronic PE.[75] Often in patients with dyspnea of unknown cause, the presence of a perfusion defect on MECT iodine map may be the only clue to the presence of chronic PE and chronic thromboembolic pulmonary hypertension (CTEPH).[75] Perfusion defects are also seen in pulmonary hypertension, with variable pattern depending on the etiology. This helps in the diagnosis and provides prognostic information. Note that pseudo-perfusion defects can be seen in a variety of pulmonary abnormalities including emphysema and in artifacts such as motion.

The perfusion defects and its relationship to CTA findings are important in determining management decisions for patients with CTEPH. If there is a perfusion defect in a segment subtended by a vessel with a clot, the patient will benefit from pulmonary endarterectomy. However, if there is a perfusion defect but no corresponding abnormality in the central pulmonary artery, it means that the disease process is centered distally at the level of microvasculature and the patient will not benefit from endarterectomy.[76] If there is no perfusion defect, but there is a central chronic embolism, it means that collateral vessels have developed to supply the lung, and hence these patients will benefit from endarterectomy.[76] MECT can also be used in the follow-up of patients with CTEPH and evaluate response to therapy.[76]

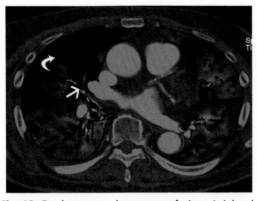

Fig. 16. Dual-energy pulmonary perfusion. Axial pulmonary blood volume (PBV) map in a patient with acute pulmonary embolism in a segmental branch (*straight arrow*) shows a wedge-shaped perfusion defect (*curved arrow*) in the anterior right upper lobe.

Perfusion of the myocardium provides the hemodynamic significance of a coronary stenosis. Using iodine maps, the perfusion can be quantified. The sensitivity of perfusion scans can be improved over single-energy perfusion CT with the use of iodine maps and low-energy VMI. High sensitivity and specificity of 96% and 98% have been described with 40-keV low-energy VMI.[77] In addition, the specificity is also increased by using high-energy VMIs, which decrease beam-hardening artifacts.[1,78] This can also be fused with 3D VR coronary angiography to get both anatomical and functional information.[36] In addition, iodine maps can also be used to improve the visualization of late iodine enhancement and quantification of extracellular volume.

ADVANCED MATERIAL DECOMPOSITION AND MULTI-CONTRAST MATERIAL IMAGING

The currently available techniques have limited ability to image more than one contrast material at a time. PCD CT provides the option of energy-selective imaging, with the availability of more than one energy bin. In addition, it also allows improved k-edge imaging, which means that an energy bin that approximates the k-edge of the element can be selected. K-edge reflects the binding energy of the electron in the inner shell of elements. Photoelectric effect increases at energies that are just above the k-shell of the material.[4] Contrast materials made of various elements can also be separated using their inherent elemental properties. One study was able to distinguish orally administered high-atomic number contrast material such as tantalum, tungsten, or rhenium from intravenously administered iodinated contrast material.[79] Iodine and barium contrast materials appear only on the iodine-equivalent images, whereas the other contrast materials appear on the water-equivalent images.[79] A combination of iodine and gadolinium can be used to simultaneously evaluate the coronary arteries and myocardial enhancement in animal models.[80]

EMERGING AND FUTURE APPLICATIONS

The development of PCD CT offers several new emerging options in vascular emerging. In addition to presumably superior multi-energy capabilities, PCD CT also has the advantage of high spatial resolution, which has several applications in vascular imaging, but beyond the scope of this article.[81,82] Nevertheless, the combination of high-resolution and superior multi-energy is tailor-made for vascular imaging. High-resolution imaging of small structures such as small vessels and vessel wall can be accomplished at low doses of iodinated contrast. In future, there is potential for improved plaque characterization using the combination of high resolution and advanced contrast materials including nanoparticles.[83] PCD CT also has lower noise and artifacts. The FDA-approved dual-source PCD also has some novel options such as Flash-ME mode, which can obtain motion-free ME images, which was not possible in previous generations of dual-source scanners at low radiation and contrast doses.[84,85] Owing to the detector-basis of this technology, cardiac and vascular scans can be obtained at higher temporal resolution and spatial registration, which was not possible in previous dual-source scanners. This allows decreased motion artifacts and improved MD.[84,85]

Novel MD algorithms are being evaluated. Recently, a "Dark-blood" technique has been described for improved assessment of the vessel wall due to increased lumen-to-wall contrast. From a post-contrast image, an region of interest (ROI) is placed in the ascending aorta, and the content of this ROI is defined as one basis material (instead of iodine), with the other basis material being water.[86] This has been shown to be useful in the evaluation of intramural hematoma and vasculitis.

Potential applications of artifical intelligence (AI) in MECT include AI-assisted reconstruction of diagnostic quality CT images from a sparser data set of a low radiation dose image acquisition.[87] AI may also be applied for the automated improvement of image quality by reducing beam-hardening artifacts and the automated reconstruction of images with monoenergetic segmentation of specific anatomic structures. Super-resolution images can be generated from routine quality images.[88] In the context of the detection and classification of pathology, MECT provides additional information not available with conventional CT that allows for the use of material attenuation decomposition plots as a form of CT fingerprinting.[89–91] The combination of these CT fingerprints and AI may allow for the automated detection and classification of certain disease entities.

CHALLENGES AND LIMITATIONS

MECT typically requires dedicated hardware, which involves additional expenditure. Dedicated training is required for radiologists and technologists. There are a multitude of scanning, postprocessing, and MD techniques, with different nomenclature, which needs standardization. An MECT protocol with automatic generation of predetermined multi-energy images (depending on the clinical indication) at the scanner console improves the workflow by freeing up the technologist to take care of other patient-related tasks. Scanning large patients (>265–285 lbs) is a challenge with many of these techniques, either due to FOV (dsDECT) or noise rapid switching dual energy CT (rsDECT) limitations. The radiologist should be aware of pitfalls and artifacts that may be seen in the MECT images.[32] The low noise and artifacts in PCD CT can be potentially useful in large patients. PCD CT has additional challenges including the tremendous increase in the number of images, which might result in storage images.

SUMMARY

DECT or MECT has several applications in vascular imaging. Low-energy VMI enhances the signal from iodinated contrast material, which can be used to lower iodinated contrast dose, improve image quality, and salvage a suboptimal scan. Iodine maps and VNC images are useful in lesion characterization, with the former also useful in the evaluation of perfusion and the latter also useful in reducing radiation dose by replacing TNC from multiphasic CTA acquisitions. MECT also provides robust bone and calcium subtraction for 3D reconstructions.

CLINICS CARE POINTS

- Increased attenutation of iodinated contrast material In low-energy VMIs improves visualization of small vessels

- Virtual non contrast and iodine maps can distinguish active extravasation of contrast material, hematoma or calcification from a contrast-enhanced CT

- High-energy VMIs reduce blooming from dense calcified plaques and stents

- DECT can accomplish a more robust bone subtraction than conventional attenuation threshold-based bone separation

- DECT can improve detection of endoleaks following EVAR and reduce radiation dose by eliminating true non-contrast acquisition

DISCLOSURES

No financial disclosure or conflict of interest.

REFERENCES

1. Kalisz K, Halliburton S, Abbara S, et al. Update on Cardiovascular Applications of Multienergy CT. Radiographics 2017;37:1955–74.
2. Siegel MJ, Kaza RK, Bolus DN, et al. White Paper of the Society of Computed Body Tomography and Magnetic Resonance on Dual-Energy CT, Part 1: Technology and Terminology. J Comput Assist Tomogr 2016;40(6):841–5.
3. Rajiah P, Parakh A, Kay F, et al. Update on Multienergy CT: Physics, principals and applications. Radiographics 2020;40(5):1284–308.
4. Leng S, Bruesewitz M, Tao S, et al. Photon-counting detector CT: System design and clinical applications of an emerging technology. Radiographics 2019; 39(3):729–43.
5. Rassouli N, Etesami M, Dhanantwari A, et al. Detector-based spectral CT with novel dual-layer technology: principles and applications. Insights imaging 2017;8(6):589–98.
6. Soesbe TC, Lewis MA, Di Y, et al. A Technique to identify isoattenuating gallstones with dual-layer spectral Ct: an ex vivo phantom study. Radiology 2019;292(2):400–6.
7. Leithner D, Wichmann JL, Vogl TJ, et al. Virtual monoenergetic imaging and iodine perfusion maps improve diagnostic accuracy of dual-energy computed tomography pulmonary angiography with suboptimal contrast attenuation. Invest Radiol 2017;42:659–65.
8. Kulkarni NM, Sahani DV, Desai GS, Kalva SP. Indirect computed tomography venography of the lower extremities using single-source dual-energy computed tomography: advantage of low-kiloelectron volt monochromatic images. J Vasc Interv Radiol 2012;23(7):879–86.
9. Ghandour A, Sher A, Rassouli N, et al. Evaluation of Virtual Monoenergetic Images on Pulmonary Vasculature Using the Dual-Layer Detector-Based Spectral Computed Tomography. J Comput Assist Tomogr 2018;42:858–65.
10. Chalian H, Kalisz K, Rassouli N, et al. Utility of virtual monoenergetic images derived from a dual-layer detector-based spectral CT in the assessment of aortic anatomy and pathology: A retrospective case control study. Clin Imaging 2018;52:292–301.
11. Yuan R, Shuman WP, Earls JP, et al. Reduced iodine load at CT pulmonary angiography with dual-energy monochromatic imaging: comparison with standard CT pulmonary angiography–a prospective randomized trial. Radiology 2012;262(1):290–7.
12. Shuman WP, O'Malley RB, Busey JM, et al. Prospective comparison of dual-energy CT aortography using 70% reduced iodine dose versus single-energy CT aortography using standard iodine dose in the same patient. Abdom Radiol (NY) 2017;42(3):759–65.
13. Carrascosa P, Capunay C, Rodriguez-Granillo GA, et al. Substantial iodine volume load reduction in CT angiography with dual-energy imaging: insights from a pilot randomized study. Int J Cardiovasc Imaging 2014;30(8):1613–20.
14. Patino M, Parakh A, Lo GC, et al. Virtual Monochromatic Dual-Energy Aortoiliac CT Angiography with Reduced Iodine Dose: A Prospective Randomized Study. AJR Am J Roentgenol 2019;212(2):467–74.
15. Leng S, Yu L, Wang J, et al. Noise reduction in spectral CT: Reducing dose and breaking the trade-off between image noise and energy bin selection. Med Phys 2011;4946–57.
16. Grant KL, Flohr TG, Krauss B, et al. Assessment of an advanced image-based technique to calculate virtual monoenergetic images from a dual-energy examination to improve contrast-to-noise ratio in examinations using iodinated contrast media. Invest Radiol 2014;49(9):586–92.
17. Albrecht MH, Trommer J, Wichmann JL, et al. Comprehensive comparison of virtual monoenergetic and linearly blended reconstruction techniques in third-generation dual-source dual-energy computed tomography angiography of the thorax and abdomen. Invest Radiol 2016;51(9):582–90.
18. Martin SS, Albrecht MH, Wichmann JL, et al. Value of a noise-optimized virtual monoenergetic reconstruction technique in dual -energy CT for planning of transcatheter aortic valve replacement. Eur Radiol 2017;27(2):705–14.
19. Weiss J, Notohamiprodjo M, Bongers M, et al. Effect of Noise-Optimized Monoenergetic Postprocessing on diagnostic accuracy for detecting incidental pulmonary embolism in portal-venous phase dual-energy computed tomography. Invest Radiol 2017; 52:142–7.
20. Godoy MC, Naidich DP, Marchiori E, et al. Single acquisition dual energy multidetector computed tomography: analysis of vascular enhancement and post processing techniques for evaluating the thoracic aorta. J Comput Assist Tomogr 2010; 34(5):670–7.
21. Patel AA, Sutphin PD, Xi Y, et al. Arterial Phase CTA Replacement by a Virtual Arterial Phase Reconstruction from a Venous Phase CTA: Preliminary Results Using Detector-Based Spectral CT. Cardiovasc Intervent Radiol 2019;42:250–9.
22. Vlahos I, Chung R, Nair A, et al. Dual-energy CT: vascular applications. AJR Am J Roentgenol 2012; 199(5 Suppl):S87–97.
23. Martin SS, Wichmann JL, Weyer H, et al. Endoleaks after endovascular aortic aneurysm repair: Improved detection with noise-optimized virtual monoenergetic dual-energy CT. Eur J Radiol 2017; 94:125–32.

24. Vlahos I, Godoy MC, Naidich DP. Dual-energy computed tomography imaging of the aorta. J Thorac Imaging 2010;25:289–300.

25. Stolzmann P, Frauenfelder T, Pfammatter T, et al. Endoleaks after endovascular abdominal aortic aneurysm repair: detection with dual-energy dual-source CT. Radiology 2008;249:682–91.

26. Ascenti G, Mazziotti S, Iamberto S, et al. Dual-energy CT for detection of endoleaks after endovasucular abdominal aortic aneurysm repair: usefulness of colored iodine overlay. AJR Am J Roentgenol 2011 Jun;196(6):1408–14.

27. Maturen KE, Kaza RK, Liu PS, et al. "Sweet spot" for endoleak detection: optimizing contrast to noise using low keV reconstructions from fast-switch kVp dual-energy CT. J Comput Assist Tomogr 2012;36:83–7.

28. Martin SS, Wichmann JL, Scholtz JE, et al. Noise-Optimized Virtual Monoenergetic Dual-Energy CT Improves Diagnostic Accuracy for the Detection of Active Arterial Bleeding of the Abdomen. J Vasc Interv Radiol 2017;28:1257–66.

29. Darras KE, McLaughlin PD, Kang H, et al. Virtual monoenergetic reconstruction of contrast-enhanced dual energy CT at 70 keV maximizes mural enhancement in acute small bowel obstruction. Eur J Radiol 2016;85(5):950–6.

30. Potretzke TA, Brace CL, Lubner MG, et al. Early small-bowel ischemia: dual-energy CT improves conspicuity compared with conventional CT in a swine model. Radiology 2015;275(1):119–26.

31. Mileto A, Ananthakrishnan L, Morgan DE, et al. Clinical implementation of dual-energy CT for gastrointestinal bleeding. AJR Am J Roentgenol 2021;217: 651–3.

32. Parakh A, Lennartz S, An C, et al. Dual-Energy CT Images: Pearls and Pitfalls. Radiographics 2021; 41(1):98–119.

33. Phan CM, Yoo AJ, Hirsch JA, et al. Differentiation of hemorrhage from iodinated contrast in different intracranial compartments using dual energy head CT. AJNR Am J Neuroradiol 2012;33(6):1088–94.

34. Potter CA, Sodickson AD. Dual energy CT in emergency neuroimaging: Added value and novel applications. Radiographics 2016;36(7):2186–95.

35. Hur J, Kim YJ, Lee H-J, et al. Cardioembolic stroke: Dual-energy cardiac CT for differentiation of left atrial appendage thrombus and circulatory stasis. Radiology 2012;263(3):688–95.

36. Machida H, Tanaka I, Fukui R, et al. Dual-Energy Spectral CT: Various Clinical Vascular Applications. Radiographics 2016;36(4):1215–32.

37. Fulton N, Rajiah P. Abdominal applications of a novel detector-based spectral CT. Curr Probl Diagn Radiol 2018;47(2):110–8.

38. Brooks RA, Di Chiro G. Beam hardening in x-ray reconstructive tomography. Phys Med Biol 1976; 21(3):390–8.

39. Pinho DF, Kulkarni NM, Krishnaraj A, et al. Initial experience with single-source dual-energy CT abdominal angiography and comparison with single-energy CT angiography: image quality, enhancement, diagnosis and radiation dose. Eur Radiol 2013;23(2):351–9.

40. Hounsfield GN. Computerized transverse axial scanning (tomography). 1. Description of system. Br J Radiol 1973;46(552):1016–22.

41. Laukamp KR, Gupta A, Grobe Hokamp N, et al. Role of spectral-detector CT in reduction of artifacts from contrast media in axillary and subclavian veins: single institution study in 50 patients. Acta Radiol 2019; 18. 284185119868904.

42. Bamberg F, Dierks A, Nikolaou K, et al. Metal artifact reduction by dual energy computed tomography using monoenergetic extrapolation. Eur Radiol 2011; 21(7):1424–9.

43. Kosmas C, Hojjati M, Young PC, et al. Dual-layer spectral computerized tomography for metal artifact reduction: small versus large orthopedic devices. Skeletal Radiol 2019;48(12):1981–90.

44. Meinel FG, Bischoff B, Zhang Q, et al. Metal artifact reduction by dual-energy computed tomography using energetic extrapolation: A systemically optimized protocol. Invest Radiol 2012;47(7):406–14.

45. Shaqdan KW, Parakh A, Kambadakone AR, et al. Role of dual energy CT to improve diagnosis of non-traumatic abdominal vascular emergencies. Abdom Radiol (NY) 2019;44(2):406–21.

46. Patino M, Prochowski A, Agarwal MD. Material separation using dual-energy CT: Current and emerging applications. Radiographics 2016;36: 1087–105.

47. Van Hedent S, Grobe Hokamp N, Kessner R, et al. Effect of virtual monoenergetic images from spectral detector computed tomography on coronary calcium blooming. J Comput assit Tomogr 2018;42(6): 912–8.

48. Hickethier T, Baessler B, Kroeger JR, et al. Monoenergetic reconstructions for imaging of coronary artery stents using spectral detector CT: In-vitro experience and comparison to conventional images. J Cardiovasc Comput Tomogr 2017;11(1):33–9.

49. Almutairi A, Al Safran Z, AlZaabi SA, et al. Dual energy CT angiography in peripheral arterial stents: optimal scanning protocols with regard to image quality and radiation dose. Quant Imaging Med Surg 2017;7(5):520–31.

50. Mangold S, Cannao PM, Schoepf UJ, et al. Impact of an advanced image-based monoenergetic reconstruction algorithm on coronary stent visualization using third generation dual-source dual-energy CT: a phantom study. Eur Radiol 2016;26:1871–8.

51. Halpern EJ, Halpern DJ, Yanof JH, et al. Is coronary stent assessment improved with spectral analysis of dual energy CT? Acad Radiol 2009;16(10):1241–50.

52. Pessis E, Campagna R, Sverzut JM, et al. Virtual monochromatic spectral imaging with fast kilovoltage switching:reduction of metal artifacts at CT. Radiographics 2013;33(2):573–83.

53. Morhard D, Fink C, Graser A, et al. Cervical and cranial computed tomographic angiography with automated bon e removal: dual energy computed tomography versus standard computed tomography. Invest Radiol 2009;44(5):293–7.

54. Deng K, Liu C, Ma R, et al. Clinical evaluation of dual energy bone removal in CT angiography of the head and neck: comparison with conventional bone-subtraction CT angiography. Clin Radiol 2009; 64(5):534–41.

55. Meyer BC, Werncke T, Hopfenmuller W, et al. Dual energy Ct of peripheral arteries: effect of automatic bone and plaque removal on image quality and grading of stenosis. Eur J Radiol 2008;68(3):414–22.

56. Sommer WH, Johnson TR, Becker CR, et al. The value of dual-energy bone removal in maximum intensity projections of lower extremity computed tomography angiography. Invest Radiol 2009;44(5): 285–92.

57. Brockmann C, Jochum S, Sadick M, et al. Dual-energy CT angiography in peripheral arterial occlusive disease. Cardiovasc Intervent Radiol 2009;32(4): 630–7.

58. Kau T, Eicher W, Reiterer C, et al. Dual-energy CT angiography in peripheral arterial occlusive disease-accuracy of maximum intensity projections in clinical routine and subgroup analysis. Eur Radiol 2011;21 98:1677–86.

59. De Santis D, De Cecco CN, Schoepf UJ, et al. Modified calcium subtraction in dual-energy CT angiography of the lower extremity runoff: impact on diagnostic accuracy for stenosis detection. Eur Radiol 2019;4783–93.

60. De Santis D, Jin KN, Schoepf UJ, et al. Heavily Calcified Coronary Arteries: Advanced Calcium Subtraction Improves Luminal Visualization and Diagnostic Confidence in Dual-Energy Coronary Computed Tomography Angiography. Invest Radiol 2018;53(2):103–9.

61. Schmid K, McSharry WO, Pameijer CH, et al. Chemical and physicochemical studies on the mineral deposits of the human atherosclerotic aorta. Atherosclerosis 1980;37(2):199–210.

62. Matsui K, Machida H, Mitsuhashi T, et al. Analysis of coronary arterial calcification components with coronary CT angiography using single-source dual-energy CT with fast tube voltage switching. Int J Cardiovasc Imaging 2015;31(3):639–47.

63. Flors L, Leiva-Salinas C, Norton PT, et al. Imaging follow-up of endovascular repair of type B aortic dissection with dual-source, dual-energy CT and late delayed-phase scans. J Vasc Interv Radiol 2014;25:435–42.

64. Flors L, Leiva-Salinas C, Norton PT, et al. Endoleak detection after endovascular repair of thoracic aortic aneurysm using dual-source dual-energy CT: suitable scanning protocols and potential radiation dose reduction. AJR Am J Roentgenol 2013;200:451–60.

65. Numburi UD, Schoenhagen P, Flamm SD, et al. Feasibility of dual-energy CT in the arterial phase: Imaging after endovascular aortic repair. AJR Am J Roentgenol 2010;195:486–93.

66. Buffa V, Solazzo A, D'Auria V, et al. Dual-source dual-energy CT: dose reduction after endovascular abdominal aortic aneurysm repair. Radiol Med 2014;119:934–41.

67. Chandarana H, Godoy MC, Vlahos I, et al. Abdominal aorta: evaluation with dual-source dual-energy multidetector CT after endovascular repair of aneurysms–initial observations. Radiology 2008;249: 692–700.

68. Lehti L, Soderberg M, Hoglund P, et al. Reliability of virtual non-contrast computed tomography angiography: comparing it with the real deal. Acta Radiol Open 2018;7. 2058460118790115.

69. Fidler JL, Gunn ML, Soto JA, et al. Society of abdominal radiology gastrointestinal bleeding disease-focused panel consensus recommendations for CTA technical parameters in the evaluation of acute overt gastrointestinal bleeding. Abdom Radiol (NY) 2019;44:2957–62.

70. Sun K, Zhao R, Han R, et al. The feasibility of combined coronary and supraaortic angiography with single high-pitch acquisition dual source CT. Angiology 2015;3:2.

71. Patel BN, Alexander L, Allen B, et al. Dual-energy CT workflow: Multi-Institutional consensus on standardization of abdominopelvic MDCT protocols. Abdom Radiol (NY) 2017;42:676–87.

72. Trabzonlu TA, Mozaffary A, Kim D, et al. Dual-energy CT evaluation of gastrointestinal bleeding. Abdom Radiol (NY) 2020;45(1):1–14.

73. Yamada Y, Jinzaki M, Okamura T, et al. Feasibility of coronary artery calcium scoring on virtual unenhanced images derived from single-source fast kVp-switching dual-energy CT angiography. J Cardiovasc Comput Tomogr 2014;8(5):391–400.

74. Moore AJE, Wachsmann J, Chamarthy MR, et al. Imaging of acute pulmonary embolism: an update. Cardiovasc Diagn Ther 2018;8(3):225–43.

75. Goerne H, Batra K, Rajiah P. Imaging of pulmonary hypertension: an update. Cardiovasc Diagn Ther 2018;8(3):270–96.

76. Rajiah P, Tanabe Y, Partovi S, et al. State of the art utility of multienergy CT in the evaluation of pulmonary vasculature. Int J Cardiovasc Imaging 2010; 35(8):1509–24.

77. Carrascosa P, Deviggiano A, de Zan M, et al. Improved discrimination of myocardial perfusion defects at low energy levels using virtual

monochromatic imaging. J Comput Assist Tomogr 2017;41(4):661–7.

78. Tanabe Y, Kurata A, Matsuda A, et al. Computed tomographic evaluation of myocardial ischemia. Jpn J Radiol 2020;38(5):411–33.

79. Soesbe TC, lewis MA, Nasr K, et al. Separating high-z oral contrast from intravascular iodine contrast in an animal model using dual-layer spectral CT. Acad Radiol 2019;26(9):1237–44.

80. Symons R, Cork TE, Lakshmanan MN, et al. Dual-contrast agent photon-counting computed tomography of the heart: initial experience. Int J Cardiovasc Imaging 2017;33(8):1253–61.

81. Wildberger JE, Alkadhi H. New Horizons in Vascular Imaging With Photon-Counting Detector CT. Invest Radiol 2023;58(7):499–504.

82. Rajendran K, Petersilka M, Henning A, et al. First clinical photon-counting detector CT system: Technical evaluation. Radiology 2022;303(1):130–8.

83. Si-Mohamed SA, Sigovan M, Hsu JC, et al. In vivo molecular K-edge imaging of atherosclerotic plaque using photon-counting CT. Radiology 2021;300(1):98–107.

84. Ahmed Z, Campeau D, Gong H, et al. High-pitch, high temporal resolution, multi-energy cardiac imaging on a dual-source photon-counting-detector CT. Med Phys 2023;50(3):1428–35.

85. Rajiah PS, Dunning CAS, Rajendran K, et al. High-Pitch Multienergy Coronary CT Angiography in Dual-Source Photon-Counting Detector CT Scanner at Low Iodinated Contrast Dose. Invest Radiol 2023. https://doi.org/10.1097/RLI.0000000000000961.

86. Rotzinger DC, Si-Mohamed SA, Shapira N, et al. "Dark-blood" Dual-energy computed tomography angiography for thoracic aortic wall imaging. Eur Radiol 2020;30(1):425–31.

87. Willemink MJ, Noel PB. The evolution of image reconstruction for CT-from filtered back projection to artificial intelligence. Eur Radiol 2019;29(5):2185–95.

88. Kawai H, Motoyama S, Sarai M, et al. Super resolution deep learning reconstruction for detection of in-stent restenosis. Circulation 2022;146:A10054.

89. Weir-McCall JR, Villines TC, Shaw LJ, et al. Highlights of the Twelfth Annual Scientific Meeting of the Society of Cardiovascular Computed Tomography. J Cardiovasc Comput Tomogr 2018;12(1):3–7.

90. Lewis MA, Soesbe TC, Ananthakrishnan L, et al. Spectral CT analysis using custom plugins for a clinical DICOM viewer. Chicago, IL: Radiological Society of North America; 2017 2017. p. 11–27.

91. Lewis MA, Soesbe TC, Do QN, et al. Spectral CT "fingerprinting" on a pre-clinical detection based spectral CT scanner: tools for exploration and examples. Chicago, IL: Radiological Society of North America; 2016 2016. p. 11–28.

Dual-Energy, Spectral and Photon Counting Computed Tomography for Evaluation of the Gastrointestinal Tract

Avinash K. Nehra, MD[a],*, Bari Dane, MD[b], Benjamin M. Yeh, MD[c], Joel G. Fletcher, MD[a], Shuai Leng, PhD[a], Achille Mileto, MD[d]

KEYWORDS

• Dual-energy CT • Photon-counting detector CT • Virtual monoenergetic images • Iodine maps
• Hepatocellular carcinoma • Pancreatic adenocarcinoma • Gastrointestinal bleeding
• Peritoneal disease

KEY POINTS

- Dual-energy computed tomography (CT) can augment the diagnostic assessment of gastrointestinal disease using energy- and material-specific image datasets.
- The combination of virtual unenhanced, low-energy monochromatic images, and iodine maps can improve detection and characterization of lesions and other abnormalities of the gastrointestinal tract.
- Novel contrast agents and photon-counting CT can further expand the role of dual-energy CT in assessment of gastrointestinal pathologies.

INTRODUCTION

Since the US Food and Drug Administration approval of the first clinical dual-source dual-energy computed tomographic (CT) platform in 2006, the dual-energy CT scanning mode has emerged as a promising tool with multiple clinical applications that have proved usefulness in the evaluation of gastrointestinal diseases.

Conventional single-energy CT is limited by relying on CT numbers (in Hounsfield units) for quantitation because different materials can show similar attenuation values. Dual-energy CT obtains simultaneous or near-simultaneous data from 2 different X-ray energy levels, thus resulting in 2 distinct energy spectra.[1] This feature allows for identification and quantification of different materials that have distinct atomic numbers and energy characteristics, resulting in material-specific datasets. For example, the closer the energy level is to the K edge of a substance such as iodine, the more the substance attenuates.[2,3] Dual-energy CT also provides energy-specific data with optimized contrast and noise characteristics.

Current applications of dual-energy CT in the abdomen and pelvis provide information about tissue composition and how tissues behave at different energies, the ability to generate virtual unenhanced datasets, and improved detection of iodine-containing substances on low-energy images. This article illustrates principles and applications of dual-energy CT relevant to the evaluation of gastrointestinal diseases.

[a] Department of Radiology, Mayo Clinic, 200 First Street Southwest, Rochester, MN 55905, USA; [b] Department of Radiology, New York University Langone Medical Center, 550 First Avenue, New York, NY 10016, USA; [c] Department of Radiology and Biomedical Imaging, University of California, 505 Parnassus Avenue, San Francisco, CA 94143, USA; [d] Department of Radiology, Virginia Mason Medical Center, 1100 9th Avenue, Seattle, WA 98101, USA
* Corresponding author.
E-mail address: nehra.avinash@mayo.edu

Radiol Clin N Am 61 (2023) 1031–1049
https://doi.org/10.1016/j.rcl.2023.06.002
0033-8389/23/© 2023 Elsevier Inc. All rights reserved.

BASICS OF DUAL-ENERGY COMPUTED TOMOGRAPHY

CT numbers, in Hounsfield Units, represent the distribution of X-ray attenuation, which depends on both electron density and atomic number of the materials.[4,5] Therefore, different materials, for example, iodine and calcium, could have similar CT numbers if the anatomic number difference is precisely offset by the density difference. This generates a limitation of standard single-energy CT, that is, images are not material-specific.

Dual-energy CT acquires 2 data sets at different beam spectra and provides more information than single-energy CT.[1,6,7] By exploring the energy dependence of attenuation properties for different materials, dual-energy CT can provide material-specific images. For the energy range of X-ray used in diagnostic CT, there are 2 main interactions, that is, photoelectric and Compton effects. With the 2 measurements in dual-energy CT, anatomic number and electron density can be solved.

As explained, the key concept of dual-energy CT is to acquire data at 2 different spectra. Various approaches have been investigated and implemented on commercial dual-energy CT scanners.[1,7] These are commonly divided into 2 categories: source-based and detector-based approaches. Source-based implementation includes dual source, kV switching (fast or slow), and split filter. Detector-based implementation includes multi-layer detector (eg, dual-layer) and photon-counting detector (details will be discussed later). Detailed description of each dual-energy CT approach, along with advantages and disadvantages, can be found in the literature, for example, AAPM TG 291 report and several review articles.[1,7–11]

Dual-Energy Computed Tomography Processing and Image Types

A major strength of dual-energy CT is that various types of images can be generated and presented adaptive to the specific clinical applications. This attributes to the 2 distinct measurements and the dual-energy processing techniques. In dual-energy CT, material density maps can be generated from the process referred to as material decomposition, which can decompose the dual-energy CT measurements into density maps of two or more so called basis materials, such as iodine, calcium, and soft tissue.[1,6,12,13] Note that these are effective density map that may or may not representing the exact true density map. For example, on a noncontrast dual-energy CT scan where iodine and soft tissue are used as basis

materials, bone and calcification could show up bright signals on the iodine map although there is no iodine contrast on board.[7]

With the material decomposition capability, another application of dual-energy CT is to generate material suppress/removal images. A classic example is to create a virtual noncontrast image from a contrast-enhanced scan.[14–19] This is achieved with removing the iodine component from the original images based on the iodine map obtained through material decomposition. Another common application is virtual non-calcium images where calcium component is removed to highlight signals behind the bone, for example, edema in the context of a bone bruise.[20–23]

Another common type of images is the so-called virtual monoenergetic (or monochromatic) images.[24–28] The X-ray beam used in the data acquisition (single- or dual-energy CT) is polychromatic. Virtual monoenergetic images can be simulated from dual-energy CT by multiplying the material density and its attenuation at a specific energy (keV) and add up all components. The attenuation coefficient at a given energy is known for each material, which can be obtained from places like NIST.[29]

Dual-energy CT can also generate electron density and atomic number, so called r–z maps.[6,30,31] From physics perspective, material decomposition can also be performed to the 2 interaction mechanisms, for example, photoelectric and Compton effects.

In addition to the quantification capabilities provided by dual-energy CT, differentiation tasks can also be observed and found useful in certain clinical applications where classification of imaging target is more important than quantification of material density, for example, renal stone differentiation and gout detection.[32–36]

Radiation Dose Considerations

A common misconception is that dual-energy CT has higher radiation dose than that of single-energy CT as 2 acquisitions are performed. On the contrary, modern dual-energy CT platforms have comparable or near-comparable radiation dose to that of single-energy CT and could be even lower radiation dose for certain applications.[37,38] In dual-energy CT, the total radiation dose is divided into the 2 measurements, each of which only gets a fraction of the total radiation dose. In addition to the various types of dual-energy CT images, it can also generate a single-energy like image by mixing/blending the 2 measurements. Therefore, it is not necessary to have higher radiation dose for dual-energy CT than single-energy CT to achieve the same image quality. In addition, lower keV virtual monoenergetic images are known to have augmented contrast characteristics compared with that of standard single-energy CT images.[26] These images, especially with the help of advanced noise reduction techniques (some of which are specifically applied in the energy domain), could have higher contrast-to-noise ratio (CNR) compared with that of single-energy CT images, thus enabling further potential for radiation dose reduction compared with single-energy CT.[39–43]

Photon Counting Detector Computed Tomography

Another method to achieve dual- and multi-energy CT is to use photon-counting detector CT.[44–47] Conventional CT detectors use scintillating materials that can interact with X-ray photons and create visible light, which is consequently converted by photodiode to generate electrical signals. This is referred to indirect conversion as 2 steps are involved to generate the final signal. These detectors work in an energy-integrating mode as the final signal is proportional to the total energy deposited by all the X-ray photons. Therefore, they are commonly referred to as energy-integrating detectors.

Photon-counting detector CT is a new technology that gained substantial research and clinical development in the last 5 years at the time of this writing, with the first commercial photon-counting detector CT hardware commercially introduced in the late 2021 (NEATOM Alpha, Siemens Healthineers, Germany).[48] Photon-counting detector CT uses a direct conversion technique where X-ray directly interacts with semi-conductors (eg, CdTe, CZT, and silicon) to create electrical signals, which counts the number of photons instead of their total energy. The signal amplitude of each photon is proportional to its energy. The way photon-counting detector CT works is that it compares the detected signal to preselected energy threshold and allocates each photon to the energy bin accordingly. Therefore, photon-counting detector CT intrinsically has multi-energy capability.

Substantial benefits of photon-counting detector CT have been demonstrated, such as reduction of electronic noise, increased CNR, radiation dose-efficient ultra-high-resolution mode, multi-energy capability, and low radiation dose.[44–46,49–52] The radiation dose-efficient ultra-high-resolution mode comes with the fact that there is no septa (dead space) among detector cells as no visible light is generated as that in energy-integrating detectors.[51] As photon-counting detector CT allocates each photon into certain energy bins based on preselected energy thresholds, it naturally provides multi-energy capability when more than one energy bin is used. It can go beyond the 2 energy bins that are usually used for traditional dual-energy CT, with 2 to 8 energy bins investigated by different systems.[47]

DUAL-ENERGY COMPUTED TOMOGRAPHY OF THE HEPATOBILIARY SYSTEM
Liver

Focal liver lesions
Dual-energy CT has demonstrated benefits in both allowing for improved visualization and characterization of liver lesions.[53,54] Virtual monoenergetic images use material decomposition to simulate images acquired as if a theoretic monoenergetic X-ray source was used, thereby increasing relative differences in iodine signal at lower energies.[55,56] Therefore, virtual monoenergetic images, particularly low-energy images (40–60 keV), can result in improved detection for both hypervascular and hypovascular liver lesions while minimizing image noise.[57] This phenomenon is afforded by the substantial increase in iodine attenuation levels with use of low-keV monochromatic images, therefore iodine signal within hypervascular lesions appear more conspicuous compared with background liver parenchyma.[57,58]

The diagnosis of hepatocellular carcinoma has been established using the Liver Imaging Reporting and Data System.[59] However, small hepatocellular carcinomas (<2 cm) may pose a diagnostic challenge due to subtle enhancement characteristics and anatomic changes within the cirrhotic liver. It has been demonstrated that the use of dual-energy 50 keV images virtual monoenergetic images resulted in increased radiologist confidence in the detection of several key imaging features of hepatocellular carcinoma, such as late arterial enhancement, enhancing capsule, and tumor washout as well as improved diagnostic confidence in the diagnosis of small hepatocellular carcinomas (<2 cm; **Figs. 1** and **2**).[60] In addition, hypovascular lesions are also more easily detectable in the portal venous phase compared with the higher-attenuating liver parenchyma at low-energy settings and studies have demonstrated improved sensitivity for the detection of hypovascular liver lesions at 50 keV compared with conventional blended images (sensitivity of 95% vs 83%, respectively).[61]

Dual-energy CT has also shown benefits for liver lesion characterization. For example, analysis of

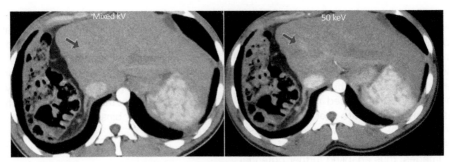

Fig. 1. A 71 year old man with hepatocellular carcinoma (HCC) (*red arrow*). Arterial phase images obtained at mixed kV and at 50 keV demonstrate hyperenhancement of the known HCC. The 50 keV DE virtual monoenergetic images increase iodine signal and may be particularly useful for detecting hypervascular neoplasms including HCC.

single-phase contrast-enhanced dual-energy CT in 55 patients demonstrated that iodine material attenuation images and iodine quantification helped improve the characterization of small incidental hypoattenuating hepatic lesions (<2 cm).[53]

Portal vein thrombosis
Iodine maps may also help to differentiate between bland thrombus from tumor thrombus, with the latter demonstrating increased uptake of iodine. When comparing iodine maps from dual-energy CT to single-energy CT-based conventional attenuation measurements, use of iodine quantification improved the characterization of portal vein thrombus in patients with hepatocellular carcinoma.[62,63]

Evaluation of hepatic tumor response
The use of iodine maps has also shown benefit in the detection of residual disease following locoregional or systemic treatment of hepatobiliary malignancies, particularly with hepatocellular carcinoma. Iodine maps obtained with dual-energy CT can improve the conspicuity of the ablation zone, and may be helpful in detecting residual viable tumor.[64,65]

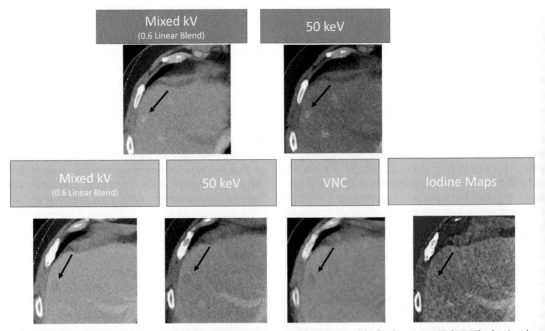

Fig. 2. Hepatocellular carcinoma (*black arrows*) in a 66 year old woman with dual-energy CT (DECT) obtained at 3 mm slices. The top row of images demonstrates arterial phase hyperenhancement and 50 keV images increase the conspicuity of enhancement. The delayed phase images (*bottom row*) demonstrate washout within the lesion that also appears more conspicuous at 50 keV images. DECT is also able to provide virtual unenhanced images as well as iodine maps.

Diffuse liver disease

An additional area currently undergoing investigation is the usefulness of dual-energy CT to evaluate for diffuse liver disease, including steatosis and iron deposition. Fat and water behave differently at low and high energies, therefore dual-energy CT vendors can utilize material decomposition algorithm with fat-water pair to quantify hepatic fat content.[66] Additional investigation has also demonstrated that the multimaterial decomposition algorithm used by dual-energy CT correlates with fat content measured using MR imaging.[67]

Liver iron quantification may also be calculated with dual-energy CT. It has been demonstrated that the virtual iron content calculated with dual-energy CT correlated with R2* and MR imaging-measured liver iron content measurements.[68]

As described, dual-energy CT imaging has shown diagnostic value in the assessment of the liver and the gallbladder. The use of low-keV monoenergetic images and iodine density maps improves the conspicuity of liver lesions. Although the assessment of liver lesion characterization, portal vein thrombosis, and evaluation of treatment response of tumors have shown clinical benefits, these continue to remain areas of ongoing research to further determine the clinical benefits.

Gallbladder

Although ultrasound is typically performed in the evaluation of gallstones, dual-energy CT may help to improve the detection of non-radiopaque gallstones on CT examinations performed for alternative indications. The use of low-keV virtual monoenergetic imaging can improve the detection of noncalcified gallstones.[69,70] An experimental model using a cholesterol–bile 2 material decomposition algorithm demonstrated an area under the ROC curve (AUC) of 0.99 for isoattenuating gallstones of all sizes in a phantom model.[71] Additionally, dual-energy CT may also provide guidance into composition of gallstones. A study using a phantom model demonstrated accurate identification of gallstones containing a high percentage of cholesterol and no calcium.[72]

Dual-Energy Computed Tomography of the Pancreas

Solid and cystic neoplasms

Pancreatic ductal adenocarcinoma typically presents a hypoattenuating and infiltrative mass due to the presence of desmoplastic response and fibrosis associated with the tumor. However, approximately 11% of lesions are isoattenuating or small, and therefore pose a diagnostic challenge with dual-phase pancreatic CT protocols.[73,74]

The use of dual-energy CT for evaluation of the pancreas utilizes low-energy monoenergetic images and iodine maps to improve the detection of pancreatic lesions, due to increased CNR.[75] A study by Noda and colleagues assessed 74 patients with pancreatic adenocarcinoma and found that virtual monoenergetic images at 40 keV demonstrated significant increase in signal-to-noise ratio (SNR) of the pancreas, tumor-to-pancreas CNR, and tumor conspicuity, in addition to high reproducibility of measuring tumor size.[76]

Iodine maps also provide high SNR and CNR, resulting in increased conspicuity due to lower attenuation in comparison to normal pancreatic parenchyma and assessment of vascular involvement.[77,78] Furthermore, dual-energy CT may be useful in evaluation of chemotherapeutic response for pancreatic adenocarcinoma.[79] Metal artifact reduction algorithms and monochromatic images at high keV (ie, 140 keV) may also help reduce streak artifact in patients with biliary stents or surgical clips.[80]

Dual-energy CT has also shown improved lesion detection for pancreatic neuroendocrine tumors (**Fig. 3**). A study by Lin and colleagues examined the detection rate of insulinomas using dual-energy CT compared with the conventional dual-phase multidetector CT and demonstrated increase in sensitivity from 69% to 96% using low-keV monoenergetic and iodine images.[81] It has been demonstrated that 55 keV monoenergetic images are preferred by radiologists for detection of neuroendocrine tumors.[82]

Recent studies have shown that dual-energy CT may be useful in further characterization of pancreatic cystic lesions (**Fig. 4**). Chu and colleagues demonstrated that iodine maps were useful in evaluating heterogeneity of cystic masses by enabling differentiation of solid and cystic components.[78] A study by Li and colleagues used iodine quantification technique to differentiate oligocystic serous cystadenomas from mucinous cystic neoplasms, with the latter characterized by higher iodine concentrations.[83]

Further prospective studies are needed to compare dual-energy CT with other modalities including MR imaging and endoscopic ultrasound to understand clinical implications.

Acute pancreatitis

Studies have suggested a higher sensitivity of dual-energy CT in diagnosis of early acute pancreatitis[84] along with diagnosing complications of pancreatitis. For example, using low-keV images allows for improved evaluation of complex

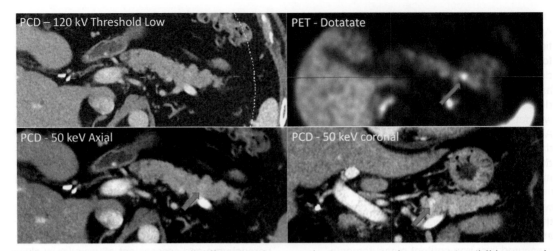

Fig. 3. A 58 year old woman with well-differentiated neuroendocrine tumor in the pancreatic tail (*blue arrows*). Dual-energy CT obtained at 120 kV with 2 mm slice thickness does not clearly demonstrate a lesion within the pancreatic tail. However, dual-energy 50 keV images of the pancreas (axial and coronal) demonstrate a small 7 mm focal area of enhancement, which correlates to known location of neuroendocrine tumor as demonstrated on Dotatate PET/CT.

pancreatic and peripancreatic collections to differentiate between necrotic debris, hematomas, or residual parenchyma with preserved enhancement.[85]

Trauma

Pancreatic trauma is associated with significant morbidity and mortality and pancreatic lacerations may be challenging to diagnose. A study by Sugrue and colleagues showed that low-energy monoenergetic images maximize CNR and increases conspicuity of lacerations to improve diagnostic confidence.[86]

DUAL-ENERGY COMPUTED TOMOGRAPHY OF THE BOWEL

Dual-energy CT-based virtual noncontrast images can replace true noncontrast images, if desired, in gastrointestinal bleeding protocols with multiphase CT and also afford confident determination of enhancement when compared with contrast-enhanced images.[87] Iodine overlay images, which are color iodine maps superimposed on grayscale virtual noncontrast images, provide excellent anatomic detail in addition to iodine visualization. Iodine map and iodine overlay images allow for clear visualization of enhancement or bleeding.[87–89] Finally, virtual monoenergetic images can be created from the source polychromatic dataset. Low-keV virtual monoenergetic images are closer to the k-edge of iodine and consequently increase iodine conspicuity,[89] whereas high-keV reconstructions can be used to overcome metallic streak artifact.[27] The utility of these dual-energy CT reconstructions in the assessment of common bowel disorders including gastrointestinal bleeding, bowel ischemia, Crohn's disease, and bowel neoplasms will be reviewed.

Gastrointestinal Bleeding

The Society of Abdominal Radiology Gastrointestinal Bleeding Disease-Focused Panel suggests a

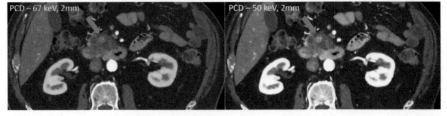

Fig. 4. An 80 year old man underwent surveillance CT for evaluation of intraductal papillary mucinous neoplasm (IPMN). CT obtained at 0.2 cm slices demonstrates a 4.7 × 3.9 × 2.7 cm complex cystic mass, with the 50 keV images best demonstrating nodular enhancement within the mass, consistent with malignant transformation of IPMN.

multiphase CT for overt gastrointestinal bleeding including a true or virtual noncontrast, late arterial phase, and portal venous or late venous phase acquisition.[88,90–92] Replacing the true with virtual noncontrast images derived from either of the other acquisitions can reduce patient radiation exposure by one-third, while still maintaining diagnostic accuracy.[87] An additional benefit of the virtual noncontrast images is that they are derived from the same acquisition as the contrast-enhanced dataset. Consequently, there is no movement of intraluminal material between virtual noncontrast, and postcontrast images as could occur with a separate true noncontrast acquisition due to peristalsis or differences in respiratory motion. Low-keV images can increase the conspicuity of contrast extravasation and areas of enhancement. Additionally, iodine overlay and iodine map images can increase conspicuity of active gastrointestinal bleeding.[93]

Active gastrointestinal bleeding is as hyperattenuating as blood pool in the arterial phase, not visible on virtual noncontrast images, and hyperattenuating in low-keV and iodine map/overlay images (**Figs. 5** and **6**). In addition, active gastrointestinal bleeding often expands or changes shape in the venous phase compared with the arterial acquisition (see **Fig. 6**). Sentinel clot will appear hyperattenuating in the arterial phase, virtual noncontrast, and low-keV images,

but will show lower attenuation than blood pool (see **Fig. 5**). Ingested hyperdense enteric contents will appear hyperattenuating on arterial phase and virtual noncontrast images (see **Fig. 6**).

Ischemic Bowel

Bowel ischemia can result from strangulation in the setting of small bowel obstruction, low-flow ischemia often affecting the descending colon, or thromboembolic disease.[94] Ischemic bowel typically displays symmetric wall thickening with mural edema and adjacent mesenteric fluid.[95,96] Hypoenhancement of the bowel wall is highly specific for bowel ischemia; however, the bowel wall may be hyper- or hypoattenuating.[96] Iodine map or iodine overlay images from dual-energy CT can increase conspicuity of these findings, facilitating confident diagnosis of bowel ischemia (**Fig. 7**), a surgical emergency.

Crohn's Disease

Crohn's disease is an inflammatory bowel disease affecting any portion of the bowel from mouth to anus. As the majority of small bowel is inaccessible by routine endoscopy, cross-sectional imaging, particularly CT enterography, is critical in the assessment of Crohn's disease activity. CT enterography findings of active inflammation include asymmetric wall thickening and hyperenhancement

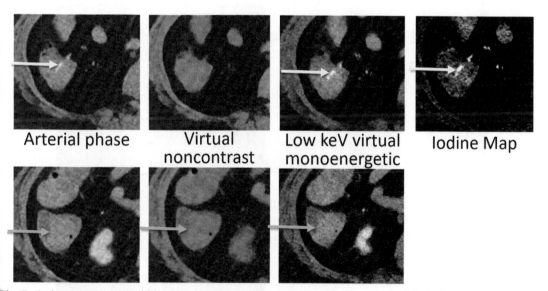

Arterial phase   Virtual noncontrast   Low keV virtual monoenergetic   Iodine Map

Fig. 5. Active gastrointestinal bleeding (*top row*) and sentinel clot (*bottom row*) with dual-energy CT. A linear hyperattenuating focus within the ascending colon (*yellow arrows*) in the arterial phase (*top left*), with high attenuation in the iodine map (*top right*) and low-keV virtual monoenergetic images, but no hyperattenuation on virtual noncontrast images is compatible with active gastrointestinal bleeding (*top row*). An adjacent sentinel clot is hyperattenuating (*blue arrows*), but less bright than blood pool, in arterial phase, virtual noncontrast, and low-keV virtual monoenergetic images (*bottom row*).

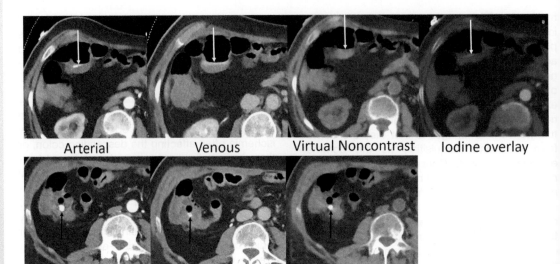

Fig. 6. Active gastrointestinal bleeding (*top row*) and hyperdense enteric contents (*bottom row*) with dual-energy CT. Virtual noncontrast images are derived from the arterial phase. Active gastrointestinal bleeding within the transverse colon (*white arrows*) appears hyperattenuating during the arterial phase, expands during the venous phase, and displays bright color in the arterial-derived iodine overlay image (*top right*). Associated sentinel clot in the virtual noncontrast image (*yellow arrow*) has lower attenuation than the contrast extravasation seen in the arterial phase. Hyperdense enteric contents (*bottom row, black arrows*) show the same hyperattenuation in arterial, venous, and virtual noncontrast images.

affecting the mesenteric more than the antimesenteric border. Additionally, the bowel typically demonstrates mural stratification with a bi- or trilaminar appearance.[97]

Dual-energy CT reconstructions including the iodine map, iodine overlay, or low-keV virtual monoenergetic images can increase the conspicuity of active inflammation[98] (**Fig. 8**). In addition,

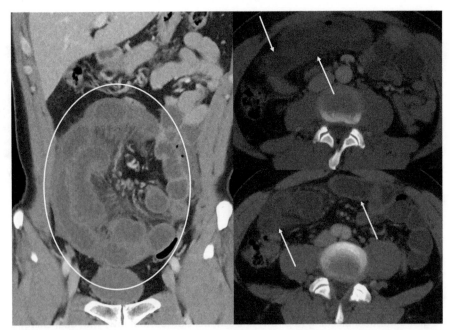

Fig. 7. Small bowel ischemia in 47 year old man presenting with acute abdominal pain. The coronal image from CT with intravenous contrast (*left*) shows dilated, fluid-filled small bowel with symmetric wall thickening, and mesenteric fluid (*oval*). Iodine overlay images (*right*) show hypoenhancement of these small bowel loops (*white arrows*) relative to normal enhancing small bowel in the left upper quadrant (*yellow arrow*). This patient had 50 cm ischemic small bowel due to a closed-loop small bowel obstruction.

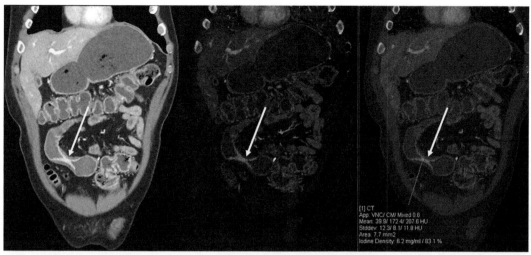

Fig. 8. Crohn's disease active inflammation with dual-energy CT. Coronal image from dual-energy CT enterography (*left*) shows ileal stricture with active inflammation (*white arrows*). Active inflammation is easily visible on iodine map (*center*) and iodine overlay (*right*) images. Region of interest measurements within the hyperdense portion of Crohn's disease affected ileal wall show iodine density of 6.2 mg/mL, 83.1% normalized to the aorta, compatible with active inflammation using previously reported iodine density thresholds.

dual- or multi-energy CT alone allows for the determination of iodine density (mg/mL), which only reflects the iodine content within each voxel. On the other hand, Hounsfield units also incorporate the intrinsic tissue attenuation.[1] Hounsfield units also vary with acquisition potential, injection flow rate, and patient size.[99] Iodine density from dual-energy CT has been shown to be a radiologic marker of Crohn's disease activity.[100–102] A 20% iodine density normalized to aortic enhancement has 100% sensitivity and 92% accuracy for active inflammation compared with histopathologic analysis.[100]

Bowel Neoplasms

Dual-energy CT reconstructions can aid the detection of bowel neoplasms. Low-keV virtual monoenergetic images increase the conspicuity of neoplasms, particularly hypervascular lesions, such as neuroendocrine tumors (**Fig. 9**). Iodine maps and overlay images can also improve detection of hypervascular lesions (see **Fig. 9**). Enhancing masses can be differentiated from hyperdense enteric contents on single-phase contrast-enhanced CT utilizing the virtual noncontrast, iodine overlay, or iodine map images (**Fig. 10**).

DUAL-ENERGY COMPUTED TOMOGRAPHY OF THE PERITONEUM AND OMENTUM

Peritoneal carcinomatosis remains a diagnostic challenge for the radiologist and referring medical and surgical oncologists. While the sensitivity is high for advanced disease, sensitivity for disease measuring 1 cm or less in size is 25% to 50%.[103] Moreover, while CT is the predominant modality used for the screening and surveillance of peritoneal disease due to its widespread use and ability to quickly scan large body regions, its performance is suboptimal compared with PET/CT or MR imaging.[104] In the past decade, there had been substantial improvements in targeted medical therapies for peritoneal disease[105] including cytoreductive surgery combined with hyperthermic intraperitoneal chemotherapy, increasing the importance of detailed anatomic imaging for surgical planning and assessment of treatment response.[106,107]

Peritoneal disease has a wide variety of imaging appearances depending upon the primary neoplasm and can range from large solid masses to small cystic implants, and the visibility of disease on CT depends not only on size, but CT number differences between peritoneal implants and surrounding structures (eg, mesenteric fat, adjacent bowel, stomach, or spleen). Numerous studies, particularly those in body MR imaging, have demonstrated that many non-cystic peritoneal implants are solid and thus show contrast enhancement, particularly if delayed phase images are attained.[108] Consequently, dual-energy CT has been hypothesized as a method to increase the visibility of peritoneal implants owing to its ability to increase iodine signal using low energy virtual monoenergetic and iodine overlay/map images.[109]

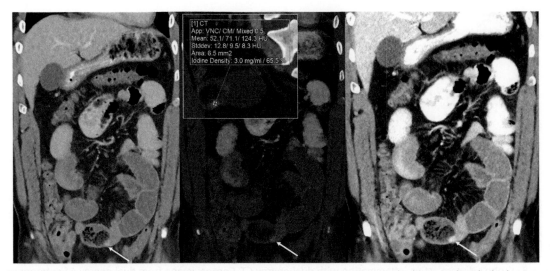

Fig. 9. Small bowel obstruction secondary to neuroendocrine tumor prospectively diagnosed with dual-energy CT. Coronal linear-blended image from CT with intravenous and positive oral contrast (*left*) shows dilated, fluid-filled small bowel, small bowel feces sign, and collapsed distal small bowel compatible with small bowel obstruction. Small enhancing lesion (*white arrows*) within small bowel at the site of transition is more conspicuous on iodine overlay (*center*) and 50 keV virtual monoenergetic images (*right*) than on the conventional reconstruction (*left*).

Dual-energy CT is beneficial in increasing the conspicuity of peritoneal metastases, particularly ovarian cancer.[110–113] A retrospective study of 50 patients with ovarian cancer showed that the mean CNR of peritoneal implants compared with adjacent anatomic surrounding (ie, ascites, bowel, liver, or spleen) was significantly greater for low-energy VMIs compared with routine CT images using filtered back projection, without or with iterative reconstruction[112] (**Fig. 11**). It has also been demonstrated that z-effective color map images, which display the effective atomic number within a pixel, can also be used to distinguish small enhancing peritoneal metastases from small mesenteric lymph nodes.[113] While these studies highlight the potential for dual-energy CT to improve detection of peritoneal metastases, prospective studies documenting improved performance using reference standards are lacking.

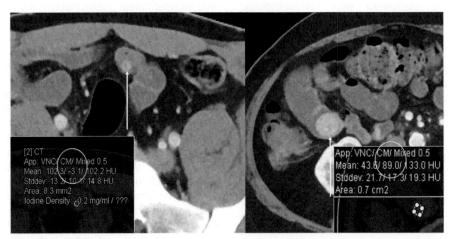

Fig. 10. Differentiation between intraluminal enhancing mass and hyperdense enteric contents on single-phase dual-energy CT enterography. Two axial images from single-phase dual-energy CT enterography examinations in different patients show round hyperdense foci within the small bowel (*arrows*). The focus on the left is nonenhancing by dual-energy analysis, compatible with hyperdense enteric contents. The lesion on the right shows 89 Hounsfield unit enhancement (*white oval*) compatible with an enhancing mass, found to be a breast cancer metastasis.

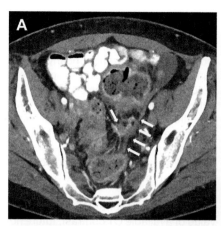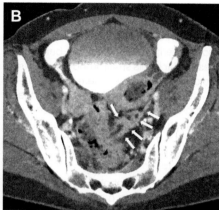

Fig. 11. A 51 year old woman with history of ovarian cancer underwent conventional CT at 100 kV using conventional single-energy CT and 2 mm slices (*A*) compared to same day research dual-energy 50 keV images, also at 2 mm using photon-counting CT (*B*). Note improved visualization of the enhancement, nodularity, and thickening along the anterior peritoneal reflection and sigmoid mesocolon (*arrows*).

Dual-energy CT can also be useful in displaying the internal structure and complexity of primary neoplasms and nodal metastases. It has been demonstrated that internal enhancing components such as thickened septations greater than 3 mm and mural nodules, which are associated with malignancy, are better visualized at low-energy virtual monoenergetic images from dual-energy CT compared with routine CT techniques[111] (**Fig. 12**). Additionally, ovarian low-grade serous carcinoma often contains calcifications from psammoma bodies, and even though these are seen in a minority of patients, calcification can be an important imaging sign suggesting its presence.[110] In this setting, low-energy virtual monoenergetic images can be used to look for enhancing tumor or nodules, and high-energy virtual monoenergetic images and virtual noncontrast images can be used to suppress iodine signal in enhancing structures and oral contrast to visualize tumor-related calcifications. Pan and colleagues examined dual-energy CT in 96 patients undergoing surgical staging for gastric cancer and found that the sensitivity for nodal metastases was improved using VMI images, and that normalized iodine concentrations correlated with tumor type.[114]

Photon-counting CT systems directly convert incident photons to electrical signals, thus offering improved spatial resolution as well as improved iodine signal and VMI images like dual-energy CT.[115] Esquivel and colleagues performed a multi-reader pilot evaluation of 21 patients with known

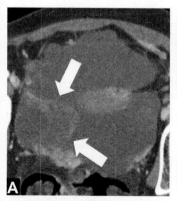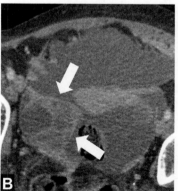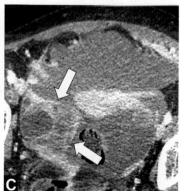

Fig. 12. A 64 year old woman with peritoneal carcinomatosis of unknown primary with bilateral adnexal masses, presumed to be drop metastases (*white arrows*). Conventional portal phase single-energy CT examination at 90 kV using 140 cc of Omnipaque 300 intravenous contrast (*A*) was followed by same-day research CT examination using a prototype photon-counting CT system (*B*) using 50 cc of Ominpaque 300 intravenous contrast, also scanned in the portal phase. Note improved enhancement to the septations of the mass using photon-counting CT at 120 kV, owing to improved signal of low-energy photons, with further increase in visualization of enhancing septations using 50 keV images (*C*) created using photon-counting energy thresholding.

peritoneal disease undergoing conventional, contrast-enhanced abdominopelvic CT followed by same-day photon-counting CT.[116] They found that confidence in peritoneal malignancy between techniques was similar in this small group of patients with advanced disease. However, there was significantly greater estimation of tumor burden about the spleen at photon-counting CT, and that disease visualization on photon-counting CT images likely improved confidence or diagnosis in head-to-head blinded comparisons in the mid-abdomen and pelvis in most cases (**Figs. 13** and **14**).

Although dual-energy and photon-counting CT can increase the conspicuity of peritoneal disease, prospective studies are warranted to demonstrate the accuracy and impact on patient care of routine of dual-energy and photon-counting CT in the imaging of peritoneal disease.

NOVEL CONTRAST AGENTS

Although CT has undergone many hardware and software revolutions, the current CT contrast agents have not changed substantively since before the invention of clinical CT in 1971. As

such, generations of radiologists have come to believe that only iodine and barium contrast agents are useful for CT imaging. Unfortunately, iodine and barium show nearly identical atomic numbers of z = 53 and 56, respectively, and their K-edges are both just below 40 keV. This similarity between iodine and barium means that the CT attenuations of these two classes of contrast agents cannot be reliably differentiated from each other at CT imaging, even with photon-counting CT scanners. We are currently limited to one "color" of contrast, regardless of which agents are used concurrently.

But just as spectral CT greatly increased the value of available CT contrast, future novel generations of non-iodine/non-barium agents promise to augment the capabilities of spectral imaging. Several studies show that spectral CT can accurately distinguish iodine and soft tissues from many compounds containing radiodense high atomic number (high-Z) elements (**Fig. 15A**), including gadolinium, tantalum, hafnium, tungsten, bismuth, ytterbium, gold, and silver. At photon-counting CT, the signal of high-Z elements that have a K-edge well above 40 keV

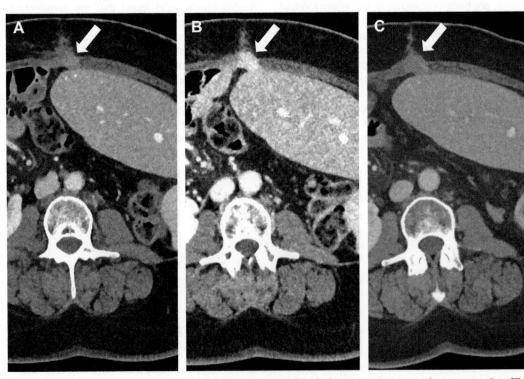

Fig. 13. A 47 year old woman with prior right hepatectomy for cholangiocarcinoma underwent routine CT (*A*) followed by research photon-counting CT examination (*B*) using identical slice thickness of 2 mm. Images show improved enhancement and conspicuity of abdominal wall metastasis extending into the peritoneal cavity adjacent to the liver capsule using 50 keV images (*B*), with the metastasis having greater signal differences compared with the adjacent abdominal wall or liver parenchyma. Subsequent follow-up examination performed 4 months later demonstrated interval growth of the metastasis (*C*).

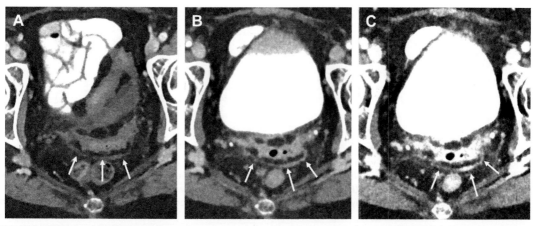

Fig. 14. A 74 year old woman with ovarian cancer underwent conventional CT at 100 kV (*A*) followed by research photon-counting detector (PCD) at 120 kV (*B*) using the same window-level setting (40/400). Note the increased signal and nodularity along the anterior peritoneal reflection at photon-counting CT (*B*). 50 keV images reconstructed from the same PCD-CT dataset shows further increase the conspicuity and signal in the small peritoneal implants along the anterior peritoneal reflection (*C*).

would be even more readily delineated from iodine and soft tissue due to the boost in attenuation of X-rays just above the K-edge (**Fig. 15**B). These high-Z contrast agents are essentially a different "color" than current iodine/barium agents and soft tissues and may be given in different compartments than iodine to obtain multi-color CT scans in a single 10 second pass of a spectral scanner. The intensity of these complementary contrast color pairs (iodine and high-Z agents) can be independently digitally selected using dual-energy CT scans to better deconstruct the anatomy of fine structures.[117–119] An example is that one agent could be given intravenously while the other orally. Alternatively, one agent could be given intravenously during the arterial phase while another in the venous phase for perfectly co-registered assessment of

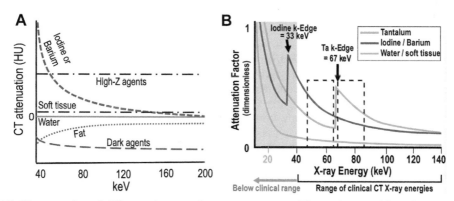

Fig. 15. (*A*) CT attenuation of different tissues and contrast agents at different keVs. Unlike soft tissue and water which have relative constant Hounsfield unit (HU) values across all keVs, current iodine and barium contrast agents show HU values that diminish rapidly with increasing keV reconstructions, and also with increasing kVp settings (not shown). As such, iodine and barium contrasts are less effective in large body parts, such as the obese abdomen, where beam hardening and use of higher kVp imaging commonly occur. On the other hand, novel high-Z contrast agents do not lose substantial CT attenuation even with hardened X-rays/high keV image reconstructions and may provide more vibrant imaging in thick body parts. Also, the difference in X-ray attenuation between high-Z and iodine contrast agents allows them to be readily differentiated from each other at multi-energy CT. (*B*) New contrast agents with high-Z elements, such as tantalum (Ta) will have k-edges well above 40 keV. Photon-counting detector CT energy bins placed just below and just above the high-Z element k-edge should allow for outstanding distinction of Ta signal from both soft tissue and iodine due to the marked increase in X-ray attenuation just above the k-edge than below.

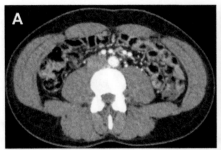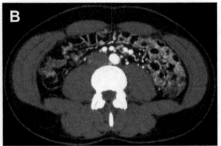

Fig. 16. (*A*) Abdominal spectral CT with IV iodine and oral dark borosilicate contrast material (DBCM) from a clinical phase 2 trial. The bowel lumen is filled material that has lower CT attenuation than fat and soft tissue, allowing for good bowel wall visualization. (*B*) Dual-energy CT color overlay shows the DBCM in purple and IV contrast in orange. These agents may be displayed together, or individually, by spectral image reconstructions.

intestinal anatomy. Although these high-Z agents are not yet in human trials, the promise of complementary color contrast agents is easy to imagine. As an example, if one "color" agent is given orally and the other "color" agent intravenously, then the etiology of extravasated contrast material such as from bowel perforation versus bleeding would be much more easily determined than if current agents were used instead. A preclinical sharp abdomen injury study showed that such scans improved the accuracy of diagnoses for both nonspecialized and specialized radiologists without the need for extensive training on double-color spectral CT interpretation.[120] A concern for the high-Z contrast agents is that, much like for iodine intravenous agents, a large amount (>30 g of the high-Z element) generally needs to be injected[121] for vivid opacification of the vasculature and capillary bed. Injection of such high doses of gadolinium chelate is expensive and raises safety concerns but nevertheless may provide good risk–benefit radio in certain clinical scenarios. Preliminary pre-clinical tests show that high-Z agents may improve the CT signal of contrast agents for thick body parts, such as the abdomen of the obese body habitus.[122] Further study and clinical translation of these agents are warranted.

Another class of spectral CT contrast agents is the dark oral agent that is made of radiolucent low-Z material, such as dark borosilicate contrast material. This class of agent has CT attenuations lower than that of water and may even be lower than that of fat. However, unlike fat, which increases in CT attenuation when imaged with higher energy X-ray spectra, and iodine, which shows marked decrease in CT attenuation with higher energy X-ray spectra, these dark oral agents may show little change in CT attenuation and can be delineated readily at spectral CT (**Fig. 16**). Preliminary studies show that these

agents can reduce CT peristalsis artifact and may improve the detection of bowel and bowel-adjacent disease at conventional CT. These agents may also reduce radiation doses required for CT scans that use automated exposure control. At spectral CT, the CT signal of dark oral contrast agents are readily differentiated from that of iodine agents.

Potentially these different classes of contrast agents may be used concurrently to generate information-rich multicolor contrast-enhanced spectral CT scans. In such spectral CT scans, the signals of the different "colors" of contrast agent can be readily separated by image reconstructions. Separation of the signals of the different color-contrast agents should enable faster and more accurate detection and staging of disease, particularly for intertwined anatomy such as bowel and blood vessels. It is hoped that such data-rich multi-contrast spectral CT scans will also improve the quality of artificial intelligence image reconstructions and image interpretations for a broad range of clinical scenarios.

SUMMARY

Through reconstruction of energy- and material-specific image datasets, dual-energy CT can expand the array of diagnostic tools for the evaluation of gastrointestinal diseases as compared with single-energy CT. The combined use of virtual unenhanced, monochromatic, and iodine overlay/iodine maps allows for improved assessment of a variety of gastrointestinal diseases. Use of virtual unenhanced images can decrease radiation dose in the context of multiphase gastrointestinal CT examinations. Emerging photon-counting CT systems and novel contrast can further expand the role of dual- and multi-energy CT techniques in the assessment of gastrointestinal diseases.

CLINICS CARE POINTS

- Dual-energy CT is beneficial in many clinical applications including detection and characterization of focal lesions as well as additional pathologies involving the liver, gallbladder, and pancreas.

- Use of low-keV virtual monoenergetic images, iodine map, and iodine overlay images allows for assessment of gastrointestinal bleeding, bowel ischemia, Crohn's disease, and bowel neoplasms.

- Photon-counting CT can increase the visibility of peritoneal disease owing to its ability to increase iodine signal.

DISCLOSURE

J.G. Fletcher is the recipient of a research grant to the institution from Siemens Healthcare GmbH, unrelated to this work. The other authors have nothing to disclose.

REFERENCES

1. McCollough CH, Leng S, Yu L, et al. Dual- and Multi-Energy CT: Principles, Technical Approaches, and Clinical Applications. Radiology 2015;276(3): 637–53.
2. Coursey CA, Nelson RC, Boll DT, et al. Dual-energy multidetector CT: how does it work, what can it tell us, and when can we use it in abdominopelvic imaging? Radiographics 2010;30(4):1037–55.
3. Rajiah P, Parakh A, Kay F, et al. Update on Multienergy CT: Physics, Principles, and Applications. Radiographics 2020;40(5):1284–308.
4. Hsieh J, SPIE. Computed tomography: principles, design, artifacts, and recent advances. SPIE; 2009.
5. Kalender WA. Computed tomography: fundamentals, system technology, image quality, applications. John Wiley & Sons; 2011.
6. Alvarez RE, Macovski A. Energy-selective reconstructions in X-ray computerized tomography. Phys Med Biol 1976;21(5):733–44.
7. McCollough CH, Boedeker K, Cody D, et al. Principles and applications of multienergy CT: Report of AAPM Task Group 291. Med Phys 2020;47(7): e881–912.
8. Forghani R, De Man B, Gupta R. Dual-energy computed tomography: physical principles, approaches to scanning, usage, and implementation: part 1. Neuroimaging Clinics 2017;27(3):371–84.
9. Grajo JR, Patino M, Prochowski A, et al. Dual energy CT in practice: basic principles and applications. Appl Radiol 2016;45(7):6–12.
10. Karcaaltincaba M, Aktas A. Dual-energy CT revisited with multidetector CT: review of principles and clinical applications. Diagn Interv Radiol 2011;17(3):181–94.
11. Graser A, Johnson TR, Chandarana H, et al. Dual energy CT: preliminary observations and potential clinical applications in the abdomen. Eur Radiol 2009;19:13–23.
12. Kalender WA, Perman WH, Vetter JR, et al. Evaluation of a prototype dual-energy computed tomographic apparatus. I. Phantom studies. Med Phys 1986;13(3):334–9.
13. Macovski A, Alvarez RE, Chan JL, et al. Energy dependent reconstruction in X-ray computerized tomography. Comput Biol Med 1976;6(4):325–36.
14. Ferda J, Novak M, Mirka H, et al. The assessment of intracranial bleeding with virtual unenhanced imaging by means of dual-energy CT angiography. Eur Radiol 2009;19(10):2518–22.
15. Graser A, Johnson TR, Hecht EM, et al. Dual-energy CT in patients suspected of having renal masses: can virtual nonenhanced images replace true nonenhanced images? Radiology 2009; 252(2):433–40.
16. Takahashi N, Hartman RP, Vrtiska TJ, et al. Dual-energy CT iodine-subtraction virtual unenhanced technique to detect urinary stones in an iodine-filled collecting system: a phantom study (PMC2705667). AJR Am J Roentgenol 2008; 190(5):1169–73.
17. Takahashi N, Vrtiska TJ, Kawashima A, et al. Detectability of urinary stones on virtual nonenhanced images generated at pyelographic-phase dual-energy CT. Radiology 2010;256(1): 184–90.
18. Ho LM, Marin D, Neville AM, et al. Characterization of adrenal nodules with dual-energy CT: can virtual unenhanced attenuation values replace true unenhanced attenuation values? AJR Am J Roentgenol 2012;198(4):840–5.
19. Mangold S, Thomas C, Fenchel M, et al. Virtual nonenhanced dual-energy CT urography with tin-filter technology: determinants of detection of urinary calculi in the renal collecting system. Radiology 2012;264(1):119–25.
20. Pache G, Krauss B, Strohm P, et al. Dual-energy CT virtual noncalcium technique: detecting posttraumatic bone marrow lesions–feasibility study. Radiology 2010;256(2):617–24.
21. Ai S, Qu M, Glazebrook KN, et al. Use of dual-energy CT and virtual non-calcium techniques to evaluate post-traumatic bone bruises in knees in the subacute setting. Skeletal Radiol 2014;43: 1289–95.

22. D'Angelo T, Albrecht MH, Caudo D, et al. Virtual non-calcium dual-energy CT: clinical applications. European radiology experimental 2021;5(1):1–13.

23. Gong H, Baffour FI, Glazebrook KN, et al. Deep learning-based virtual noncalcium imaging in multiple myeloma using dual-energy CT. Med Phys 2022;49(10):6346–58.

24. Mileto A, Nelson RC, Samei E, et al. Impact of dual-energy multi–detector row CT with virtual monochromatic imaging on renal cyst pseudoenhancement: in vitro and in vivo study. Radiology 2014;272(3):767–76.

25. Pomerantz SR, Kamalian S, Zhang D, et al. Virtual monochromatic reconstruction of dual-energy unenhanced head CT at 65-75 keV maximizes image quality compared with conventional polychromatic CT. Radiology 2013;266(1):318–25.

26. Yu L, Christner JA, Leng S, et al. Virtual monochromatic imaging in dual-source dual-energy CT: radiation dose and image quality. Med Phys 2011; 38(12):6371–9.

27. Yu L, Leng S, McCollough CH. Dual-energy CT-based monochromatic imaging. AJR Am J Roentgenol 2012;199(5 Suppl):S9–15.

28. Matsumoto K, Jinzaki M, Tanami Y, et al. Virtual monochromatic spectral imaging with fast kilovoltage switching: improved image quality as compared with that obtained with conventional 120-kVp CT. Radiology 2011;259(1):257–62.

29. Hubbell JH, Seltzer SM. X-Ray Mass Attenuation Coefficients: NIST Standard Reference Database 126. 2004; Available at: https://www.nist.gov/pml/x-ray-mass-attenuation-coefficients.

30. Goodsitt MM, Christodoulou EG, Larson SC. Accuracies of the synthesized monochromatic CT numbers and effective atomic numbers obtained with a rapid kVp switching dual energy CT scanner. Med Phys 2011;38(4):2222–32.

31. Heismann BJ, Leppert J, Stierstorfer K. Density and atomic number measurements with spectral x-ray attenuation method. J Appl Phys 2003; 94(3):2073–9.

32. Primak AN, Fletcher JG, Vrtiska TJ, et al. Noninvasive differentiation of uric acid versus non-uric acid kidney stones using dual-energy CT. Acad Radiol 2007;14(12):1441–7.

33. Primak AN, Ramirez Giraldo JC, Liu X, et al. Improved dual-energy material discrimination for dual-source CT by means of additional spectral filtration. Med Phys 2009;36(4):1359–69.

34. Glazebrook KN, Guimaraes LS, Murthy NS, et al. Identification of intraarticular and periarticular uric acid crystals with dual-energy CT: initial evaluation. Radiology 2011;261(2):516–24.

35. Qu M, Ramirez-Giraldo JC, Leng S, et al. Dual-energy dual-source CT with additional spectral filtration can improve the differentiation of non-uric acid renal stones: an ex vivo phantom study. AJR Am J Roentgenol 2011;196(6):1279–87.

36. Boll DT, Patil NA, Paulson EK, et al. Renal stone assessment with dual-energy multidetector CT and advanced postprocessing techniques: improved characterization of renal stone composition–pilot study. Radiology 2009;250(3):813–20.

37. Wichmann JL, Hardie AD, Schoepf UJ, et al. Single-and dual-energy CT of the abdomen: comparison of radiation dose and image quality of 2nd and 3rd generation dual-source CT. Eur Radiol 2017;27: 642–50.

38. Uhrig M, Simons D, Kachelrieß M, et al. Advanced abdominal imaging with dual energy CT is feasible without increasing radiation dose. Cancer Imag 2016;16:1–8.

39. Leng S, Yu L, Wang J, et al. Noise reduction in spectral CT: reducing dose and breaking the trade-off between image noise and energy bin selection. Med Phys 2011;38(9):4946–57.

40. Leng S, Yu L, Fletcher JG, et al. Maximizing iodine contrast-to-noise ratios in abdominal CT imaging through use of energy domain noise reduction and virtual monoenergetic dual-energy CT. Radiology 2015;276(2):562–70.

41. Tao S, Rajendran K, McCollough CH, et al. Material decomposition with prior knowledge aware iterative denoising (MD-PKAID). Phys Med Biol 2018; 63(19):195003.

42. Tao S, Rajendran K, Zhou W, et al. Improving iodine contrast to noise ratio using virtual monoenergetic imaging and prior-knowledge-aware iterative denoising (mono-PKAID). Phys Med Biol 2019; 64(10):105014.

43. Tao S, Rajendran K, Zhou W, et al. Noise reduction in CT image using prior knowledge aware iterative denoising. Phys Med Biol 2020;65(22):225032.

44. Leng S, Bruesewitz M, Tao S, et al. Photon-counting detector CT: system design and clinical applications of an emerging technology. Radiographics 2019;39(3):729–43.

45. Flohr T, Petersilka M, Henning A, et al. Photon-counting CT review. Phys Med 2020;79:126–36.

46. Willemink MJ, Persson M, Pourmorteza A, et al. Photon-counting CT: technical principles and clinical prospects. Radiology 2018;289(2):293–312.

47. Taguchi K, Iwanczyk JS. Vision 20/20: Single photon counting x-ray detectors in medical imaging. Med Phys 2013;40(10):100901.

48. Rajendran K, Petersilka M, Henning A, et al. First clinical photon-counting detector CT system: technical evaluation. Radiology 2022;303(1):130–8.

49. Zhou W, Lane JI, Carlson ML, et al. Comparison of a photon-counting-detector CT with an energy-integrating-detector CT for temporal bone imaging: a cadaveric study. Am J Neuroradiol 2018;39(9): 1733–8.

50. Leng S, Rajendran K, Gong H, et al. 150-μm spatial resolution using photon-counting detector computed tomography technology: technical performance and first patient images. Invest Radiol 2018;53(11):655–62.

51. Leng S, Yu Z, Halaweish A, et al. Dose-efficient ultrahigh-resolution scan mode using a photon counting detector computed tomography system. J Med Imag 2016;3(4):043504.

52. Zhou W, Bartlett DJ, Diehn FE, et al. Reduction of metal artifacts and improvement in dose efficiency using photon counting detector CT and tin filtration. Invest Radiol 2019;54(4):204.

53. Patel BN, Rosenberg M, Vernuccio F, et al. Characterization of Small Incidental Indeterminate Hypoattenuating Hepatic Lesions: Added Value of Single-Phase Contrast-Enhanced Dual-Energy CT Material Attenuation Analysis. AJR Am J Roentgenol 2018;211(3):571–9.

54. Shuman WP, Green DE, Busey JM, et al. Dual-energy liver CT: effect of monochromatic imaging on lesion detection, conspicuity, and contrast-to-noise ratio of hypervascular lesions on late arterial phase. AJR Am J Roentgenol 2014;203(3):601–6.

55. Hanson GJ, Michalak GJ, Childs R, et al. Low kV versus dual-energy virtual monoenergetic CT imaging for proven liver lesions: what are the advantages and trade-offs in conspicuity and image quality? A pilot study. Abdom Radiol (NY) 2018; 43(6):1404 12.

56. Manjunatha HC, Rudraswamy B. Study of effective atomic number and electron density for tissues from human organs in the energy range of 1 keV-100 GeV. Health Phys 2013;104(2):158–62.

57. Mileto A, Nelson RC, Samei E, et al. Dual-energy MDCT in hypervascular liver tumors: effect of body size on selection of the optimal monochromatic energy level. AJR Am J Roentgenol 2014; 203(6):1257–64.

58. Marin D, Ramirez-Giraldo JC, Gupta S, et al. Effect of a Noise-Optimized Second-Generation Monoenergetic Algorithm on Image Noise and Conspicuity of Hypervascular Liver Tumors: An In Vitro and In Vivo Study. AJR Am J Roentgenol 2016; 206(6):1222–32.

59. Chernyak V, Fowler KJ, Kamaya A, et al. Liver Imaging Reporting and Data System (LI-RADS) Version 2018: Imaging of Hepatocellular Carcinoma in At-Risk Patients. Radiology 2018;289(3):816–30.

60. Voss BA, Khandelwal A, Wells ML, et al. Impact of dual-energy 50-keV virtual monoenergetic images on radiologist confidence in detection of key imaging findings of small hepatocellular carcinomas using multiphase liver CT. Acta Radiol 2022;63(11): 1443–52.

61. Caruso D, De Cecco CN, Schoepf UJ, et al. Can dual-energy computed tomography improve visualization of hypoenhancing liver lesions in portal venous phase? Assessment of advanced image-based virtual monoenergetic images. Clin Imag 2017;41:118–24.

62. Ascenti G, Sofia C, Mazziotti S, et al. Dual-energy CT with iodine quantification in distinguishing between bland and neoplastic portal vein thrombosis in patients with hepatocellular carcinoma. Clin Radiol 2016;71(9). 938.e931-939.

63. Qian LJ, Zhu J, Zhuang ZG, et al. Differentiation of neoplastic from bland macroscopic portal vein thrombi using dual-energy spectral CT imaging: a pilot study. Eur Radiol 2012;22(10):2178–85.

64. Dai X, Schlemmer HP, Schmidt B, et al. Quantitative therapy response assessment by volumetric iodine-uptake measurement: initial experience in patients with advanced hepatocellular carcinoma treated with sorafenib. Eur J Radiol 2013;82(2): 327–34.

65. Lee SH, Lee JM, Kim KW, et al. Dual-energy computed tomography to assess tumor response to hepatic radiofrequency ablation: potential diagnostic value of virtual noncontrast images and iodine maps. Invest Radiol 2011;46(2):77–84.

66. Patel BN, Kumbla RA, Berland LL, et al. Material density hepatic steatosis quantification on intravenous contrast-enhanced rapid kilovolt (peak)-switching single-source dual-energy computed tomography. J Comput Assist Tomogr 2013;37(6): 904–10.

67. Hyodo T, Yada N, Hori M, et al. Multimaterial Decomposition Algorithm for the Quantification of Liver Fat Content by Using Fast-Kilovolt-Peak Switching Dual-Energy CT: Clinical Evaluation. Radiology 2017;283(1):108–18.

68. Luo XF, Xie XQ, Cheng S, et al. Dual-Energy CT for Patients Suspected of Having Liver Iron Overload: Can Virtual Iron Content Imaging Accurately Quantify Liver Iron Content? Radiology 2015;277(1): 95–103.

69. Lee HA, Lee YH, Yoon KH, et al. Comparison of Virtual Unenhanced Images Derived From Dual-Energy CT With True Unenhanced Images in Evaluation of Gallstone Disease. AJR Am J Roentgenol 2016;206(1):74–80.

70. Uyeda JW, Richardson IJ, Sodickson AD. Making the invisible visible: improving conspicuity of non-calcified gallstones using dual-energy CT. Abdom Radiol (NY) 2017;42(12):2933–9.

71. Soesbe TC, Lewis MA, Xi Y, et al. A Technique to Identify Isoattenuating Gallstones with Dual-Layer Spectral CT: An ex Vivo Phantom Study. Radiology 2019;292(2):400–6.

72. Bauer RW, Schulz JR, Zedler B, et al. Compound analysis of gallstones using dual energy computed tomography–results in a phantom model. Eur J Radiol 2010;75(1):e74–80.

73. Lee ES, Lee JM. Imaging diagnosis of pancreatic cancer: a state-of-the-art review. World J Gastroenterol 2014;20(24):7864–77.

74. Prokesch RW, Chow LC, Beaulieu CF, et al. Isoattenuating pancreatic adenocarcinoma at multidetector row CT: secondary signs. Radiology 2002;224(3):764–8.

75. Macari M, Spieler B, Kim D, et al. Dual-source dual-energy MDCT of pancreatic adenocarcinoma: initial observations with data generated at 80 kVp and at simulated weighted-average 120 kVp. AJR Am J Roentgenol 2010;194(1):W27–32.

76. Noda Y, Goshima S, Kaga T, et al. Virtual monochromatic image at lower energy level for assessing pancreatic ductal adenocarcinoma in fast kV-switching dual-energy CT. Clin Radiol 2020; 75(4):320.e317–23.

77. Bhosale P, Le O, Balachandran A, et al. Quantitative and Qualitative Comparison of Single-Source Dual-Energy Computed Tomography and 120-kVp Computed Tomography for the Assessment of Pancreatic Ductal Adenocarcinoma. J Comput Assist Tomogr 2015;39(6):907–13.

78. Chu AJ, Lee JM, Lee YJ, et al. Dual-source, dual-energy multidetector CT for the evaluation of pancreatic tumours. Br J Radiol 2012;85(1018):e891–8.

79. Noda Y, Goshima S, Miyoshi T, et al. Assessing Chemotherapeutic Response in Pancreatic Ductal Adenocarcinoma: Histogram Analysis of Iodine Concentration and CT Number in Single-Source Dual-Energy CT. AJR Am J Roentgenol 2018;211(6):1221–6.

80. Pessis E, Campagna R, Sverzut JM, et al. Virtual monochromatic spectral imaging with fast kilovoltage switching: reduction of metal artifacts at CT. Radiographics 2013;33(2):573–83.

81. Lin XZ, Wu ZY, Tao R, et al. Dual energy spectral CT imaging of insulinoma-Value in preoperative diagnosis compared with conventional multidetector CT. Eur J Radiol 2012;81(10):2487–94.

82. Hardie AD, Picard MM, Camp ER, et al. Application of an Advanced Image-Based Virtual Monoenergetic Reconstruction of Dual Source Dual-Energy CT Data at Low keV Increases Image Quality for Routine Pancreas Imaging. J Comput Assist Tomogr 2015;39(5):716–20.

83. Li C, Lin X, Hui C, et al. Computer-Aided Diagnosis for Distinguishing Pancreatic Mucinous Cystic Neoplasms From Serous Oligocystic Adenomas in Spectral CT Images. Technol Cancer Res Treat 2016;15(1):44–54.

84. Martin SS, Trapp F, Wichmann JL, et al. Dual-energy CT in early acute pancreatitis: improved detection using iodine quantification. Eur Radiol 2019;29(5):2226–32.

85. Murray N, Darras KE, Walstra FE, et al. Dual-Energy CT in Evaluation of the Acute Abdomen. Radiographics 2019;39(1):264–86.

86. Sugrue G, Walsh JP, Zhang Y, et al. Virtual monochromatic reconstructions of dual energy CT in abdominal trauma: optimization of energy level improves pancreas laceration conspicuity and diagnostic confidence. Emerg Radiol 2021;28(1):1–7.

87. Sun H, Hou XY, Xue HD, et al. Dual-source dual-energy CT angiography with virtual non-enhanced images and iodine map for active gastrointestinal bleeding: image quality, radiation dose and diagnostic performance. Eur J Radiol 2015;84(5):884–91.

88. Guglielmo FF, Wells ML, Bruining DH, et al. Gastrointestinal Bleeding at CT Angiography and CT Enterography: Imaging Atlas and Glossary of Terms. Radiographics 2021;41(6):1632–56.

89. Trabzonlu TA, Mozaffary A, Kim D, et al. Dual-energy CT evaluation of gastrointestinal bleeding. Abdom Radiol (NY) 2020;45(1):1–14.

90. Fidler JL, Gunn ML, Soto JA, et al. Society of abdominal radiology gastrointestinal bleeding disease-focused panel consensus recommendations for CTA technical parameters in the evaluation of acute overt gastrointestinal bleeding. Abdom Radiol (NY) 2019;44(9):2957–62.

91. Wells ML, Hansel SL, Bruining DH, et al. CT for Evaluation of Acute Gastrointestinal Bleeding. Radiographics 2018;38(4):1089–107.

92. Soto JA, Park SH, Fletcher JG, et al. Gastrointestinal hemorrhage: evaluation with MDCT. Abdom Imag 2015;40(5):993–1009.

93. Shaqdan KW, Parakh A, Kambadakone AR, et al. Role of dual energy CT to improve diagnosis of non-traumatic abdominal vascular emergencies. Abdom Radiol (NY) 2019;44(2):406–21.

94. Fulwadhva UP, Wortman JR, Sodickson AD. Use of Dual-Energy CT and Iodine Maps in Evaluation of Bowel Disease. Radiographics 2016;36(2):393–406.

95. Barmase M, Kang M, Wig J, et al. Role of multidetector CT angiography in the evaluation of suspected mesenteric ischemia. Eur J Radiol 2011;80(3):e582–7.

96. Fernandes T, Oliveira MI, Castro R, et al. Bowel wall thickening at CT: simplifying the diagnosis. Insights Imaging 2014;5(2):195–208.

97. Bruining DH, Zimmermann EM, Loftus EV Jr, et al. Consensus Recommendations for Evaluation, Interpretation, and Utilization of Computed Tomography and Magnetic Resonance Enterography in Patients With Small Bowel Crohn's Disease. Radiology 2018;286(3):776–99.

98. Dua A, Sharma V, Gupta P. Dual energy computed tomography in Crohn's disease: a targeted review. Expert Rev Gastroenterol Hepatol 2022;16(8):699–705.

99. Li Y, Li Y, Jackson A, et al. Comparison of virtual unenhanced CT images of the abdomen under

different iodine flow rates. Abdom Radiol (NY) 2017;42(1):312–21.

100. Dane B, Sarkar S, Nazarian M, et al. Crohn Disease Active Inflammation Assessment with Iodine Density from Dual-Energy CT Enterography: Comparison with Histopathologic Analysis. Radiology 2021;301(1):144–51.

101. Dane B, Duenas S, Han J, et al. Crohn's Disease Activity Quantified by Iodine Density Obtained From Dual-Energy Computed Tomography Enterography. J Comput Assist Tomogr 2020;44(2): 242–7.

102. Dane B, Kernizan A, O'Donnell T, et al. Crohn's disease active inflammation assessment with iodine density from dual-energy CT enterography: comparison with endoscopy and conventional interpretation. Abdom Radiol (NY) 2022;47(10):3406–13.

103. Coakley FV, Choi PH, Gougoutas CA, et al. Peritoneal metastases: detection with spiral CT in patients with ovarian cancer. Radiology 2002;223(2): 495–9.

104. van 't Sant I, Engbersen MP, Bhairosing PA, et al. Diagnostic performance of imaging for the detection of peritoneal metastases: a meta-analysis. Eur Radiol 2020;30(6):3101–12.

105. Lheureux S, Braunstein M, Oza AM. Epithelial ovarian cancer: Evolution of management in the era of precision medicine. CA Cancer J Clin 2019;69(4):280–304.

106. Bartlett DJ, Thacker PG Jr, Grotz TE, et al. Mucinous appendiceal neoplasms: classification, imaging, and HIPEC. Abdom Radiol (NY) 2019; 44(5):1686–702.

107. Nougaret S, Addley HC, Colombo PE, et al. Ovarian carcinomatosis: how the radiologist can help plan the surgical approach. Radiographics 2012;32(6):1775–800 [discussion: 1800-1773].

108. Low RN, Sigeti JS. MR imaging of peritoneal disease: comparison of contrast-enhanced fast multiplanar spoiled gradient-recalled and spin-echo imaging. AJR Am J Roentgenol 1994;163(5): 1131–40.

109. Agrawal MD, Pinho DF, Kulkarni NM, et al. Oncologic applications of dual-energy CT in the abdomen. Radiographics 2014;34(3):589–612.

110. Amante S, Santos F, Cunha TM. Low-grade serous epithelial ovarian cancer: a comprehensive review and update for radiologists. Insights Imaging 2021;12(1):60.

111. Benveniste AP, de Castro Faria S, Broering G, et al. Potential Application of Dual-Energy CT in Gynecologic Cancer: Initial Experience. AJR Am J Roentgenol 2017;208(3):695–705.

112. Kim TM, Kim SY, Cho JY, et al. Utilization of virtual low-keV monoenergetic images generated using dual-layer spectral detector computed tomography for the assessment of peritoneal seeding from ovarian cancer. Medicine (Baltim) 2020;99(23): e20444.

113. Zorzetto G, Coppola A, Molinelli V, et al. Spectral CT in peritoneal carcinomatosis from ovarian cancer: a tool for differential diagnosis of small nodules? Eur Radiol Exp 2022;6(1):45.

114. Pan Z, Pang L, Ding B, et al. Gastric cancer staging with dual energy spectral CT imaging. PLoS One 2013;8(2):e53651.

115. Esquivel A, Ferrero A, Mileto A, et al. Photon-Counting Detector CT: Key Points Radiologists Should Know. Korean J Radiol 2022;23(9):854–65.

116. Esquivel A, Inoue A, Takahashi H, et al. Head-to-head comparison of photon-counting and conventional CT in patients with peritoneal disease. 108th Scientific Assembly and Annual Meeting of the Radiological Society of North America. Chicago, IL: RSNA; 2022.

117. Cormode DP, Si-Mohamed S, Bar-Ness D, et al. Multicolor spectral photon-counting computed tomography: in vivo dual contrast imaging with a high count rate scanner. Sci Rep 2017;7(1):4784.

118. Soesbe TC, Lewis MA, Nasr K, et al. Separating High-Z Oral Contrast From Intravascular Iodine Contrast in an Animal Model Using Dual-Layer Spectral CT. Acad Radiol 2019;26(9):1237–44.

119. Yeh BM, FitzGerald PF, Edic PM, et al. Opportunities for new CT contrast agents to maximize the diagnostic potential of emerging spectral CT technologies. Adv Drug Deliv Rev 2017;113:201–22

120. Mongan J, Rathnayake S, Fu Y, et al. Extravasated contrast material in penetrating abdominopelvic trauma: dual-contrast dual-energy CT for improved diagnosis–preliminary results in an animal model. Radiology 2013;268(3):738–42.

121. Mongan J, Rathnayake S, Fu Y, et al. In vivo differentiation of complementary contrast media at dual-energy CT. Radiology 2012;265(1):267–72.

122. Lambert JW, Sun Y, Stillson C, et al. An Intravascular Tantalum Oxide-based CT Contrast Agent: Preclinical Evaluation Emulating Overweight and Obese Patient Size. Radiology 2018;289(1): 103–10.

Dual-Energy Computed Tomography Applications in the Genitourinary Tract

Mayur K. Virarkar, MD[a], Achille Mileto, MD[b],
Sai Swarupa R. Vulasala, MD[c],*, Lakshmi Ananthakrishnan, MD[d],
Priya Bhosale, MD[e]

KEYWORDS

- DECT • Genitourinary tract • Renal stone • Trauma • Incidentaloma

KEY POINTS

- DECT can differentiate the uric acid from non-uric acid renal calculi.
- DECT characterizes the incidentaloma and is cost- effective than multiphasic CT or MRI.
- DECT has an advantage of minimizing the radiation dose by eliminating the need for true nonenhnaced images.

INTRODUCTION

Material differentiation based on conventional single-energy CT (SECT) is solely based on X-ray attenuation measured in Hounsfield units (HUs), which is an arbitrary unit using the attenuation of water as a benchmark.[1] Two materials with similar attenuation coefficients (eg, iodine and calcium) may display similar HUs, even though they have different elemental compositions and mass-attenuation coefficients.[2] This limitation can be overcome by imaging tissues using 2 different X-ray energy levels—an imaging concept that is referred to as *dual-energy CT* (DECT). The basic principle of DECT heavily relies on leveraging the photoelectric interactions of materials with high atomic numbers and electron density, such as iodine, calcium, or iron.[3] Materials attenuate the X-ray beam to a greater extent when the energy of an incident photon is close to the K-edge value of that given atom. The K-edge value increases with higher atomic number values, and DECT uses this feature to differentiate the components of the matter based on different attenuation achievable at high-energy and low-energy levels—usually 140 and 80 kV, respectively.[2] Based on the unique K-edge values of the tissues, DECT can perform material decomposition by creating material-specific (ie, virtual unenhanced images [VUEs], iodine maps, and effective atomic number images) and energy-specific images (eg, virtual monoenergetic images). At the time of this writing, there are 6 DECT scanner implementations available on the imaging market, including dual-source DECT (ds-DECT), rapid kilovoltage switching DECT (rs-DECT), rapid kilovoltage switching DECT with deep learning (rsdl-DECT), dual-layer DECT (dl-DECT), split-filter DECT (sf-DECT), and rotate-rotate DECT (rr-DECT) (**Fig. 1**).

Each DECT system has different technical specifications, with some differences in utilization mostly based on the patient's weight or circumference.[2] For instance, the ds-DECT system has coverage limitations due to the smaller field-of-view

[a] Department of Radiology, University of Florida College of Medicine, Clinical Center, C90, 2nd Floor, 655 West 8th Street, Jacksonville, FL 32209, USA; [b] Department of Radiology, Mayo Clinic, Mayo Building West, 2nd Floor, 200 First Street SW, Rochester, MN, 55905, USA; [c] Department of radiology, University of Florida College of Medicine, Clinical Center, C90, 2nd Floor, 655 West 8th Street, Jacksonville, FL, 32209, USA; [d] Department of Radiology, UT Southwestern Medical Center, 5323 Harry Hines Boulevard, Dallas, TX 75390, USA; [e] Department of Diagnostic Radiology, Division of Diagnostic Imaging, The University of Texas MD Anderson Cancer Center, 1515 Holcombe Boulevard, Unit 1479, Houston, TX 77030, USA
* Corresponding author.
E-mail address: vulasalaswarupa@gmail.com

Radiol Clin N Am 61 (2023) 1051–1068
https://doi.org/10.1016/j.rcl.2023.05.007

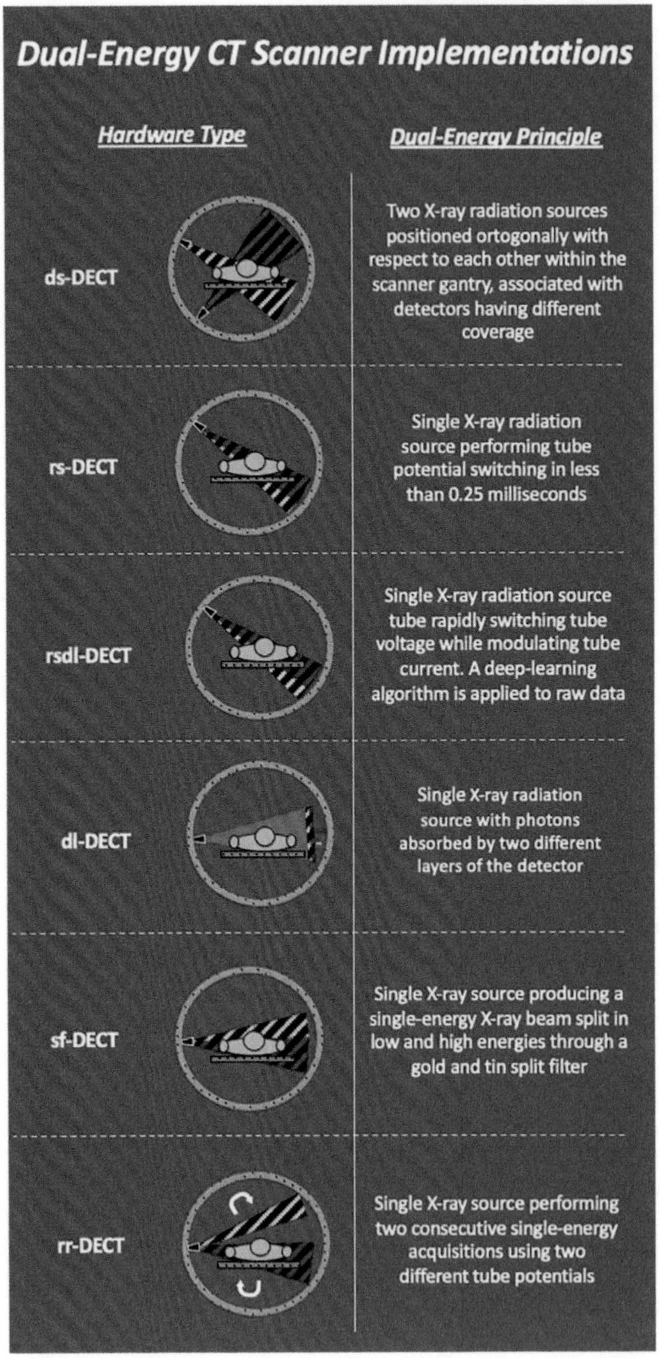

Dual-Energy CT Scanner Implementations

Hardware Type	Dual-Energy Principle
ds-DECT	Two X-ray radiation sources positioned ortogonally with respect to each other within the scanner gantry, associated with detectors having different coverage
rs-DECT	Single X-ray radiation source performing tube potential switching in less than 0.25 milliseconds
rsdl-DECT	Single X-ray radiation source tube rapidly switching tube voltage while modulating tube current. A deep-learning algorithm is applied to raw data
dl-DECT	Single X-ray radiation source with photons absorbed by two different layers of the detector
sf-DECT	Single X-ray source producing a single-energy X-ray beam split in low and high energies through a gold and tin split filter
rr-DECT	Single X-ray source performing two consecutive single-energy acquisitions using two different tube potentials

Fig. 1. Commercially available DECT scanner implementations with dual-energy acquisition principles. ds-DECT, dual-source dual-energy CT; rs-DECT, rapid kilovoltage switching dual-energy CT; rsdl-DECT, rapid kilovoltage switching dual-energy CT with deep learning; dl-DECT, dual layer dual-energy CT; sf-DECT, split-filter dual-energy CT; rr-DECT, rotate-rotate dual-energy CT.

determined by a 36-cm detector; however, this system enables tube current modulation operated in dual-energy mode, and the tube voltage of the low and high energy X-ray tubes (scanning pair) can be changed.[2] Of note, higher scanning pairs (ie, 150/90 kV, usually with tin filtration) can be selected to improve photon penetration when scanning patients weighing more than 260 lbs (117 Kg). On the contrary, the rs-DECT is equipped with a full 50-cm field-of-view resulting in no coverage limitations. However, this implementation does not allow tube current or dual-energy scanning pair variation when scanning in dual-energy mode, which is the reason why it is recommended to image patients weighing more than 260 lbs using the single-energy mode with this system.[2] The rsdl-DECT has similar hardware features as the rs-DECT, with the addition of spectral analysis enabled by deep learning reconstruction applied to raw data. This system also allows for tube current modulation. The dl-DECT has virtually no coverage or patient weight limitations; however, its degree of spectral separation is lower than either ds-DECT or rs-DECT systems. Because of the use of a gold and tin split filter, the sf-DECT system has a lower degree of spectral separation between the 2 energy spectra.[2] The rr-DECT scanners use 2 consecutive single-energy scans at 2 different tube potential values (ie, 130–140 kV and 80 kV); however, this implementation type is limited by spatial and temporal misregistration.[2]

By implementing material-specific and energy-specific postprocessing techniques, DECT can provide a noninvasive characterization of renal stones and render expanded ability for characterization of incidental lesions that would otherwise remain incompletely characterized based on a routine SECT examination. In addition, the synthesis of VUEs using DECT enables one to eliminate the acquisition of true nonenhanced images, thus potentially decreasing radiation doses during multiphasic genitourinary computed tomography (CT) examination protocols.[4,5] Herein, we review the diagnostic use of DECT in the assessment of genitourinary diseases, with emphasis on its role in renal stone characterization, incidental renal and adrenal lesion characterization, retroperitoneal trauma, radiation dose and contrast media dose reduction and cost-effectiveness potential. We also discuss future perspectives of the DECT scanning mode, including the use of novel contrast injection strategies and photon-counting detector CT.

DUAL-ENERGY COMPUTED TOMOGRAPHY: RADIATION DOSE REDUCTION AND COST EFFECTIVENESS

DECT can be incorporated in the setting of genitourinary protocols in different ways. A basic requirement for seamless incorporation of DECT in daily radiology practice is radiation dose neutrality of modern DECT scanners and acquisition modes. Most DECT systems are fully radiation dose neutral at the time of this writing; most clinical scans in dual-energy mode deliver the same radiation dose as the equivalent SECT clinical protocols. DECT can be incorporated during any study phase of a given clinical protocol. However, accumulating evidence has shown that if DECT is used in one phase of a multiphase protocol, the nephrographic (multiphasic renal CT) or venous (ie, adrenal CT protocol) phases yield diagnostic-quality

material decomposition with the synthesis of optimal-quality VUE images and iodine maps. DECT clinical protocols have yielded radiation dose reductions of 30% to 50% for multiphasic protocols, respectively when true unenhanced (TUE) images are omitted.[6]

Growing evidence suggests the diagnostic value and cost-effectiveness of single-phase DECT examinations incorporating multiple postprocessing techniques in comparison with multiphasic CT or MR for abdominal incidentaloma characterization. Multiple studies indicate that single-phase DECT may be more cost-effective for the evaluation of small incidental renal lesions as compared with traditional multiphasic CT or MR.[7–10] In particular, cost-effectiveness analysis, clinical-based and payer-based analysis, as well as impact analysis studies have highlighted that DECT has lower costs per patient than traditional multiphasic approaches, while also providing higher diagnostic effectiveness, including the decreased need for additional imaging or follow-up after an incidental renal lesion is discovered on the initial index DECT examination.[7,8]

DUAL-ENERGY COMPUTED TOMOGRAPHY: UROLITHIASIS

Urolithiasis is one of the most common causes of acute and recurrent flank pain in men aged 20 to 30 years.[11] It affects 12% to 14% of men and 6% of women during their lifetime, with a high recurrence rate of 50% to 75% in 5 to 20 years.[12] An unenhanced SECT acquisition is the clinical standard of care for the evaluation of patients with urolithiasis, with sensitivity and specificity in the range of 95% to 98% and 96% to 100%, respectively.[12]

Renal stones are usually composed of calcium oxalate, calcium phosphate, or uric acid (UA), observed in 70%, 20%, or 8% of cases, respectively.[13] In addition to the identification and localization of urolithiasis, the knowledge of stone composition can be factored for subsequent treatment. In particular, UA stones can be managed conservatively using medical therapy with a success rate of 70% to 80%,[14] whereas struvite stones require extracorporeal shockwave lithotripsy. Cystine and calcium stones are usually treated with percutaneous lithotripsy or ureteroscopic removal. SECT has shown the potential to reliably differentiate among different renal stone types in phantom studies.[12,15,16] Of note, UA stones have been shown to attenuate a polychromatic X-ray beam, usually in the 200 to 400 HU range, whereas calcium oxalate stones attenuate in the range of 600 to 1200 HU. However, SECT has notable limitations for renal stone differentiation in patients due to considerable overlap in HU values.[12,15,16]

DECT has a unique ability to noninvasively differentiate UA from non-UA stones. Sensitivity, specificity, positive predictive value, and negative predictive value of SECT and DECT in differentiating UA from non-UA stones have been demonstrated to be 94%, 72%, 64%, 96% versus 100%, 94%, 100%, and 96%, respectively.[11] DECT evaluation for urolithiasis can be performed with an acquisition in the DE mode for the entire urinary system (ie, from the top of the kidneys to the urinary bladder).[17] Alternatively, after acquiring a low-dose unenhanced SECT of the abdomen and pelvis, a small field-of-view DECT acquisition targeted to the location of the stone of interest can be performed to minimize radiation exposure. Of note, the latter approach can yield an effective radiation dose in the range of 3.4 to 5.3 mSv.[18] Radiation exposure to patients can be further optimized with many DECT systems by modulation of the tube current.[19]

Following image acquisition, postprocessing can be performed using either 2-material or 3-material decomposition algorithms depending on the type of DECT technology. Using ds-DECT systems, images are reconstructed using a 3-material decomposition algorithm to analyze the stone composition and display their composition on color-coded material-specific images. Of note, the DECT attenuation index is calculated from the image data. The DECT attenuation index is the ratio of CT numbers on low-energy and high-energy images and is determined by the spectral separation and difference in atomic numbers. The atomic numbers of UA stones are in a narrow range (6.84–7.01), whereas those of non-UA stones are in a wider range (10.78–15.56). This difference enables DECT to distinguish between UA and non-UA stones. The DECT attenuation indices of UA, cystine, and calcium oxalate/phosphate stones are approximately less than 1.13, 1.13 to 1.24, and greater than 1.24, respectively,[20] resulting in sensitivity and specificity of 100% and 94%, respectively, in identifying UA stones and an accuracy of 94% in differentiating UA and non-UA stones.[11,21] The addition of a tin filter to the high-energy spectra may allow the subcategorization of non-UA stones based on their DECT attenuation indices.[22] Once the DECT attenuation index of a given renal stone is mathematically computed by the postprocessing software, renal stones are color-coded as red or blue using the ds-DECT implementation, depending if the composition is UA or non-UA (Figs. 2 and 3), respectively.[23] The rs-DECT and dl-DECT systems use 2-material

decomposition algorithms.[2] UA stones are generally visualized on both material-specific iodine-density and water-density images, whereas non-UA stones are visualized only on material-specific water-density images.

In patients undergoing contrast-enhanced DECT examination, several studies have shown that VUE images allow detection of renal calculi in the absence of true unenhanced (TUE) images (Fig. 4).[24–27] A recent study showed that VUE could detect most renal stones, although with slightly lower diagnostic performance compared with TUE images (ie, approximate accuracy: 79% vs 93%) due to the imprecise subtraction of stones smaller than 3 mm.[26] Two primary considerations affecting visualization of renal calculi on VUE images include stone size and attenuation. Small calculi (ie, <3 mm in size), especially those with lower attenuation, can be often obscured due to image smoothing and algorithmic mis-subtraction (algorithm mistakes part of the calculus for iodine) occurring during the reconstruction process of VUE images.

DUAL-ENERGY COMPUTED TOMOGRAPHY: RENAL MASS EVALUATION

Most renal masses are incidentally detected in routine practice on contrast-enhanced scans performed for unrelated clinical indications. A renal lesion with unenhanced attenuation greater than 20 HU or venous phase attenuation greater than 30 HU is considered indeterminate and may require further workup using either a renal mass MR examination or a dedicated multiphasic CT protocol with the inclusion of TUE images, resulting in additional cost, time, and patient anxiety.[28–30] One study reviewing a large cohort of patients scanned in the emergency department showed that 5% of patients had indeterminate renal lesions on contrast-enhanced CT, and 51% of those lesions could be definitively characterized as benign using DECT data.[10] Owing to the unique feature of synthesizing material-specific and energy-specific datasets, DECT can aid in characterizing incidental renal masses even in the absence of TUE images, thus potentially eliminating the need for additional imaging. By leveraging the unique spectral behavior of iodine at low-energy and high-energy levels, DECT allows the user to identify, subtract, or selectively display and quantify iodinated contrast. Using material-specific datasets, iodine can be spectrally erased in VUE images, or selectively represented, in iodine maps, either in a gray-scale scheme or in a color-coded fashion with different color palettes.[28–31] These image series can be achieved

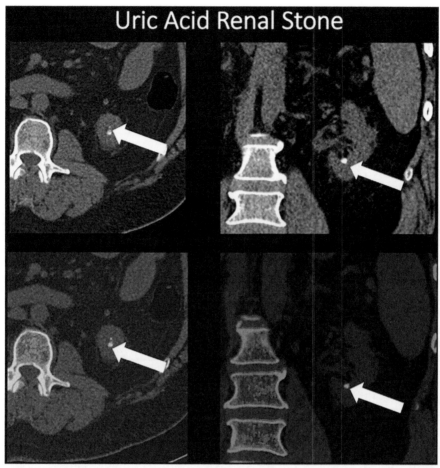

Fig. 2. Conventional gray-scale (*top row*) and material-specific (*bottom row*) axial and coronal dsDECT images in a patient with nonobstructive left renal collecting system UA stone (*arrow*) based on material decomposition analysis.

using either 3-material (ie, ds-DECT) or 2-material decomposition (ie, rs-DECT, dl-DECT) algorithms depending on the DECT system used.

Multiple studies have shown that VUE images represent a good approximation of TUE images for nonenhanced baseline renal mass evaluation (Fig. 5).[26,28,31] Cumulative evidence indicates that attenuation values of VUE images correlate well with those of TNE images with errors in the range of 3 to 10 HU.[26,28,31] The similarity in attenuation values represents the basis for use of VUE in lieu of TUE images when the latter is unavailable.[26,32] A recent study evaluated the use of dl-DECT in patients with renal cell carcinoma and reported that the CT value, image noise, and signal-to-noise ratio of TUE and VUE images are similar.[33] This study recommended the reconstruction of VUE images from the excretory phase and virtual monoenergetic images from the nephrographic phase for optimal renal mass evaluation. The radiation dose was reduced by 50% when the

conventional techniques were replaced by VUE and virtual monoenergetic images.[33] A more recent study demonstrated the similarity in attenuation of VUE and TUE images for both enhancing solid masses and nonenhancing avascular cysts (Fig. 6).[26] In this study, VUE images from multiple study phases were reconstructed and compared with TUE images, concluding that VUE images obtained from the nephrographic phase render diagnostic-quality levels closest to TUE images.[34] Using VUE images instead of TUE may reduce the radiation dose by 30% to 50% and may negate inaccuracies in quantification secondary to spatial misregistration occurring with multiphase acquisition protocols.[28] In comparing VUE to TUE images for renal mass characterization, cumulative evidence indicates that VUE is slightly inferior to TUE images, with the sensitivity and specificity of VUE being 79% and 90%, respectively, whereas those of TUE being 85% and 97%, respectively.[35] The lower diagnostic yield of VUE compared with

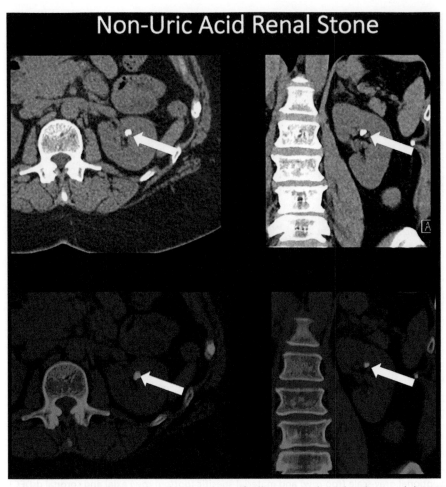

Fig. 3. Conventional gray-scale (*top row*) and material-specific (*bottom row*) axial and coronal dsDECT images in a patient with nonobstructive left renal collecting system non-UA stone (*arrow*) based on material decomposition analysis.

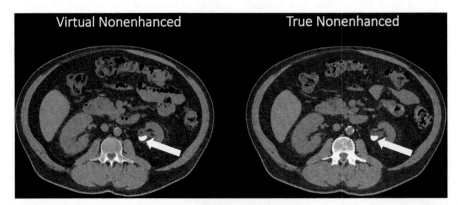

Fig. 4. Side-by-side comparison between virtual nonenhanced and true nonenhanced images in a patient with nonobstructive urolithiasis (*arrow*) within the left collecting system. Although the conspicuity of the renal stone is similar between the 2 image sets, the virtual nonenhanced image has a smoother appearance with decreased conspicuity of the aortic calcifications.

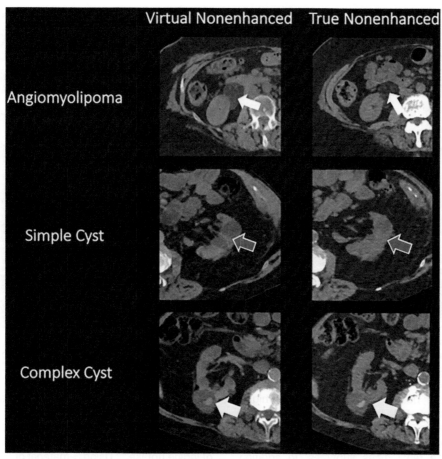

Fig. 5. Side-by-side comparison between virtual nonenhanced and true nonenhanced images in patients with different renal mass types, including renal angiomyolipoma (*white arrows*) and simple (*red arrows*) and complex cysts (*yellow arrows*). Note the smoother appearance of virtual nonenhanced as compared with true nonenhanced images.

TUE images is primarily due to the algorithmic smoothening occurring during the reconstruction of VUE images, resulting in the smoothed appearance of organ boundaries, diminutive appearance of calcifications, or inadequate subtraction of iodine contrast.

In addition to using VUE images, DECT material-specific datasets can be helpful for renal mass evaluation using iodine maps. Incidental renal masses can be characterized as either nonenhancing cysts or enhancing solid lesions based on their appearance on iodine maps. Specifically, nonenhancing cysts seem as devoid of iodine signal on iodine maps (Fig. 7), whereas enhancing solid masses show varying degrees of uptake of iodine contrast within (Fig. 8). Owing to limitations of the material decomposition algorithms, calcifications or hemorrhage can be erroneously visualized as spuriously high signal on iodine maps. To help recognize these pitfalls, it is recommended that iodine maps are interpreted side-by-side with VUE images. Iodine quantification (in milligrams of iodine per milliliter) can be performed on iodine maps and potentially be used as a measure of renal mass vascularity instead of HU measurements when TUE images are not available.[36] Multiple diagnostic thresholds ranging between 0.5 and 3.0 mgI/mL with varying diagnostic accuracy have been suggested in multiple studies to differentiate nonenhancing cysts from enhancing solid masses (conceptually similar to the traditional 20-HU attenuation change between TUE and postcontrast images), with differences depending on different patient populations and DECT systems.[6,36] Along the same application principle, multiple studies have shown that quantification of iodine content can successfully differentiate the usually indolent and hypovascular papillary subtype of renal cell carcinoma from the more common and potentially aggressive clear

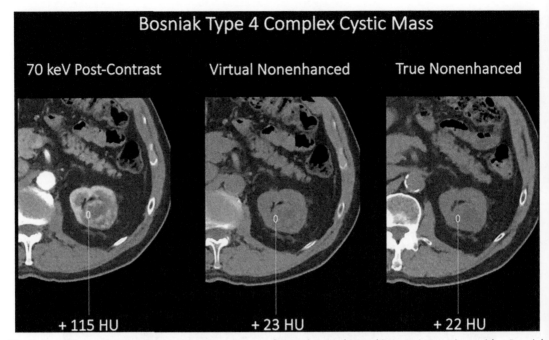

Fig. 6. Renal lesion characterization based on the use of virtual nonenhanced images in a patient with a Bosniak type 4 complex cystic mass. Note the similarity in attenuation between virtual and true nonenhanced images, despite the smoother appearance of the former.

cell subtype based on the significantly higher iodine content of the latter.[37–43] However, it is unclear whether DECT has any advantage over a conventional multiphasic SECT examination to characterize renal mass subtypes. In addition, attenuation values or iodine content of renal cell carcinoma can greatly overlap with other solid renal tumors, including oncocytomas or lipid-poor angiomyolipomas.

Recently, effective atomic number and fat content estimation have been suggested as additional quantitative biomarkers for the renal mass assessment.[44,45] Effective atomic number maps

can be obtained by contrast-enhanced DECT data, and use of this dataset may yield an additional biomarker of iodine content within renal masses based on theoretical electronic signatures of iodine uptake.[44] Using 3-material or 2-material-decomposition analysis, intralesion fat within renal masses can be quantified and used to isolate fat-containing renal masses, such as renal angiomyolipoma and clear-cell renal cell carcinoma.[45] A more recent study proposed the combined use of iodine maps and fat density images to quantify microscopic fat in solid renal masses with the goal of distinguishing clear-cell renal carcinoma

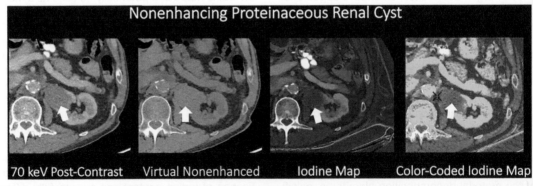

Fig. 7. Renal lesion characterization based on the combined use of virtual nonenhanced images and iodine maps in a patient with a nonenhancing proteinaceous cyst (*arrow*) within the left kidney. Note that the lesion is iso-attenuating to the kidney parenchyma on virtual nonenhanced images and shows a devoid-of-iodine signal on iodine maps.

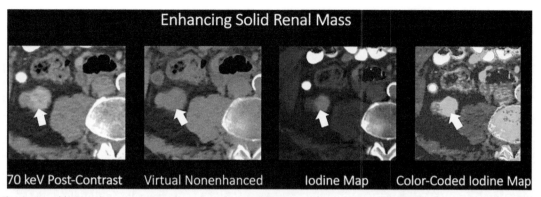

Enhancing Solid Renal Mass

70 keV Post-Contrast   Virtual Nonenhanced   Iodine Map   Color-Coded Iodine Map

Fig. 8. Renal lesion characterization based on the combined use of virtual nonenhanced images and iodine maps in a patient with an enhancing solid mass (*arrow*) originating from the right kidney lower pole. Note that the lesion is isointense to the right kidney on virtual nonenhanced images and shows an intralesion iodine signal on iodine maps.

from other solid renal lesion types.[38] This study found that the presence of intralesion fat quantified using DECT fat density images yielded high specificity (ie, up to approximately 94%) for diagnosis of clear cell renal carcinoma.[38] This type of approach underscores the emerging need for multiparametric assessment of renal masses incorporating other factors, including quantification of materials other than only iodine (eg, fat and calcium content within clear-cell renal cell carcinoma or iron content as a surrogate of hemosiderin storages within papillary renal cell carcinoma[46]), tumor heterogeneity and necrosis, lesion size, and growth rate to more closely reflect on CT the continuum phenotypic spectrum among different solid lesion types. Finally, it should be noted that the use of material-specific DECT quantification techniques in clinical practice is currently limited by the emerging wide variability of quantification across different DECT systems and additional postprocessing time.[47-50]

Another way DECT can help working up incidental renal masses is through energy-specific datasets. Using contrast-enhanced DECT data, monoenergetic image series at individual kiloelectron energy levels (keV) can be synthesized, similar to the use of a theoretical monoenergetic X-ray, which would be less susceptible to beam-hardening and energy-shifting phenomena.[51] High-energy (70 keV or higher) monoenergetic images can be used to decrease the magnitude of the pseudoenhancement phenomenon, which might lead to the misclassification of small intraparenchymal renal cysts as solid neoplasms, potentially requiring further imaging workup.[51] In particular, high-energy (70 keV or higher) monoenergetic images are less prone to pseudoenhancement than conventional polychromatic 120 kVp images.[52] Another feature available using DECT monoenergetic images is

real-time interrogation across different energy levels using multienergy spectral curves. Regions of interest drawn within a renal mass and the neighboring renal parenchyma allow the graphical display of comparative spectral behavior. Non–iodine-containing avascular cysts yield flat spectral curves across the whole explored monoenergetic spectrum. In contrast, iodine-containing renal masses show an upward curve toward gradually lower energy levels, similar to the renal parenchyma (**Fig. 9**).

A novel area of emerging interest using DECT is estimating quantitative biomarkers that may help predict response to treatment in patients with advanced or metastatic renal cell carcinoma. Specifically, iodine content and effective atomic number values may be used for prognostication in patients with metastatic renal cell carcinoma.[53] A recent study reported that high baseline iodine content and effective atomic number values on dl-DECT are good prognostic markers of treatment response in metastatic renal cell carcinoma, independent of tumor histology, treatment group, or International Metastatic Renal Cell Carcinoma Database Consortium risk score.[54] The calculated iodine content and effective atomic number values may assist in monitoring the response of the tumors to anticancer therapies, such as vascular endothelial growth factor and mammalian target of rapamycin inhibitors.[53] Recent studies also demonstrated that dynamic contrast-enhanced CT-derived parameters, such as blood volume and blood flow correlate well with iodine content and effective atomic number derived from dl-DECT, indicating favorable treatment response and survival rates in metastatic renal cell carcinoma.[53,55-57] Another useful application in patients with renal cell carcinoma or small solid renal masses is represented by the use of DECT material-specific datasets in the assessment of

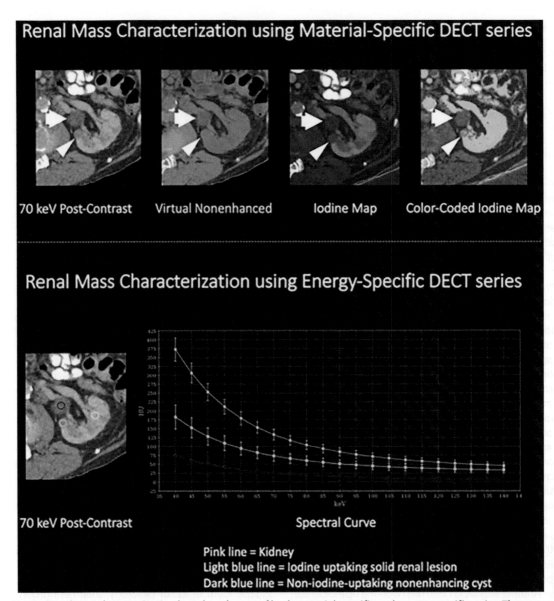

Fig. 9. Renal mass characterization based on the use of both material-specific and energy-specific series. The upper part of the figure shows that the 2 lesions with the left kidney can be characterized as a nonenhancing cyst (*arrow*) and enhancing mass (*arrowhead*) based on devoid of iodine signal and intralesion iodine signal on iodine maps (*arrowhead*, manifested by low grade signal similar to the enhancing renal medulla on grayscale iodine map and color signal on color-coded iodine map), respectively. The lower part of the figure shows that the 2 lesions can be characterized as a nonenhancing cyst (dark blue region of interest and corresponding *line* on the graph) and enhancing mass (light blue region of interest and corresponding *line* on the graph) based on a near-flat curve across the whole monoenergetic spectrum and an upward curve at low monoenergetic levels, respectively.

treatment zones after percutaneous renal interventions, such as cryoablation. The use of VUE images and iodine maps as replacement of multiphasic renal protocols with the inclusion of TUE images may help decrease radiation exposure following solid lesion ablation while also allowing distinction between posttreatment hematoma and small solid recurrences, which is not readily feasible using a SECT examination lacking TUE images.[58]

COMPUTED TOMOGRAPHY UROGRAM WITH DUAL-ENERGY COMPUTED TOMOGRAPHY

Hematuria is the most common indication for referral for a CT urogram. Urinary calculi, solid renal masses, and urothelial lesions constitute the most common causes of hematuria. SECT urography protocols incorporate the acquisition of TUE to detect and measure urinary calculi and contrast-enhanced images during the nephrographic and delayed phases to evaluate for renal masses, ureteral pathology, and infections. Regardless of the CT scanning mode, the use of the split bolus CT urogram technique can decrease radiation exposure to patients by injecting contrast at different time intervals and acquiring the images with simultaneous contrast-enhancement of renal parenchyma and opacification of the excretory system.[59] DECT can potentially further decrease radiation exposure during CT urogram by eliminating the acquisition of TUE images. It has been reported that the combined use of the split bolus technique and DECT with the use of VUE in lieu of TUE images allows prompt identification of most commonly encountered causes of hematuria (Fig. 10),[60] while facilitating an approximately 50% radiation dose reduction.[59]

Urinary calculi detection on excretory phase imaging can be challenging due to the densely opacified urine (>740 HU), resulting in streak artifacts and beam-hardening.[27] Postprocessing algorithms may extract the VUE images from either the nephrographic or urographic phases of a contrast-enhanced DECT examination. However, it cannot be overemphasized that there are limitations when using VUE images to detect and measure urinary calculi. Specifically, the generation of VUE images from excretory phase images can often be unreliable due to image artifacts related

to the breakdown of the material decomposition techniques occurring with extremely dense iodinated urine. Even with diagnostic-quality subtraction of iodine from the collecting system, urinary calculi can be subtracted along with the contrast to varying degrees.[25] For this reason, it is recommended to synthesize VUE images from conventional nephrographic images,[26] which may restrict the use of the split bolus technique with DECT.

DUAL-ENERGY COMPUTED TOMOGRAPHY FOR ADRENAL LESION EVALUATION

Due to the widespread use of cross-sectional imaging, the incidental visualization of adrenal lesions has increased, being estimated to be in up to 3% to 8% of patients.[61] Although most adrenal nodules are adenomas, one must exclude the possibility of primary neoplasm or metastatic disease, especially in patients with a history of solid organ malignancy.[62] Standard of care CT workup of adrenal nodules is carried out with a washout protocol entailing the acquisition of TUE images, contrast-enhanced venous, and delayed (10–15 minutes) phase images. Adenomas can be identified by nonenhanced attenuation of less than 10 HU, absolute and relative contrast washout values greater than 60% and greater than 40%, respectively.[63]

The foremost advantage of using DECT for incidental adrenal nodules evaluation is based on the use of VUE images reconstructed from contrast-enhanced data when TUE images are

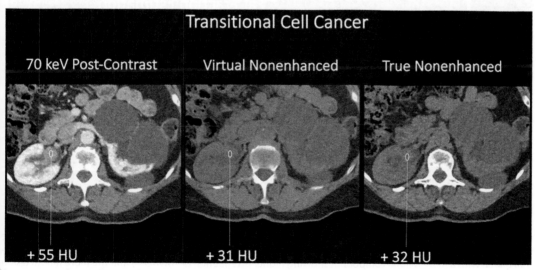

Fig. 10. Use of virtual nonenhanced images reconstructed from a CT urogram examination in a patient referred for hydronephrosis seen on outside ultrasound. A solid low-level enhancing mass is seen within the right renal pelvis with similarity in attenuation between virtual nonenhanced and true nonenhanced images, enabling a diagnosis of transitional cell tumor.

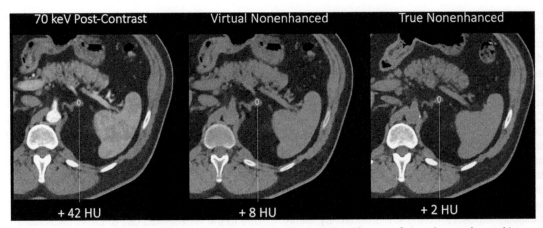

Fig. 11. Example of incidental adrenal nodule characterization based on the use of virtual nonenhanced images reconstructed from postcontrast DECT data. Note the 6 HU attenuation difference between virtual nonenhanced and true nonenhanced images.

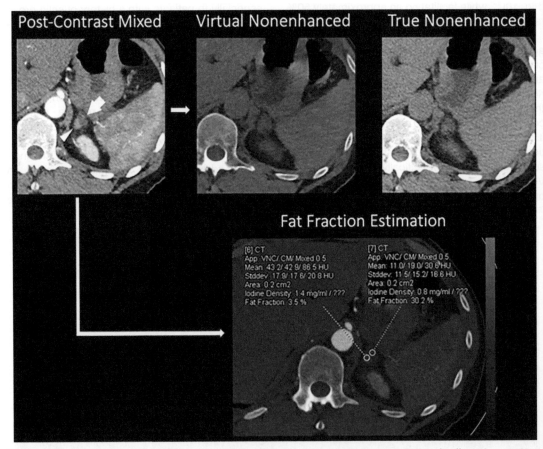

Fig. 12. DECT-based diagnosis of adrenal collision tumor in a patient with metastatic renal cell carcinoma. Note the presence of 2 coexisting lesion types initially seen on the postcontrast mixed DECT image within the left adrenal gland, with a more medial component showing higher attenuation (*arrowhead*) and the more lateral lesion component with lower attenuation (*arrow*). Similar to the true nonenhanced image, the virtual nonenhanced image can identify the 2 components. DECT-based fat content estimation further confirms that the more medial tissue with higher attenuation has negligible fat content, whereas the more lateral component displays higher fat content, which is suggestive of an adenoma.

not available[64] (**Fig. 11**). There are, however, some differences in measured attenuation values between TUE and VUE images. A recent study demonstrated that VUE images tend to overestimate adrenal adenoma attenuation by an average of 11HU compared with TUE images. However, it has been suggested that the characterization of adrenal lesions based on the ratio of iodine density to VUE attenuation has superior sensitivity (95% vs 85%) and equivalent specificity (95% vs 96%) to the TUE images.[61] More recent studies suggest another way to differentiate adenomas from nonadenomas potentially is by using fat fraction measurements based on contrast-enhanced DECT data (**Fig. 12**).[65]

RETROPERITONEAL TRAUMA

If adopted as the routine scanning mode in the emergency department, DECT can aid in promptly identifying critical findings in the setting of blunt abdominal trauma. Through the combined use of material-specific and energy-specific image series, DECT can help characterize sequelae of abdominal trauma and increase the conspicuity of traumatic injuries.[66] VUE images can be beneficial in working up high-density posttraumatic lesions such as adrenal or renal hematomas. Similar to other DECT applications, one cannot overemphasize the need for side-by-side use of VUE images and iodine maps, especially for differentiating hematomas versus laceration and hematomas with active extravasation.[66] In addition, low-keV images can pinpoint small grade 1 to 2 renal parenchymal lacerations, which may be less conspicuous on conventional polychromatic SECT images.[66]

RENAL SPARING, CONTRAST MEDIA REDUCTION, AND EXAMINATION— RECOVERY WITH DUAL-ENERGY COMPUTED TOMOGRAPHY

With the increasing incidence of renal dysfunction and, more recently, the global shortage of iodinated contrast stockpiles, finding new strategies to decrease iodinated contrast utilization has become of clinical relevance. Modern DECT systems offer different strategies to reduce the iodine load administered to the patient by either adopting a lower kV acquisition mode or by reconstructing low-keV monoenergetic images.

A renal-sparing CT technique combining a weight-based contrast volume reduction with patient width-based low tube potential selection and bolus-tracking has recently been developed.[67] This novel size-based contrast reduction algorithm has shown the capability of iodine dose reductions

on the order of 50% while achieving diagnostic-quality in 95% of examinations.[67]

Low-keV monoenergetic images represent an alternative way to substantially decrease the iodine load administrated to patients while rendering diagnostic-quality examinations. It has been shown that the use of DECT-based 50-keV monoenergetic images enables one to reduce the amount of iodinated contrast up to 50% during CT urograms while still obtaining image quality within an acceptable diagnostic range.[68] By the same principle, low-keV monoenergetic images can be used to retrospectively recover examination quality whenever the administered contrast bolus is suboptimal (eg, in cases of extravasation or lower amount of iodine administered). Under these circumstances, a caveat is that higher noise levels typically occur on low-keV images, which may be detrimental for specific tasks such as detecting small hypoattenuating liver lesions.[69]

DUAL-ENERGY COMPUTED TOMOGRAPHY FOR GYNECOLOGIC MALIGNANCIES

Ovarian cystic masses can be classified as simple or complex based on certain observed features on low-keV images.[70] Thickened septations of more

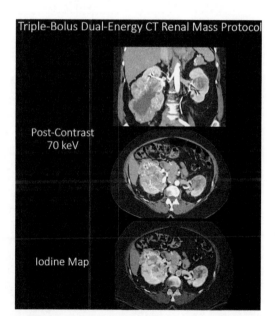

Fig. 13. Use of the triple-bolus injection technique in a patient with hereditary renal cell carcinoma syndrome and bilateral solid renal masses. Note that the triple-bolus injection technique renders within the same acquisition simultaneous contrast-opacification of the arterial and venous vasculature along with parenchymal contrast-enhancement and collecting system contrast excretion, which can be used for staging and surgical planning.

than 3 mm, papillary projections, and intramural nodularity suggest malignant tumor behavior and are best appreciated on low-keV images after contrast administration.[70,71] In addition to morphologic characteristics, the effective atomic number, iodine content, and water content allow for differentiation between malignant and benign ovarian tumors.[72] A study by Elsherif and colleagues reported that the iodine concentration 9.74 or greater is concerning for malignant ovarian tumors with a sensitivity and specificity of 81% and 73%, respectively.[72] An effective atomic number of 8.16 or greater is observed in malignant ovarian tumors, and it has a sensitivity and

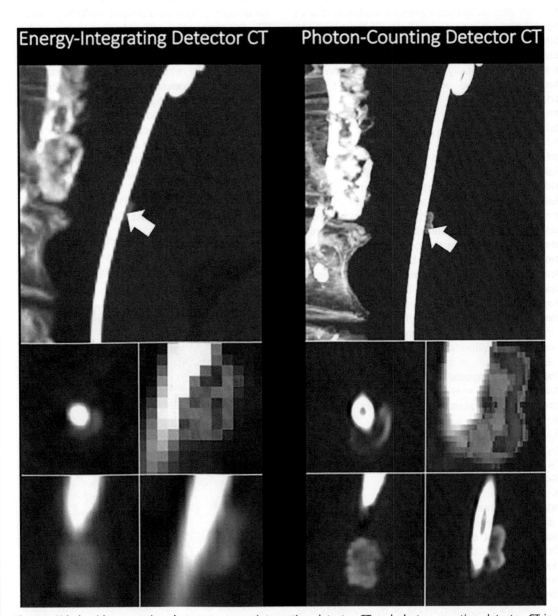

Fig. 14. Side-by-side comparison between energy-integrating detector CT and photon-counting detector CT in the detection of small stone fragments following ureteroscopy, stone extraction, and urinary stent insertion. There is a cluster of tiny stone fragments alongside the ureteric stent (*arrow*) that were nearly missed on the initial examination performed using the energy-integrating detector CT, whereas they were readily visualized on the following scan using the photon-counting detector CT. In addition, an in-house Mayo Clinic CT Clinical Innovation Center (Rochester, MN) solution using qSAS 1.3 color-coding applied to axial and coronal images shows the different coexisting components within the stone conglomerate alongside the urinary stent. qSAS, semi-automated software system. (*Courtesy of* A Ferrero, Ph.D., Rochester, MN.)

specificity of 85% and 73%, respectively.[72] Conversely, the water content of 1013.92 mg/cm³ or greater differentiates benign and malignant tumors with a sensitivity of 80% and specificity of 83%.[72]

DECT is also useful for accurate ovarian cancer staging before debulking surgery by visualizing the subdiaphragmatic, perihepatic, and perisplenic tumor implants.[71] These areas are routinely not inspected during the debulking laparotomy and can be easily missed, which might affect the disease prognosis.[70] Implants have variable imaging appearance including calcification, soft tissue, or fluid attenuation. Due to this heterogeneity, a combination of material attenuation and monochromatic low-keV images assists better in the detection.[70,73] Scatterplots based on attenuation help differentiate cystic and solid implants and enhance conspicuity. On the material decomposition dataset, noncalcified implants are better seen with iodine-enhanced images, whereas the calcified implants can be observed with water-enhanced images. Among patients with uterine sarcoma, hepatic metastases are more common and can be easily missed on routine portal venous phase imaging because they have similar attenuation to the normal hepatic parenchyma.[71] The low-keV images of DECT improve the contrast resolution between the hepatic parenchyma and metastases.

FUTURE APPLICATIONS

The radiation dose optimization potential of DECT in the evaluation of genitourinary diseases can be further expanded by using novel injection techniques, such as the triple-bolus technique.[74,75] This injection technique represents an applicative expansion of the split bolus with the addition of a third injection, overall yielding within the same acquisition the opacification of renal arteries and aorta, renal veins, and IVC, as well as renal collecting system (Fig. 13).

Owing to improved spectral separation, increased iodine signal, and noise suppression, photon-counting detector CT can further expand the DECT application spectrum, including increasing the potential for contrast media reduction, improving quality of DECT material-specific and energy-specific datasets, quantification accuracy, and low-contrast lesion detection.[76] Furthermore, the higher spatial resolution afforded by photon-counting detector CT can be beneficial in more accurate renal stone detection and characterization compared with energy-integrating detector CT.[24] Potential applications of photon-counting detector CT include the detailed visualization of a cluster of tiny stones that are usually averaged as a single large stone on energy-integrating detector CT, or the depiction of small stone fragments alongside ureteric stents that are commonly nearly missed on examinations performed using energy-integrating detector CT (Fig. 14).[24,77] A potentially impactful application of photon-counting detector CT is represented by single-acquisition multiphase imaging, whereby 2 different contrast agents with varying compartments of distribution are administered at the same time, and DECT-based postprocessing renders synthesis of different study phases based on different distribution compartments (eg, blood pool and interstitial), and VUE images are created from spectral extraction of both contrast agents.[78] Deep-learning image reconstruction techniques can further augment the quality of DECT datasets and quantification properties.[79]

SUMMARY

The use of DECT has the potential to improve the diagnostic evaluation of genitourinary diseases. DECT can enable the characterization of genitourinary pathology beyond the diagnostic possibilities of SECT, including renal stone composition and incidental lesions diagnosis while also providing expanded avenues for radiation dose reduction and improved cost-effectiveness as compared with multiphasic CT or MR examinations. Novel injection protocols and the advent of photon-counting detector CT may further augment the diagnostic potential of the dual-energy scanning mode for the evaluation of the genitourinary tract.

CLINICS CARE POINTS

- DECT can reliably differentiate UA from non-UA urinary calculi.

- Urinary calculi as small as 3 mm can be reliably detected and measured using virtual nonenhanced images from contrast-enhanced DECT data.

- DECT is useful in characterizing incidental renal or adrenal lesions that would otherwise remain indeterminate on single-phase contrast-enhanced SECT examinations.

- DECT can be more cost-effective than multiphasic CT or MR examinations for incidentaloma characterization.

- Through the omission of true nonenhanced images, DECT can decrease radiation exposure during multiphasic examinations.

DECLARATION OF INTEREST

None.

ACKNOWLEDGMENTS

None.

REFERENCES

1. Vernuccio F, Meyer M, Mileto A, et al. Use of Dual-Energy Computed Tomography for Evaluation of Genitourinary Diseases. Urol Clin North Am 2018; 45(3):297–310.

2. Patino M, Prochowski A, Agrawal MD, et al. Material Separation Using Dual-Energy CT: Current and Emerging Applications. Radiographics 2016;36(4): 1087–105.

3. Jepperson MA, Cernigliaro JG, Sella D, et al. Dual-energy CT for the evaluation of urinary calculi: image interpretation, pitfalls and stone mimics. Clin Radiol 2013;68(12):e707–14.

4. Virarkar MK, Vulasala SSR, Gupta AV, et al. Virtual Non-contrast Imaging in The Abdomen and The Pelvis: An Overview. Semin Ultrasound CT MR 2022;43(4):293–310.

5. Vulasala SSR, Wynn GC, Hernandez M, et al. Dual-Energy Imaging of the Chest. Semin Ultrasound CT MR 2022;43(4):311–9.

6. Kaza RK, Ananthakrishnan L, Kambadakone A, et al. Update of Dual-Energy CT Applications in the Genitourinary Tract. Am J Roentgenol 2017;208(6):1185–92.

7. Patel BN, Boltyenkov AT, Martinez MG, et al. Cost-effectiveness of dual-energy CT versus multiphasic single-energy CT and MRI for characterization of incidental indeterminate renal lesions. Abdom Radiol (NY) 2020;45(6):1896–906.

8. Pourvaziri A, Mojtahed A, Hahn PF, et al. Renal lesion characterization: clinical utility of single-phase dual-energy CT compared to MRI and dual-phase single-energy CT. Eur Radiol 2022. https://doi.org/10.1007/s00330-022-09106-6.

9. Itani M, Bresnahan BW, Rice K, et al. Clinical and Payer-Based Analysis of Value of Dual-Energy Computed Tomography for Workup of Incidental Abdominal Findings. J Comput Assist Tomogr 2019;43(4):605–11.

10. Wortman JR, Shyu JY, Fulwadhva UP, et al. Impact Analysis of the Routine Use of Dual-Energy Computed Tomography for Characterization of Incidental Renal Lesions. J Comput Assist Tomogr 2019;43(2):176–82.

11. Bonatti M, Lombardo F, Zamboni GA, et al. Renal stones composition in vivo determination: comparison between 100/Sn140 kV dual-energy CT and 120 kV single-energy CT. Urolithiasis 2017;45(3):255–61.

12. Kambadakone AR, Eisner BH, Catalano OA, et al. New and evolving concepts in the imaging and management of urolithiasis: urologists' perspective. Radiographics 2010;30(3):603–23.

13. Saita A, Bonaccorsi A, Motta M. Stone composition: where do we stand? Urol Int 2007;79(Suppl 1):16–9.

14. Ngo TC, Assimos DG. Uric Acid nephrolithiasis: recent progress and future directions. Rev Urol 2007;9(1):17–27.

15. Bellin MF, Renard-Penna R, Conort P, et al. Helical CT evaluation of the chemical composition of urinary tract calculi with a discriminant analysis of CT-attenuation values and density. Eur Radiol 2004;14(11):2134–40.

16. Motley G, Dalrymple N, Keesling C, et al. Hounsfield unit density in the determination of urinary stone composition. Urology 2001;58(2):170–3.

17. Lazar M, Ringl H, Baltzer P, et al. Protocol analysis of dual-energy CT for optimization of kidney stone detection in virtual non-contrast reconstructions. Eur Radiol 2020;30(8):4295–305.

18. Thomas C, Patschan O, Ketelsen D, et al. Dual-energy CT for the characterization of urinary calculi: In vitro and in vivo evaluation of a low-dose scanning protocol. Eur Radiol 2009;19(6):1553–9.

19. Rajiah P, Parakh A, Kay F, et al. Update on Multienergy CT: Physics, Principles, and Applications. Radiographics 2020;40(5):1284–308.

20. Hidas G, Eliahou R, Duvdevani M, et al. Determination of renal stone composition with dual-energy CT: in vivo analysis and comparison with x-ray diffraction. Radiology 2010;257(2):394–401.

21. Spek A, Strittmatter F, Graser A, et al. Dual energy can accurately differentiate uric acid-containing urinary calculi from calcium stones. World J Urol 2016; 34(9):1297–302.

22. Qu M, Ramirez-Giraldo JC, Leng S, et al. Dual-energy dual-source CT with additional spectral filtration can improve the differentiation of non-uric acid renal stones: an ex vivo phantom study. AJR Am J Roentgenol 2011;196(6):1279–87.

23. Nourian A, Ghiraldi E, Friedlander JI. Dual-Energy CT for Urinary Stone Evaluation. Curr Urol Rep 2020;22(1):1.

24. Marcus RP, Fletcher JG, Ferrero A, et al. Detection and Characterization of Renal Stones by Using Photon-Counting-based CT. Radiology 2018; 289(2):436–42.

25. Takahashi N, Vrtiska TJ, Kawashima A, et al. Detectability of urinary stones on virtual nonenhanced images generated at pyelographic-phase dual-energy CT. Radiology 2010;256(1):184–90.

26. Xiao JM, Hippe DS, Zecevic M, et al. Virtual Unenhanced Dual-Energy CT Images Obtained with a Multimaterial Decomposition Algorithm: Diagnostic Value for Renal Mass and Urinary Stone Evaluation. Radiology 2021;298(3):611–9.

27. McCoombe K, Dobeli K, Meikle S, et al. Sensitivity of virtual non-contrast dual-energy CT urogram for detection of urinary calculi: a systematic review

and meta-analysis. Eur Radiol 2022. https://doi.org/10.1007/s00330-022-08939-5.

28. Meyer M, Nelson RC, Vernuccio F, et al. Virtual Unenhanced Images at Dual-Energy CT: Influence on Renal Lesion Characterization. Radiology 2019;291(2):381–90.

29. Herts BR, Silverman SG, Hindman NM, et al. Management of the Incidental Renal Mass on CT: A White Paper of the ACR Incidental Findings Committee. J Am Coll Radiol 2018;15(2):264–73.

30. Dunnick NR. Renal cell carcinoma: staging and surveillance. Abdom Radiol (NY) 2016;41(6):1079–85.

31. Graser A, Johnson TR, Hecht EM, et al. Dual-energy CT in patients suspected of having renal masses: can virtual nonenhanced images replace true nonenhanced images? Radiology 2009;252(2):433–40.

32. Toia GV, Mileto A, Wang CL, et al. Quantitative dual-energy CT techniques in the abdomen. Abdom Radiol (NY) 2022;47(9):3003–18.

33. Zhang X, Zhang G, Xu L, et al. Utilisation of virtual non-contrast images and virtual mono-energetic images acquired from dual-layer spectral CT for renal cell carcinoma: image quality and radiation dose. Insights Imaging 2022;13(1):12.

34. Lin YM, Chiou YY, Wu MH, et al. Attenuation values of renal parenchyma in virtual noncontrast images acquired from multiphase renal dual-energy CT: Comparison with standard noncontrast CT. Eur J Radiol 2018;101:103–10.

35. Hines JJ, Eacobacci K, Goyal R. The Incidental Renal Mass- Update on Characterization and Management. Radiol Clin North Am 2021;59(4):631–46.

36. Chandarana H, Megibow AJ, Cohen BA, et al. Iodine Quantification With Dual-Energy CT: Phantom Study and Preliminary Experience With Renal Masses. Am J Roentgenol 2011;196(6):W693–700.

37. Zarzour JG, Milner D, Valentin R, et al. Quantitative iodine content threshold for discrimination of renal cell carcinomas using rapid kV-switching dual-energy CT. Abdom Radiol (NY) 2017;42(3):727–34.

38. Mileto A, Marin D, Alfaro-Cordoba M, et al. Iodine quantification to distinguish clear cell from papillary renal cell carcinoma at dual-energy multidetector CT: a multireader diagnostic performance study. Radiology 2014;273(3):813–20.

39. Marcon J, Graser A, Horst D, et al. Papillary vs clear cell renal cell carcinoma. Differentiation and grading by iodine concentration using DECT-correlation with microvascular density. Eur Radiol 2020;30(1):1–10.

40. Udare A, Walker D, Krishna S, et al. Characterization of clear cell renal cell carcinoma and other renal tumors: evaluation of dual-energy CT using material-specific iodine and fat imaging. Eur Radiol 2020;30(4):2091–102.

41. Dai C, Cao Y, Jia Y, et al. Differentiation of renal cell carcinoma subtypes with different iodine quantification methods using single-phase contrast-enhanced dual-energy CT: areal vs. volumetric analyses. Abdom Radiol (NY) 2018;43(3):672–8.

42. Çamlıdağ İ, Nural MS, Danacı M, et al. Usefulness of rapid kV-switching dual energy CT in renal tumor characterization. Abdom Radiol (NY) 2019;44(5):1841–9.

43. Meyer M, Nelson RC, Vernuccio F, et al. Comparison of Iodine Quantification and Conventional Attenuation Measurements for Differentiating Small, Truly Enhancing Renal Masses From High-Attenuation Nonenhancing Renal Lesions With Dual-Energy CT. AJR Am J Roentgenol 2019;213(1):W26–37.

44. Mileto A, Allen BC, Pietryga JA, et al. Characterization of Incidental Renal Mass With Dual-Energy CT: Diagnostic Accuracy of Effective Atomic Number Maps for Discriminating Nonenhancing Cysts From Enhancing Masses. AJR Am J Roentgenol 2017;209(4):W221–30.

45. Walker D, Udare A, Chatelain R, et al. Utility of material-specific fat images derived from rapid-kVp-switch dual-energy renal mass CT for diagnosis of renal angiomyolipoma. Acta Radiol 2021;62(9):1263–72.

46. Takahashi H, Kawashima A, Inoue A, et al. Hemosiderin deposition in papillary renal cell carcinoma and its potential to mask enhancement on MRI: analysis of 110 cases. Eur Radiol 2020;30(11):6033–41.

47. Lennartz S, Pisuchpen N, Parakh A, et al. Virtual Unenhanced Images: Qualitative and Quantitative Comparison Between Different Dual-Energy CT Scanners in a Patient and Phantom Study. Invest Radiol 2022;57(1):52 61.

48. Lennartz S, Parakh A, Cao J, et al. Longitudinal reproducibility of attenuation measurements on virtual unenhanced images: multivendor dual-energy CT evaluation. Eur Radiol 2021;31(12):9240–9.

49. Cai LM, Hippe DS, Zamora DA, et al. A Method for Reducing Variability Across Dual-Energy CT Manufacturers in Quantification of Low Iodine Content Levels. AJR Am J Roentgenol 2022;218(4):746–55.

50. Mileto A, Barina A, Marin D, et al. Virtual Monochromatic Images from Dual-Energy Multidetector CT: Variance in CT Numbers from the Same Lesion between Single-Source Projection-based and Dual-Source Image-based Implementations. Radiology 2016;279(1):269–77.

51. Yu L, Leng S, McCollough CH. Dual-energy CT-based monochromatic imaging. AJR Am J Roentgenol 2012;199(5 Suppl):S9–15.

52. Jung DC, Oh YT, Kim MD, et al. Usefulness of the virtual monochromatic image in dual-energy spectral CT for decreasing renal cyst pseudoenhancement: a phantom study. AJR Am J Roentgenol 2012;199(6):1316–9.

53. Hellbach K, Sterzik A, Sommer W, et al. Dual energy CT allows for improved characterization of response to antiangiogenic treatment in patients with metastatic renal cell cancer. Eur Radiol 2017;27(6):2532–7.

54. Drljevic-Nielsen A, Donskov F, Mains JR, et al. Prognostic Utility of Parameters Derived From Pretreatment Dual-Layer Spectral-Detector CT in Patients With Metastatic Renal Cell Carcinoma. AJR Am J Roentgenol 2022;218(5):867–76.

55. Mains JR, Donskov F, Pedersen EM, et al. Dynamic contrast-enhanced computed tomography as a potential biomarker in patients with metastatic renal cell carcinoma: preliminary results from the Danish Renal Cancer Group Study-1. Invest Radiol 2014; 49(9):601–7.

56. Mains JR, Donskov F, Pedersen EM, et al. Dynamic Contrast-Enhanced Computed Tomography-Derived Blood Volume and Blood Flow Correlate With Patient Outcome in Metastatic Renal Cell Carcinoma. Invest Radiol 2017;52(2):103–10.

57. Mains JR, Donskov F, Pedersen EM, et al. Use of patient outcome endpoints to identify the best functional CT imaging parameters in metastatic renal cell carcinoma patients. Br J Radiol 2018;91(1082): 20160795.

58. Park SY, Kim CK, Park BK. Dual-energy CT in assessing therapeutic response to radiofrequency ablation of renal cell carcinomas. Eur J Radiol 2014;83(2):e73–9.

59. Manoharan D, Sharma S, Das CJ, et al. Split bolus dual-energy CT urography after urine dilution: a one-stop shop for detection and characterisation of urolithiasis. Clin Radiol 2020;75(8):643.e11–8.

60. Hansen C, Becker CD, Montet X, et al. Diagnosis of urothelial tumors with a dedicated dual-source dual-energy MDCT protocol: preliminary results. AJR Am J Roentgenol 2014;202(4):W357–64.

61. Nagayama Y, Inoue T, Oda S, et al. Adrenal Adenomas versus Metastases: Diagnostic Performance of Dual-Energy Spectral CT Virtual Noncontrast Imaging and Iodine Maps. Radiology 2020;296(2): 324–32.

62. Mayo-Smith WW, Song JH, Boland GL, et al. Management of Incidental Adrenal Masses: A White Paper of the ACR Incidental Findings Committee. J Am Coll Radiol 2017;14(8):1038–44.

63. Cao J, Lennartz S, Parakh A, et al. Dual-layer dual-energy CT for characterization of adrenal nodules: can virtual unenhanced images replace true unenhanced acquisitions? Abdom Radiol (NY) 2021; 46(9):4345–52.

64. Connolly MJ, McInnes MDF, El-Khodary M, et al. Diagnostic accuracy of virtual non-contrast enhanced dual-energy CT for diagnosis of adrenal adenoma: A systematic review and meta-analysis. Eur Radiol 2017;27(10):4324–35.

65. Martin SS, Weidinger S, Czwikla R, et al. Iodine and Fat Quantification for Differentiation of Adrenal Gland Adenomas From Metastases Using Third-Generation Dual-Source Dual-Energy Computed Tomography. Invest Radiol 2018;53(3):173–8.

66. Wortman JR, Uyeda JW, Fulwadhva UP, et al. Dual-Energy CT for Abdominal and Pelvic Trauma. Radiographics 2018;38(2):586–602.

67. Iyer VR, Ehman EC, Khandelwal A, et al. Image quality in abdominal CT using an iodine contrast reduction algorithm employing patient size and weight and low kV CT technique. Acta Radiol 2020;61(9):1186–95.

68. Shuman WP, Mileto A, Busey JM, et al. Dual-Energy CT Urography With 50% Reduced Iodine Dose Versus Single-Energy CT Urography With Standard Iodine Dose. AJR Am J Roentgenol 2019;212(1):117–23.

69. Mileto A, Ananthakrishnan L, Morgan DE, et al. Clinical Implementation of Dual-Energy CT for Gastrointestinal Imaging. AJR Am J Roentgenol 2021;217(3): 651–63.

70. Benveniste AP, de Castro Faria S, Broering G, et al. Potential application of dual-energy CT in gynecologic cancer: initial experience. Am J Roentgenol 2017;208(3):695–705.

71. Daoud T, Sardana S, Stanietzky N, et al. Recent Imaging Updates and Advances in Gynecologic Malignancies. Cancers 2022;14(22):5528.

72. Elsherif S, Zheng S, Ganeshan D, et al. Does dual-energy CT differentiate benign and malignant ovarian tumours? Clin Radiol 2020;75(8):606–14.

73. Amante S, Santos F, Cunha TM. Low-grade serous epithelial ovarian cancer: a comprehensive review and update for radiologists. Insights into Imaging 2021;12(1):1–12.

74. Manoharan D, Netaji A, Das CJ, et al. Iodine Parameters in Triple-Bolus Dual-Energy CT Correlate With Perfusion CT Biomarkers of Angiogenesis in Renal Cell Carcinoma. AJR Am J Roentgenol 2020; 214(4):808–16.

75. Manoharan D, Sharma S, Das CJ, et al. Single-Acquisition Triple-Bolus Dual-Energy CT Protocol for Comprehensive Evaluation of Renal Masses: A Single-Center Randomized Noninferiority Trial. AJR Am J Roentgenol 2018;211(1):W22–32.

76. Rajendran K, Petersilka M, Henning A, et al. First Clinical Photon-counting Detector CT System: Technical Evaluation. Radiology 2022;303(1):130–8.

77. Ferrero A, Gutjahr R, Halaweish AF, et al. Characterization of Urinary Stone Composition by Use of Whole-body, Photon-counting Detector CT. Acad Radiol 2018;25(10):1270–6.

78. Leng S, Bruesewitz M, Tao S, et al. Photon-counting Detector CT: System Design and Clinical Applications of an Emerging Technology. Radiographics 2019;39(3):729–43.

79. Fukutomi A, Sofue K, Ueshima E, et al. Deep learning image reconstruction to improve accuracy of iodine quantification and image quality in dual-energy CT of the abdomen: a phantom and clinical study. Eur Radiol 2022. https://doi.org/10.1007/s00330-022-09127-1.

Pediatric Applications of Dual-Energy Computed Tomography

Valeria Peña-Trujillo, MD[a,b,c,1], Sebastian Gallo-Bernal, MD[a,b,c,1], Erik L. Tung, MD[b,c], Michael S. Gee, MD, PhD[a,b,c,*]

KEYWORDS

- Dual-energy CT (DECT) • Pediatrics • Radiation dose • High-pitch CT

KEY POINTS

- Dual-energy computed tomography (DECT) scanners acquire 2 sets of data at different energy levels, allowing for better material characterization and unique image reconstructions, while maintaining as low as reasonably achievable radiation doses.
- DECT Image optimization algorithms leverage the image properties of high- and low-energy acquisitions to improve image contrast and iodine conspicuity and mitigate the impact of metal artifacts.
- Material decomposition algorithms elucidate the concentration and distribution of different materials in the body based on their attenuation characteristics, allowing for the generation of virtual unenhanced images, iodine maps, and iodine overlay images.
- DECT pediatric applications are far-reaching, extending into thoracic, cardiovascular, urologic, oncologic, and gastrointestinal imaging.
- Pediatric DECT can reduce radiation doses, accelerate image acquisition, and improve motion robustness when compared with traditional single-energy computed tomography.

INTRODUCTION

Multidetector computed tomography (CT) has revolutionized medicine and has become one of the cornerstones of modern radiology practice. Technical advances have greatly improved CT access, image quality, and acquisition time in pediatric and adult patients; as a result, the annual number of CT scans performed in the United States has risen steadily over the past 20 years. Although much attention in the medical and lay literature has focused on ionizing radiation risks of CT in children,[1,2] current concerns associated with the potential acute and long-term risks related to magnetic resonance (MR) imaging performed under general anesthesia have renewed the interest in novel pediatric CT applications that

can image nonsedated patients at low-radiation doses.[3–6] Although MR imaging remains a valuable diagnostic tool in the pediatric population owing to its lack of ionizing radiation and high soft tissue contrast, the need for general anesthesia in young children undergoing MR imaging poses significant challenges, including increased cost, logistical complexity, and potential medical risk. At the same time, novel CT hardware- and software-based techniques have allowed for remarkable progress in reducing radiation doses and acquisition times while maintaining diagnostic quality.

Traditionally, CT has been performed using a single-energy source, which produces a polychromatic radiograph beam.[7] Although all clinical scanners produce images using a wide range of photon

[a] Division of Pediatric Imaging, Massachusetts General Hospital, 55 Fruit Street, Boston, MA 02114, USA;
[b] Department of Radiology, Massachusetts General Hospital, 55 Fruit Street, Boston, MA 02114, USA;
[c] Department of Radiology, Harvard Medical School, Boston, MA, USA
[1] These authors contributed equally to this article.
* Corresponding author.
E-mail address: msgee@mgh.harvard.edu
Twitter: @valeria_pt22 (V.P.-T.); @SebGal1230 (S.G.-B.); @ErikTungMD (E.L.T.); @Mike_Gee8 (M.S.G.)

Radiol Clin N Am 61 (2023) 1069–1083
https://doi.org/10.1016/j.rcl.2023.05.006

energies, the peak maximum energy is prespecified by the operator. Deciding the optimal prespecified photon energy for conventional CT is challenging and implies a constant tradeoff between contrast, noise, and radiation dose. When a conventional high (ie, 120 kilovoltage peak [kVp]) energy spectrum is used, many elements with different atomic numbers (ie, iodine and calcium) may display similar attenuation values.[7] On the other hand, although low-photon energy scans (ie, <90 kVp) allow for reduced radiation doses and increased iodine conspicuity, they result in noisier images.

Dual-energy computed tomography (DECT) provides benefits of both high- and low-energy spectra scans without significantly increasing the radiation burden. DECT scanners acquire 2 sets of data at different energy levels for each voxel, allowing for better material characterization and unique image reconstructions that enhance image analysis.[8] As a result, this technique has been widely adopted in adult clinical practice, and its use in the evaluation of children has been extensively reported.[9,10] This article aims to review the current role of DECT in pediatric imaging, focusing on available reconstruction techniques and specific pediatric applications.

DUAL-ENERGY COMPUTED TOMOGRAPHY TECHNOLOGIES AND CONFIGURATIONS

Each vendor has different hardware configurations for DECT as well as diverse approaches for imaging postprocessing. Current configurations include dual-source systems, single-source dual-layer detectors, and single-source rapid kilovoltage switching (**Fig. 1**) Although detailed descriptions of these configurations are outside the scope of this article, they are summarized in **Table 1**.[9]

DUAL-ENERGY COMPUTED TOMOGRAPHY IMAGING POSTPROCESSING: RECONSTRUCTION TECHNIQUES

Currently, several Food and Drug Administration–approved reconstruction algorithms are available on different platforms and offered by different vendors.[11] The most relevant DECT postprocessing algorithms used in pediatric radiology can be grouped into the following types: image optimization algorithms and material decomposition algorithms (**Fig. 2**).[8,12]

Image optimization algorithms

Image optimization algorithms, including virtual monoenergetic images (VMI) and metal artifact reduction protocols, were designed to leverage the image properties of high- and low-energy

acquisitions to improve image quality and mitigate the impact of artifacts. In this reconstruction, the Hounsfield units for each voxel are extrapolated using a mathematical algorithm that blends data from each energy acquisition to simulate the attenuation values of a single-energy computed tomography (SECT) image.[12,13] After reconstruction, radiograph energy of these VMIs is reported in kiloelectron volts (keV) instead of kVp. Reconstructed VMI energies typically range from 40 to 200 keV, and the operator can select a specific hypothetical energy level to reconstruct the images.[14]

The advantage of VMI is the capacity to leverage both noise reduction associated with high-energy spectrum and enhanced iodine attenuation of the low-energy spectrum to generate images optimized for different clinical indications.[15] Lower monochromatic energy (40–70 keV) reconstructions are particularly useful under low-contrast conditions given the increased radiograph attenuation of iodine at these energies. Comparative studies have shown that low-kiloelectron-volt images improve the visualization of subtle contrast enhancement compared with standard SECT while allowing for substantial radiation dose and contrast volume reductions.[15–17]

Conversely, high-energy data (>140 keV) have significantly less noise and contrast conspicuity compared with low-energy data. The primary benefit of high monochromatic energy reconstructions is the reduction of artifacts associated with high-attenuation materials, such as metal implants.[9] Metal materials are commonly found in pediatric patients who require osteosynthetic material owing to fractures, bar placement for correction of pectus excavatum, or a spinal fusion for scoliosis.[18] Metal-related artifacts comprise the photon starvation and beam-hardening effects. The beam-hardening effect results from the selective attenuation of low-energy photons, allowing only high-energy photons to reach the detector.[18] In practice, beam hardening produces streaking (dark bands) and cupping adjacent to the metal implants. Photon starvation is caused by a complete attenuation of all photons, causing zero transmission projections.[7] By preferentially removing low-energy photons that contribute to beam hardening, high-energy spectra VMI improves image quality and allows better visualization of the metallic implant and surrounding tissues (**Fig. 3**).[18,19]

Material decomposition algorithms

Material decomposition algorithms compare data from different photon energy levels to identify the

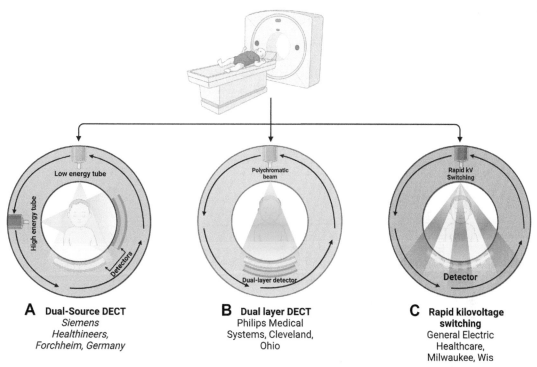

Fig. 1. The 3 commercially available configurations for DECT. (*A*) Dual source-dual-energy system. (*B*) Single-energy dual-layer detector systems. (*C*) Single-source rapid kilovoltage switching systems. (Created with BioRender.com.)

concentration and distribution of different materials in the body based on their elemental configuration and attenuation characteristics.[8] A map of this material-specific information can be generated by modeling the relative dependence of the photoelectric and Compton interaction processes.[9]

Material decomposition algorithms allow the generation of virtual unenhanced images (VUI), iodine maps, and iodine overlay images.[9] Other material decomposition images are available for select clinical applications, including calcium/bone subtraction for CT angiography, lung ventilation and perfusion studies, and renal stone characterization (**Fig. 4**).[20–22]

VUI can eliminate the need for noncontrast imaging in multiphase CT protocols, reducing total study times and significantly decreasing the total radiation dose given to the child.[9] With knowledge of the relative contribution of iodine within each voxel, VUI can be generated by subtracting the attenuation contributed by iodine from the entire image. Although infrequently used in pediatric radiology, unenhanced images can aid in diagnosing renal lesions and distinguishing calcifications versus contrast enhancement in the workup of lesions with calcified components. For example, VUIs can help to identify calcifications within common childhood tumors, including teratomas, neuroblastomas, or hepatoblastomas.

Iodine maps allow for quantitative and qualitative assessment of contrast concentration within the body. This information is valuable for determining the vascularity of a lesion, evaluating tumor burden and treatment response, characterizing organ perfusion, and identifying areas of infarction.[11,22] Quantified iodine can be expressed either as Hounsfield units or concentration units (milligrams of iodine per milliliter). However, given that exact thresholds have not been described and iodine concentrations greatly vary between vendors, the analysis of iodine concentrations in iodine maps is better performed qualitatively by comparing normal and abnormal tissues.[9]

DUAL-ENERGY COMPUTED TOMOGRAPHY–SPECIFIC PEDIATRIC CONSIDERATIONS AND APPLICATIONS
Radiation Dose Reduction and Low Kilovoltage Scanning

Radiation exposures associated with contrast-enhanced chest, abdominal, and pelvic DECT in children are equal to or less than those of an equivalent SECT.[10,23,24] Overall hardware optimization,

Table 1
Dual-energy computed tomography configurations: advantages and disadvantages in pediatric radiology

DECT Technique	Manufacturer	Description	Advantages	Disadvantages
Dual-source	Siemens Healthineers, Forchheim, Germany	• Two radiograph sources and 2 detectors are mounted on a single radiograph gantry • Each radiograph tube operates independently at high (140–150 kVp) and low energies (70–80 kVp) • Allows simultaneous acquisition of the 2 energy spectra with close spatial registration	• Enhance spectral separation, improve signal-to-noise ratio, and decrease radiation doses[9,24] • Achieve high-pitch images without gaps and decreases acquisition time	• Smaller tube size and field of view for the high-energy detector, which may not adequately evaluate peripheral structures in older or obese children[9,11]
Single-source rapid kilovoltage switching system	General Electric Healthcare, Milwaukee, WI, USA	• A single radiograph tube that alternates between high and low tube voltages and a single fast-response receiver[13] • Data are collected twice for every projection, and the short time interval between the 2 energy beams provides near-simultaneous acquisition	• Full field of view (50 cm) • Good temporal registration between both energy spectra	• Lack of tube current modulation[9] • Inherently limited photon output at low voltages resulting in noisier images • Require higher voltages (and thus higher doses) to achieve diagnostic-quality images[8]
Single-source dual-layer detector	Philips Medical Systems, Cleveland, OH, USA	• A single polychromatic radiograph beam produces a wide energy spectrum, and 2 layers of detectors simultaneously collect low- and high-energy data • The radiograph tube has a 120-kW generator with tube voltages ranging from 80 to 140 kVp (with 120 kVp routinely used in children)	• Constant acquisition of spectral images for all patients, eliminating the requirement to prospectively select patients	• Higher overlap of the energy spectrum leading to decreased spectral separation • Tube currents cannot be modified independently

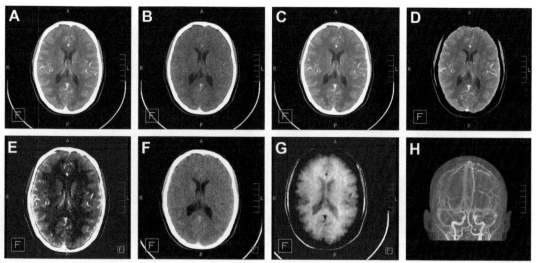

Fig. 2. Representative DECT postprocessing images of the head of a healthy 16-year-old girl. (*A*) Low-energy images (100 kV). (*B*) High-energy images (150 kV). (*C*) VMIs at 65 keV. (*D*) Automatic bone removal technique. (*E*) Iodine map. (*F*) VUIs. (*G*) Calcium subtraction algorithm. (*H*) 3D digital angiography.

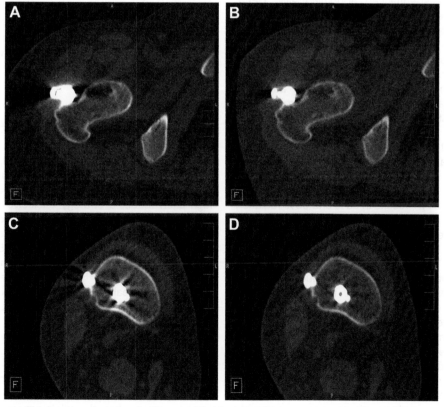

Fig. 3. Low- and high-energy images of a 12-year-old girl who underwent open reduction and internal fixation of the right femur after a traumatic fracture. A dedicated low-dose metal suppression protocol was used with dual-energy acquisition at 100 (*A* and *C*) and 140 kV (*B* and *D*). Axial DECT images at high energy (*B* and *D*) reduce metallic implant-associated beam-hardening artifacts.

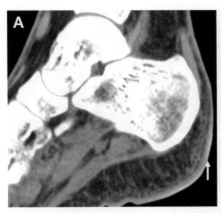
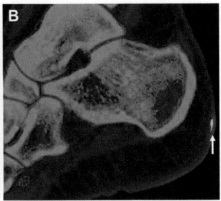

Fig. 4. Material decomposition algorithms. (*A*) Sagittal standard and (*B*) color-coded postprocessed CT images in a 17-year-old male patient with right heel pain. There is high-density soft tissue associated with skin thickening of the posterior aspect of the heel (*yellow arrow*), arising approximately 3 cm distal to the Achilles tendon insertion. There is coloration of this area on the dual-energy reformatted images used for detecting calcium urate, suggestive of crystal deposition (*white arrow*). Monosodium urate deposition is depicted in green. Blue and purple coloration represents cortical bone and trabecular bone, respectively.

including improved detector efficiency, has allowed further radiation dose reductions with most DECT systems. For example, Siegel and colleagues[25] found that regardless of effective diameter, contrast-enhanced abdominopelvic DECT can be performed with an equal or lower dose and similar image quality in children compared with SECT scans.

Using only low kilovoltage peak (≤80 kVp) on both radiograph sources of dual-source computed tomography (DSCT) scanners is an additional exciting radiation-dose reduction approach.[26] At a constant tube current, the radiation dose is proportional to the square of the tube voltage, implying that minor tube voltage variations lead to substantial radiation dose changes.[2,27] For example, when all additional parameters remain constant, reducing tube voltage from 120 kV to 100 kV or 80 kV results in 33% and 65% radiation dose reductions, respectively.[28,29] Although low kilovoltage peak decreases radiation exposure, it invariably leads to increased image noise and artifacts via increased quantum mottle. Optimal implementation of tube voltage reduction for radiation dose improvement therefore involves consideration of multiple clinical variables, such as the specific clinical question and the patient's anthropometric measurements. The degree of image noise associated with low-energy photons highly depends on patient size. In small patients (usually under 10 years of age), photons require significantly less energy to penetrate the different body tissues, and low tube voltages can provide sufficient image quality with only modest increases in tube current or exposure time, thus leading to overall dose reduction.[2,10]

CONTRAST-DOSE REDUCTION

Owing to the higher attenuation of iodine contrast at lower tube voltages, an additional advantage of low-kilovoltage DSCT is the possibility of decreasing iodinated contrast doses and injection rates.[10,29] This strategy is especially beneficial in patients at high risk of contrast-induced nephropathy and in newborns or infants with fragile peripheral vascular accesses that can only receive a low-contrast volume and injection rates.[29,30]

Fast, motion-robust studies: high-pitch

One strategy to perform fast CT imaging in awake pediatric patients is to increase the pitch, which is defined as the table distance traveled per gantry rotation divided by beam collimation. In ultra-high-pitch mode, a strategy exclusive to DSCT scanners, further decreases in image acquisition time are achieved by increasing the table pitch to greater than 3 and table speed up to 450 mm/s. This creates motion-robust images using significantly less radiation.[31,32] Motion tolerance is particularly appealing in pediatric radiology, as many children cannot remain still for extended periods of time.[3] Similarly, young children and children with intellectual disabilities may be unable to follow breathing instructions, resulting in motion artifacts that degrade image quality.[31,32]

The drawbacks of faster table movement include data gaps and undersampling, which tend to occur when the pitch increases above 1.0. Consequently, standard CTs are limited to a pitch of less than 1.5 to protect image quality. DSCT, however, can achieve high pitch without image gaps owing to the presence of 2 radiograph sources (Fig. 5). Both radiograph tubes are set to the same voltage to accomplish this, precluding the use of concomitant dual-energy technique. Using this strategy, fast and high-quality evaluations of the thorax and abdomen have been achieved in children. Bodelle and colleagues[31] used high-pitch DSCT to image the pediatric chest in less than 0.5 seconds in a free-breathing technique with excellent image quality and lower radiation exposure than a conventional-pitch protocol.

Specific pediatric clinical applications

Cardiovascular Imaging

DECT is an efficient and noninvasive method for evaluating congenital and acquired cardiac and vascular abnormalities.[33,34] It provides a detailed morphologic assessment of the coronary arteries and great vessels as well as a functional assessment of the heart (myocardium, valves, and so forth).[35] In the last few years, DECT angiography has been widely adopted to evaluate congenital cardiac (ie, Ebstein anomaly, tetralogy of Fallot,

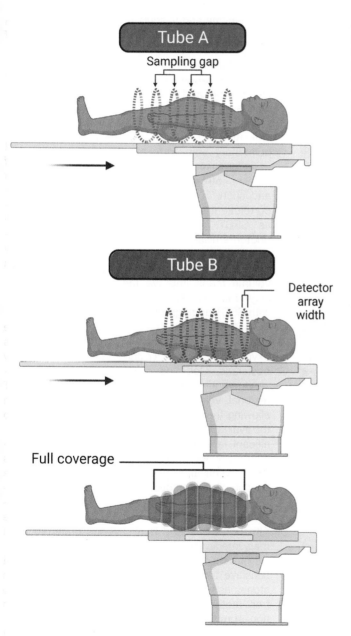

Fig. 5. Ultrahigh-pitch and dual-source systems. When a higher pitch is used, sampling gaps occur owing to incomplete 360° data sampling. Sampling gaps can be avoided in dual-source scans through simultaneous and independent data acquisition by each tube (tubes A and B), which are set to the same voltage. (Created with BioRender.com.)

transposition of great arteries)[34,35] and vascular (aortic coarctation, arteritis, and so forth) anomalies given its capacity for high-quality 3-dimensional (3D) reconstructions that permit a high-fidelity topographic depiction and facilitate surgical planning (**Fig. 6**).[36]

DECT material decomposition algorithms are instrumental in evaluating cardiac and vascular conditions. By using DECT spectral decomposition, high-quality bone-subtracted 3D vascular images can be generated to provide direct visualization and precise structural assessment of vasculature.[9] In addition, DECT-enabled iodine quantification and distribution assessments allow for evaluation of myocardial and lung perfusion and the identification of ischemic or hypoperfused areas.[35] DECT can provide simultaneous assessment of both systemic and pulmonary arterial systems, which is beneficial in the evaluation of congenital heart diseases associated with

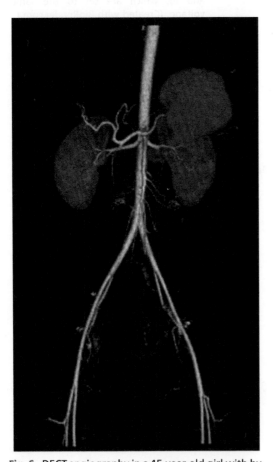

Fig. 6. DECT angiography in a 15-year-old girl with hypertension. Coronal angiogram with automated bone subtraction allows for better characterization of the abdominal aorta and its branches. The study showed no vascular abnormality.

abnormal pulmonary arteries[9] (**Fig. 7**). For example, Zucker and colleagues[37] demonstrated the feasibility of chest DECT angiography as a successful alternative for preoperative planning in pulmonary artery reconstruction. This study showed that DECT-derived pulmonary perfused blood volume or iodine maps clearly depict regional deficits in lung perfusion and serve as a qualitative and quantitative prognostic biomarker that correlates with more severe pulmonary artery obstruction.[37]

Lung assessment

DECT enables a complete evaluation of the lung parenchyma and vasculature in a single acquisition, reducing radiation exposure compared with multiphase SECT. High-energy photon data provide detailed images of the lung and mediastinal structures, whereas low-energy data accurately estimate blood distribution within the lung parenchyma aiding in identification of perfusion defects.[38,39] Currently, the most common indication for chest DECT in children is suspected pulmonary embolism, although it can also be used for assessing pulmonary hypertension, pulmonary atresia, arteriovenous malformations, and such.[38,40] DECT has shown a satisfactory correlation with other imaging techniques, such as SECT, scintigraphy, and SPECT (single-photon emission computed tomography), in patients with pulmonary emboli (**Fig. 8**).[41] Several studies have shown that DECT perfusion blood volume maps improve the sensitivity of small segmental and subsegmental emboli compared with SECT angiography.[39,42]

Another potential use of DECT is ventilation assessment using a mixture of stable xenon and oxygen. In a study of 17 children with bronchiolitis obliterans, Goo and colleagues[20] showed that xenon ventilation DECT could accurately display regional ventilation defects on inspiratory CT, allowing the omission of an expiratory phase for the evaluation of air trapping. This resulted in a significant radiation dose reduction while providing high-resolution anatomic information. However, DECT ventilation assessment is not routinely used in clinical practice.[9,42]

Kidney stone characterization

Although ultrasound is usually the preferred primary imaging modality for suspected nephrolithiasis in children, noncontrast CT is the most sensitive technique to detect kidney or ureteral stones as well as possible complications derived from ureteral obstruction. In the pediatric population, common kidney stones include calcium oxalate and calcium phosphate, struvite, cysteine,

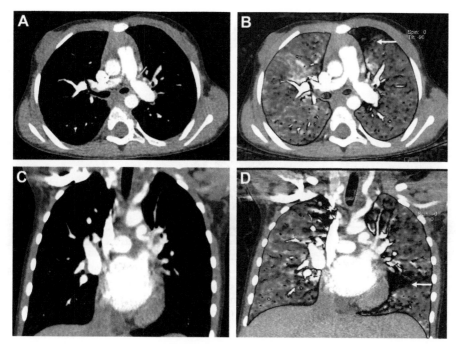

Fig. 7. DECT in a 3-year-old girl with a history of congenital left pulmonary artery stenosis. (*A*) Axial and (*C*) coronal blended contrast material–enhanced images showing severe stenosis of the left pulmonary artery (*yellow arrows*). (*B*) Axial and (*D*) coronal pulmonary blood volume showing heterogeneous perfusion of the right lung, with multiple parenchymal defects (*white arrows*). Qualitatively, there is hypoperfusion of the left lung compared with the right lung.

and uric acid.[9,43] Although a crude estimate of stone composition can be done from the stone CT attenuation values, there is significant overlap among different stone subtypes.[44] Accurately identifying and characterizing urinary stones is critical, as treatment regimens differ significantly based on the stone type, location, and size.[45]

One of the first applications of DECT in pediatric radiology was differentiating the chemical composition of urinary calculi (**Fig. 9**). Multiple studies

have demonstrated the value of DECT material decomposition algorithms to differentiate urinary stones composition accurately.[46] Through analysis of the radiograph attenuation profile of the predominant materials within urinary stones, the presence or absence of uric acid stones could be accurately elucidated.[45] With DSCT, non–uric acid stones can be further categorized into cystine, struvite, calcium oxalate, and hydroxyapatite stones by applying additional tin filtration to

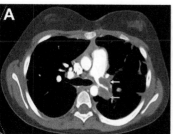
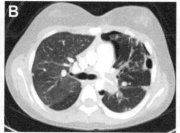
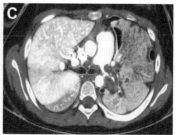

Fig. 8. Contrast-enhanced DECT in a 13-year-old girl with a previous history of metastatic osteosarcoma. (*A*) Axial blended images show a large partially occlusive thrombus at the origin of the left main pulmonary artery (*white arrow*) and a large hilar mass with soft tissue density and internal calcifications (*yellow arrow*). The mass appears contiguous with the central and left pulmonary arteries filling defect, suggestive of tumor thrombus. (*B*) Axial images in lung window showing a moderate left pneumothorax, likely secondary to bronchopleural fistula from metastatic disease (*yellow arrowheads*). (*C*) Perfusion blood volume images showing mismatched perfusion defects in the left lower lobe, left upper lobe, and right middle lobe.

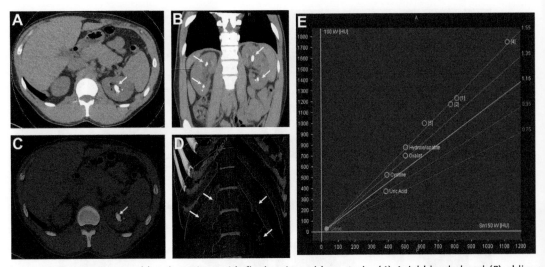

Fig. 9. DECT in an 18-year-old male patient with flank pain and hematuria. (*A*) Axial blended and (*B*) oblique maximum intensity pixel images show bilateral kidney stones (*arrows*), the largest measuring up to 17 mm. (*C*) Color-coded and (*D*) 3D postprocessed images using material decomposition algorithms show non–uric acid and calcium-containing composition. (*E*) Dual-energy ratio graph demonstrates that the kidney stones have attenuation values consistent with hydroxyapatite.

the high-energy radiograph beam.[9,47] One limitation is that material decomposition has limited utility in stones smaller than 3 mm.[45,48] However, this limitation may not be clinically relevant, as stones of this size usually pass spontaneously with conservative therapy alone.

Oncologic imaging

Children with cancer are at risk for high accumulative radiation doses, not only from inherent radiation associated with oncologic therapy but also from repeated cross-sectional imaging. Prolonged scanning times and short imaging intervals contribute to this radiation exposure. DECT can alleviate this issue by allowing for the characterization and staging of malignancies, treatment planning, and evaluation of therapy response with radiation doses less than SECT.[22,49,50]

Because of the slight attenuation differences between various soft tissues, SECT can have limited reliability in distinguishing benign lesions, active tumors, treated diseases, and healthy surrounding tissues (**Fig. 10**). DECT addresses this limitation by providing tissue-specific images and iodine concentration maps using material decomposition algorithms. By increasing iodine conspicuity as a surrogate for vascularity, iodine maps can assist in tumor characterization and staging[51] and increase the sensitivity for detecting small hypervascular lesions and distant metastases.

DECT has been used effectively for radiotherapy planning and offers unique benefits over

conventional SECT for this purpose.[52–54] To estimate the tissue absorbed dose, most radiation therapy systems convert the Hounsfield Units of CT into electron densities for photon therapy or proton stopping-power ratios for proton therapy.[17,55] However, this conversion may lead to errors, especially in estimating the electron densities, as tissues with equal or similar CT attenuations may have significantly different electron densities. In addition, as the proton stopping-power ratio strongly depends on the electron density per the Bethe formula, an accurate calculation is crucial to minimize the effects of uncertainty in the beam pathway.[17] By providing accurate spectral information, DECT allows for better tissue characterization for radiation therapy planning, and several studies have demonstrated that electron densities and proton stopping-power ratios can be estimated using DECT with excellent accuracy.[56,57]

Another advantage of DECT in pediatric radiation therapy is the possibility of acquiring VMI. Traditionally, radiation therapy planning required the acquisition of multiphase SECT with a pre-contrast acquisition for dose calculation and a contrast-enhanced acquisition to aid in tumor delineation. Unfortunately, contrast-enhanced SECT images often lead to erroneous calculations, as iodine distorts the native attenuation of tissues.[17,58] Ates and colleagues[17] identified DECT as a superior alternative, suggesting that radiotherapy miscalculations associated with contrast media, total study durations, and overall

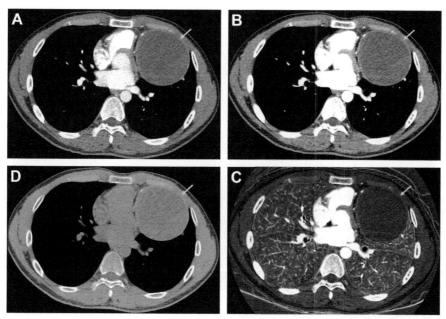

Fig. 10. Contrast-enhanced DECT in an 18-year-old male patient presenting with wheezing and cough. (*A*) Axial high-energy (140 kV), (*B*) low-monoenergetic, and (*C*) VUIs showing an indeterminate round, well-circumscribed mass with attenuation greater than simple fluid within the left mid to lower anterior thoracic cavity (*yellow arrow*). (*D*) Iodine maps suggest absent enhancement, most consistent with a benign mass, such as a congenital unilocular hemorrhagic or proteinaceous cystic lesion.

radiation doses could be significantly reduced with DECT.

Finally, DECT iodine-specific images may be a potential surrogate method for assessing treatment response and tumor viability.[49,51] Traditionally, tumor response has been based on serial examinations of tumor size. However, tumor size–based criteria may not accurately assess antineoplastic response in the era of immunotherapy and antiangiogenics, as these therapies may not cause dramatic changes in tumor volume.[22] DECT-based iodine assessment can improve treatment response assessment by characterizing lesion vascularity.[59] Successful antineoplastic therapy reduces tumor perfusion and thus intralesional iodine content on contrast-enhanced imaging, which can be effectively evaluated with DECT-generated iodine maps.[60,61] In addition, material decomposition algorithms can differentiate treatment-associated fibrosis from viable residual tumors, further aiding in tumor response assessment.[9]

Gastrointestinal applications

DECT is valuable in evaluating disease activity and detecting complications in patients with inflammatory bowel diseases (IBD). DECT provides the same information as traditional SECT enterography in IBD evaluation, including disease location and extension, evaluation of mucosal enhancement, fat stranding, and abscess presence. However, DECT enterography enhances IBD evaluation with iodine maps, which offer improved disease characterization.[62,63] As a surrogate marker and objective index of tissue perfusion and inflammation, iodine concentration and distribution help to characterize disease activity by detecting differences in bowel-wall perfusion.[62,63] For example, Lee and colleagues[64] discovered that small changes in bowel-wall iodine distribution related to active Crohn disease were most conspicuous on low-energy (40 keV) VMI. In this study, DECT improves the sensitivity and negative predictive value of active disease compared with conventional polychromatic images.

Growing evidence supports that DECT low-energy VMI (40–50 keV) and iodine maps may improve the assessment and stratification of appendicitis. Iodine maps can increase the conspicuity of subtle bowel-wall enhancement alterations that might otherwise be difficult to visualize using SECT.[65,66] In early nonperforated appendicitis, DECT shows increased transmural iodine content representing wall hyperemia and inflammation.[67] On the other hand, in later appendicitis stages, there is a focal or diffuse loss of bowel-wall enhancement and absence of transmural iodine.[67]

DUAL-ENERGY COMPUTED TOMOGRAPHY FUTURE DIRECTIONS: PHOTON-COUNTING COMPUTED TOMOGRAPHY SYSTEMS

Unlike traditional CT scanners that measure and integrate the total energy deposited during a measurement interval, photon counting (PC) detectors can register the interactions of individual photons and count their exact number and energy levels individually.[68] The simultaneous acquisition of individual photons in different energies allows for spectrally resolved measurements and material decomposition. This simultaneous acquisition could allow for DECT capabilities, including the acquisition of VMIs and iodine maps, to be easily computed in any study, removing the need to select patients prospectively. The smaller size and higher surface area of PC detectors compared with standard energy-integrating detectors also significantly improve spatial resolution.[68,69]

Several PC-CT applications are particularly advantageous to pediatric patients.[69] The improved spatial resolution and contrast-to-noise ratio allow for better basal image quality and significantly lower image noise, facilitating further dose reductions. PC systems can either improve spatial resolution at an equivalent radiation dose and image noise to traditional scanners, or lower radiation doses while maintaining equivalent spatial resolution and noise. It is estimated that PC-CT could reduce radiation doses by approximately 30% to 60%, depending on the imaging protocol and clinical question.[68,70] Although the benefits of PC are exciting, this technology is not yet widely adopted in clinical practice, and further research is needed to validate its potential benefits in pediatric radiology.

SUMMARY

DECT imaging is an excellent approach for acquiring fast, high-quality images while maintaining ALARA (as low as reasonably achievable) radiation doses in children. It exploits the properties of both high- and low-energy scans, generating spectrally resolved images, which, in combination with state-of-the-art postprocessing algorithms, have resulted in novel and exciting pediatric radiology applications. Image optimization and material decomposition algorithms allow for detailed characterization of tissues while concurrently shortening the examination time and reducing the radiation dose. Further advancements in data processing, as well as the ongoing development of PC scanners, will lead to further improvements in image quality, scanning times, and radiation doses.

CLINICS CARE POINTS

- Dual-energy computed tomography scanners acquire 2 sets of data at different energy levels, allowing for better material characterization and unique image reconstructions, while maintaining as low as reasonably achievable radiation doses.

- Dual-energy computed tomography Image optimization algorithms leverage the image properties of high- and low-energy acquisitions to improve image contrast and iodine conspicuity and mitigate the impact of metal artifacts.

- Material decomposition algorithms elucidate the concentration and distribution of different materials in the body based on their attenuation characteristics, allowing for the generation of virtual unenhanced images, iodine maps, and iodine overlay images.

- Dual-energy computed tomography pediatric applications are far-reaching, extending into thoracic, cardiovascular, urologic, oncologic, and gastrointestinal imaging.

- Pediatric dual-energy computed tomography can reduce radiation doses, accelerate image acquisition, and improve motion robustness when compared with traditional single-energy computed tomography.

DISCLOSURE

The authors have nothing to disclose.

REFERENCES

1. Miglioretti DL, Johnson E, Williams A, et al. The use of computed tomography in pediatrics and the associated radiation exposure and estimated cancer risk. JAMA Pediatr 2013;167(8):700.
2. Gottumukkala Rv, Kalra MK, Tabari A, et al. Advanced CT techniques for decreasing radiation dose, reducing sedation requirements, and optimizing image quality in children. Radiographics 2019;39(3):709–26.
3. Gallo-Bernal S, Bedoya MA, Gee MS, et al. Pediatric magnetic resonance imaging: faster is better. Pediatr Radiol 2022. https://doi.org/10.1007/s00247-022-05529-x.
4. Paterson N, Waterhouse P. Risk in pediatric anesthesia. Paediatr Anaesth 2011;21(8):848–57.
5. Andropoulos DB, Greene MF. Anesthesia and developing brains - implications of the FDA warning. N Engl J Med 2017;376(10):905–7.

6. Flick RP, Katusic SK, Colligan RC, et al. Cognitive and behavioral outcomes after early exposure to anesthesia and surgery. Pediatrics 2011;128(5): e1053–61.

7. Odedra D, Narayanasamy S, Sabongui S, et al. Dual energy CT physics—a primer for the emergency radiologist. Frontiers in Radiology 2022;2. https://doi.org/10.3389/fradi.2022.820430.

8. Johnson TRC. Dual-energy CT: general principles. Am J Roentgenol 2012;199(5_supplement):S3–8.

9. Siegel MJ, Ramirez-Giraldo JC. Dual-energy CT in children: imaging algorithms and clinical applications. Radiology 2019;291(2):286–97.

10. Tabari A, Gee MS, Singh R, et al. Reducing radiation dose and contrast medium volume with application of dual-energy CT in children and young adults. Am J Roentgenol 2020;214(6):1199–205.

11. Mileto A, Ananthakrishnan L, Morgan DE, et al. Clinical implementation of dual-energy CT for gastrointestinal imaging. Am J Roentgenol 2021;217(3). https://doi.org/10.2214/AJR.20.25093.

12. Nair JR, Burrows C, Jerome S, et al. Dual energy CT: a step ahead in brain and spine imaging. Br J Radiol 2020;93(1109).

13. Forghani R, de Man B, Gupta R. Dual-energy computed tomography. Neuroimaging Clin N Am 2017;27(3). https://doi.org/10.1016/j.nic.2017.03.002.

14. Albrecht MH, Vogl TJ, Martin SS, et al. Review of clinical applications for virtual monoenergetic dual-energy CT. Radiology 2019;293(2):260 71.

15. Yu L, Christner JA, Leng S, et al. Virtual monochromatic imaging in dual-source dual-energy CT: Radiation dose and image quality. Med Phys 2011; 38(12). https://doi.org/10.1118/1.3658568.

16. Kim TM, Choi YH, Cheon JE, et al. Optimal kiloelectron volt for noise-optimized virtual monoenergetic images of dual-energy pediatric abdominopelvic computed tomography: preliminary results. Korean J Radiol 2019;20(2). https://doi.org/10.3348/kjr.2017.0507.

17. Ates O, ho Hua C, Zhao L, et al. Feasibility of using post-contrast dual-energy CT for pediatric radiation treatment planning and dose calculation. Br J Radiol 2021;94(1118). https://doi.org/10.1259/bjr.20200170.

18. Bamberg F, Dierks A, Nikolaou K, et al. Metal artifact reduction by dual energy computed tomography using monoenergetic extrapolation. Eur Radiol 2011; 21(7). https://doi.org/10.1007/s00330-011-2062-1.

19. Kim C, Kim D, Lee KY, et al. The optimal energy level of virtual monochromatic images from spectral CT for reducing beam-hardening artifacts due to contrast media in the thorax. Am J Roentgenol 2018;211(3). https://doi.org/10.2214/AJR.17.19377.

20. Goo HW, Yang DH, Hong SJ, et al. Xenon ventilation CT using dual-source and dual-energy technique in children with bronchiolitis obliterans: correlation of xenon and CT density values with pulmonary function test results. Pediatr Radiol 2010;40(9). https://doi.org/10.1007/s00247-010-1645-3.

21. Meyer M, Nelson RC, Vernuccio F, et al. Virtual unenhanced images at dual-energy CT: influence on renal lesion characterization. Radiology 2019; 291(2). https://doi.org/10.1148/radiol.2019181100.

22. Siegel MJ, Bhalla S, Cullinane M. Dual-energy CT material decomposition in pediatric thoracic oncology. Radiol Imaging Cancer 2021;3(1). https://doi.org/10.1148/rycan.2021200097.

23. Siegel MJ, Curtis WA, Ramirez-Giraldo JC. Effects of dual-energy technique on radiation exposure and image quality in pediatric body CT. Am J Roentgenol 2016;207(4):826–35.

24. Primak AN, Giraldo JCR, Eusemann CD, et al. Dual-source dual-energy CT with additional tin filtration: dose and image quality evaluation in phantoms and in vivo. Am J Roentgenol 2010;195(5). https://doi.org/10.2214/AJR.09.3956.

25. Siegel MJ, Mhlanga JC, Salter A, et al. Comparison of radiation dose and image quality between contrast-enhanced single- and dual-energy abdominopelvic computed tomography in children as a function of patient size. Pediatr Radiol 2021;51(11): 2000–8.

26. Leyendecker P, Faucher V, Labani A, et al. Prospective evaluation of ultra-low-dose contrast-enhanced 100-kV abdominal computed tomography with tin filter: effect on radiation dose reduction and image quality with a third-generation dual-source CT system. Eur Radiol 2019;29(4):2107–16.

27. Nagayama Y, Oda S, Nakaura T, et al. Radiation dose reduction at pediatric CT: use of low tube voltage and iterative reconstruction. Radiographics 2018;38(5):1421–40.

28. Yu L, Bruesewitz MR, Thomas KB, et al. Optimal tube potential for radiation dose reduction in pediatric CT: principles, clinical implementations, and pitfalls. Radiographics 2011;31(3):835–48.

29. Sigal-Cinqualbre AB, Hennequin R, Abada HT, et al. Low-Kilovoltage multi–detector row chest CT in adults: feasibility and effect on image quality and iodine dose. Radiology 2004;231(1):169–74.

30. Nakayama Y, Awai K, Funama Y, et al. Abdominal CT with low tube voltage: Preliminary observations about radiation dose, contrast enhancement, image quality, and noise. Radiology 2005;237(3):945–51.

31. Bodelle B, Fischbach C, Booz C, et al. Free-breathing high-pitch 80 kVp dual-source computed tomography of the pediatric chest: Image quality, presence of motion artifacts and radiation dose. Eur J Radiol 2017;89. https://doi.org/10.1016/j.ejrad.2017.01.027.

32. Tabari A, Patino M, Westra SJ, et al. Initial clinical experience with high-pitch dual-source CT as a rapid technique for thoraco-abdominal evaluation in awake

infants and young children. Clin Radiol 2019;74(12). https://doi.org/10.1016/j.crad.2019.08.021.

33. Goo HW. State-of-the-Art CT imaging techniques for congenital heart disease. Korean J Radiol 2010; 11(1):4.

34. Godoy MCB, Naidich DP, Marchiori E, et al. Basic principles and postprocessing techniques of dual-energy CT: illustrated by selected congenital abnormalities of the thorax. J Thorac Imaging 2009;24(2): 152–9.

35. Schicchi N, Fogante M, Esposto Pirani P, et al. Third-generation dual-source dual-energy CT in pediatric congenital heart disease patients: state-of-the-art. Radiol Med 2019;124(12). https://doi.org/10.1007/s11547-019-01097-7.

36. Schulz B, Kuehling K, Kromen W, et al. Automatic bone removal technique in whole-body dual-energy CT angiography: performance and image quality. Am J Roentgenol 2012;199(5). https://doi.org/10.2214/AJR.12.9176.

37. Zucker EJ, Kino A, Schmiedeskamp H, et al. Feasibility and utility of dual-energy chest CTA for preoperative planning in pediatric pulmonary artery reconstruction. Int J Cardiovasc Imaging 2019; 35(8). https://doi.org/10.1007/s10554-019-01602-z.

38. Lu GM, Zhao Y, Zhang LJ, et al. Dual-energy CT of the lung. Am J Roentgenol 2012;199(5_supplement):S40–53.

39. Weidman EK, Plodkowski AJ, Halpenny DF, et al. Dual-energy CT angiography for detection of pulmonary emboli: incremental benefit of iodine maps. Radiology 2018;289(2):546–53.

40. Goo HW. Initial experience of dual-energy lung perfusion CT using a dual-source CT system in children. Pediatr Radiol 2010;40(9):1536–44.

41. Thieme SF, Becker CR, Hacker M, et al. Dual energy CT for the assessment of lung perfusion—Correlation to scintigraphy. Eur J Radiol 2008;68(3). https://doi.org/10.1016/j.ejrad.2008.07.031.

42. Goo HW. Dual-energy lung perfusion and ventilation CT in children. Pediatr Radiol 2013;43(3). https://doi.org/10.1007/s00247-012-2465-4.

43. Karmazyn B, Frush DP, Applegate KE, et al. CT with a computer-simulated dose reduction technique for detection of pediatric nephroureterolithiasis: comparison of standard and reduced radiation doses. Am J Roentgenol 2009;192(1):143–9.

44. Weisenthal K, Karthik P, Shaw M, et al. Evaluation of kidney stones with reduced–radiation dose CT: progress from 2011–2012 to 2015–2016—Not There Yet. Radiology 2018;286(2):581–9.

45. Park J, Chandarana H, Macari M, et al. Dual-energy computed tomography applications in uroradiology. Curr Urol Rep 2012;13(1). https://doi.org/10.1007/s11934-011-0226-9.

46. McCollough CH, Leng S, Yu L, et al. Dual- and multi-energy CT: principles, technical approaches, and clinical applications. Radiology 2015;276(3). https://doi.org/10.1148/radiol.2015142631.

47. Leng S, Huang A, Cardona JM, et al. Dual-energy CT for quantification of urinary stone composition in mixed stones: a phantom study. Am J Roentgenol 2016;207(2). https://doi.org/10.2214/AJR.15.15692.

48. Kaza RK, Ananthakrishnan L, Kambadakone A, et al. Update of dual-energy CT applications in the genitourinary tract. Am J Roentgenol 2017;208(6). https://doi.org/10.2214/AJR.16.17742.

49. Agrawal MD, Pinho DF, Kulkarni NM, et al. Oncologic applications of dual-energy CT in the abdomen. Radiographics 2014;34(3). https://doi.org/10.1148/rg.343135041.

50. Simons D, Kachelrieß M, Schlemmer HP. Recent developments of dual-energy CT in oncology. Eur Radiol 2014;24(4). https://doi.org/10.1007/s00330-013-3087-4.

51. de Cecco CN, Darnell A, Rengo M, et al. Dual-energy CT: Oncologic applications. Am J Roentgenol 2012;199(5_supplement). https://doi.org/10.2214/AJR.12.9207.

52. ho Hua C, Shapira N, Merchant TE, et al. Accuracy of electron density, effective atomic number, and iodine concentration determination with a dual-layer dual-energy computed tomography system. Med Phys 2018;45(6). https://doi.org/10.1002/mp.12903.

53. Kamps SE, Otjen JP, Stanescu AL, et al. Dual-energy CT of pediatric abdominal oncology imaging: private tour of new applications of CT technology. Am J Roentgenol 2020;214(5). https://doi.org/10.2214/AJR.19.22242.

54. Noid G, Zhu J, Tai A, et al. Improving structure delineation for radiation therapy planning using dual-energy CT. Front Oncol 2020;10. https://doi.org/10.3389/fonc.2020.01694.

55. van Elmpt W, Landry G, Das M, et al. Dual energy CT in radiotherapy: current applications and future outlook. Radiother Oncol 2016;119(1). https://doi.org/10.1016/j.radonc.2016.02.026.

56. Xie Y, Ainsley C, Yin L, et al. Ex vivo validation of a stoichiometric dual energy CT proton stopping power ratio calibration. Phys Med Biol 2018;63(5). https://doi.org/10.1088/1361-6560/aaae91.

57. Bär E, Lalonde A, Royle G, et al. The potential of dual-energy CT to reduce proton beam range uncertainties. Med Phys 2017;44(6). https://doi.org/10.1002/mp.12215.

58. Lalonde A, Xie Y, Burgdorf B, et al. Influence of intravenous contrast agent on dose calculation in proton therapy using dual energy CT. Phys Med Biol 2019; 64(12). https://doi.org/10.1088/1361-6560/ab1e9d.

59. Liang H, Zhou Y, Zheng Q, et al. Dual-energy CT with virtual monoenergetic images and iodine maps improves tumor conspicuity in patients with pancreatic ductal adenocarcinoma. Insights Imaging 2022; 13(1). https://doi.org/10.1186/s13244-022-01297-2.

60. Lee SH, Lee JM, Kim KW, et al. Dual-energy computed tomography to assess tumor response to hepatic radiofrequency ablation. Invest Radiol 2011;46(2). https://doi.org/10.1097/RLI.0b013e3181 f23fcd.

61. Wei X, Cao R, Li H, et al. Dual-energy CT iodine map in predicting the efficacy of neoadjuvant chemotherapy for hypopharyngeal carcinoma: a preliminary study. Sci Rep 2022;12(1). https://doi.org/10.1038/s41598-022-25828-5.

62. de Kock I, Delrue L, Lecluyse C, et al. Feasibility study using iodine quantification on dual-energy CT enterography to distinguish normal small bowel from active inflammatory Crohn's disease. Acta radiol 2019;60(6). https://doi.org/10.1177/028418511 8799508.

63. Singh R, Rai R, Mroueh N, et al. Role of dual energy computed tomography in inflammatory bowel disease. Seminars Ultrasound, CT MRI 2022;43(4). https://doi.org/10.1053/j.sult.2022.03.008.

64. Lee SM, Kim SH, Ahn SJ, et al. Virtual monoenergetic dual-layer, dual-energy CT enterography: optimization of keV settings and its added value for Crohn's disease. Eur Radiol 2018;28(6):2525–34. https://doi.org/10.1007/s00330-017-5215-z.

65. Lev-Cohain N, Sosna J, Meir Y, et al. Dual energy CT in acute appendicitis: value of low mono-energy. Clin Imaging 2021;77. https://doi.org/10.1016/j.clinimag.2021.04.007.

66. Topel C, Onur MR, Akpinar E, et al. Low tube voltage increases the diagnostic performance of dual-energy computed tomography in patients with acute appendicitis. Diagn Interventional Radiol 2019;25(4). https://doi.org/10.5152/dir.2019.18567.

67. Murray N, Darras KE, Walstra FE, et al. Dual-energy CT in evaluation of the acute abdomen. Radiographics 2019;39(1). https://doi.org/10.1148/rg.2019180087.

68. Willemink MJ, Persson M, Pourmorteza A, et al. Photon-counting CT: technical principles and clinical prospects. Radiology 2018;289(2):293–312. https://doi.org/10.1148/radiol.2018172656.

69. Cao J, Bache S, Schwartz FR, et al. Pediatric applications of photon-counting detector CT. Am J Roentgenol 2022. https://doi.org/10.2214/AJR.22.28391.

70. Rajendran K, Petersilka M, Henning A, et al. First clinical photon-counting detector CT System: technical evaluation. Radiology 2022;303(1). https://doi.org/10.1148/radiol.212579.

Leveraging Dual-Energy Computed Tomography to Improve Emergency Radiology Practice

Craig May, MD*, Aaron Sodickson, MD, PhD

KEYWORDS

- Dual-energy CT • Emergency radiology • Intracranial hemorrhage • Occult fracture • Cholelithiasis
- Pyelonephritis • Bowel ischemia • Gastrointestinal bleeding

KEY POINTS

Benefits of dual-energy computed tomography include

- Iodine identification to aid the detection of GI bleeding, bowel ischemia, and subtle perfusion defects of pyelonephritis.
- Characterization capabilities to differentiate calcium from hemorrhage in the brain, ingested bowel contents from contrast extravasation, intrinsically hyperattenuating from enhancing renal masses.
- Aid in identifying occult pathologies such as invisible gallstones or bone marrow edema in occult fractures.

In an era of overflowing emergency departments, tightening operating margins, surging demand for diagnostic imaging, and—as a result—ever-increasing caseloads placed on already-taxed emergency radiologists, it has become of utmost importance that radiology departments exploit every technical advantage possible to optimize accuracy and efficiency. Dual-energy computed tomography (DECT) is one such tool, offering an array of postprocessing algorithms that can improve lesion detection and differentiation and hasten diagnosis, all while sparing patients extraneous imaging studies and the costs inherent to them (Table 1).[1] This article uses a case-based approach to demonstrate indispensable applications of DECT in the emergency department (ED), the comparative advantages of dual-energy over conventional CT, and how DECT can be used to solve common diagnostic dilemmas encountered in the ED reading room.

CASE 1: IDENTIFYING INTRACRANIAL HEMORRHAGE

Non-contrast head CT is ubiquitous in the ED, ordered for patients with head trauma, altered mental status, or symptoms of stroke. Although many intra- and extra-axial bleeds are easily spotted, small hyperattenuating foci of calcium and hemorrhage are not easily differentiated, and volume averaging can obscure subtle hemorrhages, particularly subdural hematomas underlying the calvarium. Here, DECT can help.

Consider the case of an elderly woman with a history of prior stroke who presented to the emergency department after falling and striking her head on the sidewalk (Fig. 1). At the time of presentation, the patient's neurologic examination was nonfocal, but the extent of lacerations to her head and face suggested moderate blunt force

Department of Radiology, Brigham and Women's Hospital, 75 Francis Street, Boston, MA 02115, USA
* Corresponding author.
E-mail address: cdmay@bwh.harvard.edu

Radiol Clin N Am 61 (2023) 1085–1096
https://doi.org/10.1016/j.rcl.2023.06.003
0033-8389/23/© 2023 Elsevier Inc. All rights reserved.

Table 1
Details of commonly used dual-energy postprocessed series

Applicable Protocols	Postprocessing Algorithm	Output Image Series	Imaging Planes	Thickness × Internal	Relevant Case
Non-contrast head	Bone removal	Bone-subtracted calvarium	Axial and coronal	3 × 2 mm	Case 1
	Calcium three-material decomposition (** Not FDA-approved)	Calcium overlay Virtual non-calcium	Axial	3 × 3 mm	
Contrast-enhanced abdomen/pelvis (including computed tomography angiogram [CTA])	Iodine three-material decomposition	Iodine overlay Virtual non-contrast	Axial and coronal	3 × 2 mm	Cases 2–7
	Virtual monoenergetic	50 keV	Axial	1.5 × 1 mm	Case 5
All musculoskeletal (MSK) protocols (and trauma spine reformats)	Calcium three-material decomposition	Bone marrow edema overlay after trabecular bone subtraction	Axial, coronal, and sagittal	3 × 2 mm	Case 8

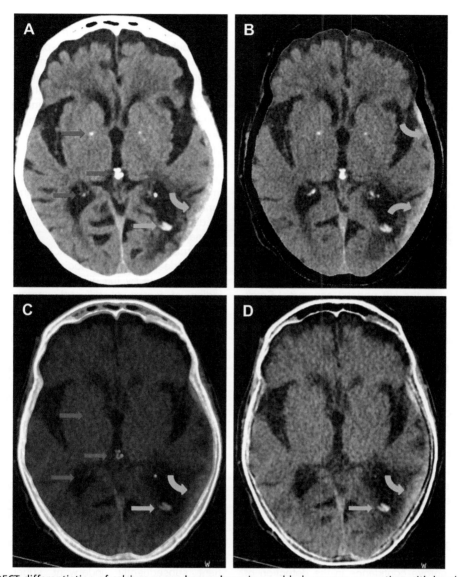

Fig. 1. DECT differentiation of calcium versus hemorrhage in an elderly woman presenting with head trauma. Conventional image (*A*) demonstrates multiple hyperattenuating foci in the choroid plexus, the pineal gland, the basal ganglia (*red arrows*), and in the occipital horn of the left lateral ventricle (*blue arrow*). There is also a subdural hematoma along the left temporoparietal convexity (*curved blue arrow*). Bone-subtraction images (*B*) remove the confounding attenuation of the calvarium, improving visualization of the full extent of the underlying subdural hematoma (*curved blue arrows*), as compared with the conventional image (*A*). Calcific foci (*red arrows*) appear orange on the color-coded calcium overlay image (*C*) and disappear on the virtual noncalcium (VNCa) image (*D*). In contrast, areas of hemorrhage (*blue arrows*) do not color-code on the calcium overlay image (*C*) and persist on the VNCa image (*D*).

injury. As such, head CT was obtained to assess possible intracranial hemorrhage.

The conventional CT image demonstrates, in addition to parieto-occipital encephalomalacia from her prior stroke, multiple hyperattenuating foci. Experience tells us that the choroid plexus, pineal, and basal ganglia foci likely represent calcification. However, does the intraventricular focus

in the occipital horn represent additional choroid plexus calcification or blood products, putting the patient at risk for hydrocephalus? Such unanswered questions are a source of much consternation for patients and providers alike. Enter dual-energy CT.

Dual-energy acquisition affords us three-material decomposition postprocessing algorithms that quantify the relative contributions of characteristic constituent materials—most commonly iodine or calcium—to the attenuation of each voxel. In head trauma, three-material decomposition can be used to separate each voxel into its constituent calcium and non-calcium components.[2–4] Calcium overlay images can be created that superimpose color-coded calcium content on the top of gray scale virtual non-calcium (VNCa) content in a manner akin to PET/CT fusion images. Doing so helps differentiate hyperattenuation related to calcium from that of hemorrhage: Calcium is displayed in color on the overlay images but disappears on the VNCa images, whereas hemorrhage remains uncolored on the overlay images and persists on the VNCa images.[2,3,5,6] Returning to Fig. 1, the occipital horn density is clearly intraventricular hemorrhage.

There is also the matter of the subdural hematoma overlying the left parietal convexity. Small subdural hematomas can be easily missed on conventional images immediately subjacent to the overlying dense calvarium. DECT bone subtraction algorithms are tuned to null the attenuation of cortical bone and can be used to improve detection and characterization of subdural hematomas (or other lesions immediately adjacent to bone), as demonstrated in Fig. 1.[3,6]

Fully automated DECT postprocessing at our institution sends the most useful postprocessed series to PACS—including axial calcium overlay and matching VNCa images and axial and coronal plane bone subtraction images—with every noncontrast head CT. As such, these additional image series are available when needed without any additional technologist or radiologist postprocessing effort. When required, they allow for rapid differentiation of hemorrhage from calcification and improve confidence in the detection of challenging small subdural hematomas.

CASES 2 AND 3: GASTROINTESTINAL BLEEDING: DIFFERENTIATING BLOOD FROM BISMUTH

Similar functionality can be used to aid assessment of active gastrointestinal bleeding (GIB). Conventional protocols intended to assess for GIB most commonly use non-contrast, angiographic, and delayed venous phase scans. Active arterial GIB manifests as contrast extravasation within the bowel lumen that is absent on the non-contrast phase, appears on the arterial phase, and grows in volume and changes in morphology on the venous phase. Evaluation relies on careful comparison between scan phases to identify the typical behavior of ongoing intraluminal bleeding. DECT

simplifies evaluation, facilitating identification of intraluminal iodine based on its characteristic DECT behavior, even on a single-phase scan.

The presentation of an elderly individual with a history of diverticulitis neatly illustrates this capability (Fig. 2). This patient came to the emergency department with two episodes of abnormally dark-colored stool followed by increasingly frequent bowel movements accompanied by bright red blood per rectum. Given the suspicion of ongoing lower gastrointestinal (GI) bleeding, a CT angiogram was performed. Conventional arterial phase imaging shows intraluminal hyperattenuating material in the distal transverse colon that expands on delayed phase imaging, diagnostic of an active arterial bleed.

Alternatively, one can exploit DECTs three-material decomposition of iodine to aid diagnosis. Made possible by the differential attenuation by iodine of x-rays of different energies, three-material decomposition segregates each voxel's attenuation into the quantity of iodine and non-iodine components that would account for the observed x-ray attenuation at low and high energies. This iodine content can be artificially removed to create a virtual non-contrast (VNC) image or can be highlighted in an iodine overlay image that displays the iodine content in color, superimposed on the gray scale VNC image.[1,7,8] Using these techniques, the intraluminal hyperattenuating focus in this case is definitively characterized as iodine from a single post-contrast scan, because it color-codes on the iodine overlay image and disappears from the VNC image.[1,9] In our practice, not only does use of these DECT images speed interpretation but creation of VNC images also obviates the need for a true non-contrast scan phase, reducing radiation exposure. This patient subsequently underwent super-selective mesenteric angiography and embolization of the middle colic branch of the superior mesenteric artery (SMA).

As a counterpoint, consider the case of a 52-year-old patient with a history of gastric adenocarcinoma and gastric bypass who presented with worsening abdominal pain and severe anemia (Fig. 3). In this patient, a routine portal venous phase CT scan in the ED demonstrated hyperattenuating material adjacent to the jejuno-jejunal anastomosis. From a single post-contrast scan phase, it is typically not possible to determine whether intraluminal hyperattenuation indicates GI bleeding or ingested material. The inherent ability of DECT to definitively characterize iodine content comes to the rescue in this scenario. On the iodine overlay image, the intraluminal hyperattenuating focus does not color-code as iodine; on VNC

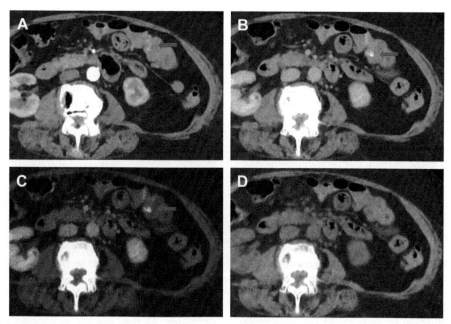

Fig. 2. Multiphase contrast-enhanced CT angiogram in a patient presenting with melena and hematochezia. The conventional arterial phase image (*A*) shows a serpiginous hyperattenuating intraluminal focus within the transverse colon (*red arrow*), which expands on the venous phase conventional image (*B*), as expected for active contrast extravasation. Dual-energy postprocessing of the venous phase demonstrates that this iodine content color codes as orange on the iodine overlay image (*C*) and disappears on the virtual non-contrast (VNC) image (*D*).

images, the focus persists. It is thus proven not to represent iodine content, ruling out active GIB. Instead, one can confidently ascribe the finding to ingested material without the need for additional multiphasic imaging, saving the patient from diagnostic uncertainty, and with it the potential for further imaging and radiation exposure.[8,9]

For these reasons, as part of every contrast-enhanced abdominal CT, we routinely send axial and coronal plane iodine overlay images and

matching VNC images. Postprocessing is fully automated, making these images available for problem-solving when needed, without adding workflow burden to our busy technologists or radiologists.

CASE 4: BOWEL: DEAD OR ALIVE?

DECT can facilitate diagnosing other subtle intestinal abnormalities such as ischemia that might otherwise be clinically challenging or take time to

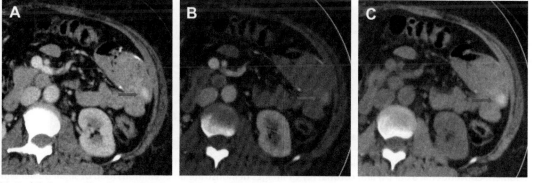

Fig. 3. (*A*) Conventional portal venous phase contrast-enhanced CT in a patient with a history of gastric adenocarcinoma and bypass with severe anemia. An intraluminal hyperattenuating focus (*red arrow*) is seen adjacent to the jejuno-jejunal anastomosis, raising suspicion for active GI bleeding. However, dual-energy postprocessing demonstrates that this focus does not in fact contain any color-coded iodine content on the iodine overlay image (*B*) and persists on the VNC image (*C*), conclusively ruling out iodine content from a single-phase post-contrast scan. This instead represents ingested material, with a characteristic appearance of ingested bismuth.

manifest on conventional imaging when time is of the essence. Time is bowel, after all. This capability is aptly illustrated in the case of an 84-year-old gentleman on Eliquis who presented with diffuse abdominal pain and a tympanitic abdomen, where the use of DECT almost certainly decreased the latency between presentation and surgery (**Fig. 4**).

Here, conventional CT imaging demonstrates an edematous small bowel loop with associated mesenteric engorgement, but no compelling findings of bowel ischemia/infarction: There is no pneumatosis, portal venous gas, or evidence of perforation. One would be hard pressed to convince a surgeon that the offending loop of small bowel shows differential hypoenhancement to suggest diminished perfusion. On conventional imaging, bowel wall hypoenhancement can be masked by mural hemorrhage, as may be found in ischemic bowel (especially in patients who are anticoagulated as this one was). Alone, a small bowel obstruction or ileus could be expectantly managed given its propensity to spontaneously

resolve with decompression and bowel rest.[10,11] To do so in those with unrecognized ischemic bowel, however, risks perforation that can be life-threatening, particularly in an elderly individual.

Dual-energy iodine images once again prove decisive. The bowel loop in question contains no colored iodine content in its walls, in contrast to adjacent avidly enhancing bowel loops, indicating focal bowel ischemia, possibly secondary to distal branch mesenteric embolus.[9,12] A finding that was at best indeterminate on conventional CT becomes unequivocally emergent with dual-energy. Subsequently at surgery, this patient had 20 cm of infarcted small bowel resected. In this capacity, dual-energy facilitates identification of malperfused bowel and reduces potential ischemic time. In doing so, it may also reduce the risk of complication in addition to the length (and cost) of the patient's hospital stay.[1] Our surgery colleagues frequently request that we review the iodine DECT images with them in cases of bowel pathology, as they quickly recognized its clinical added value after our implementation.

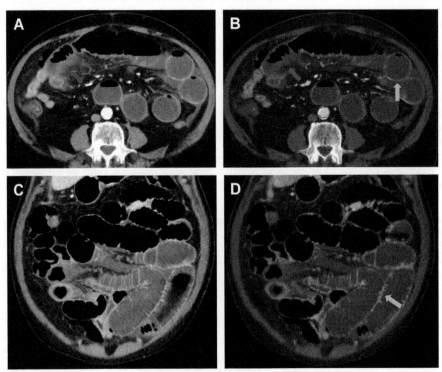

Fig. 4. Ischemic bowel in an 84-year-old gentleman who presented with diffuse abdominal pain and a tympanitic abdomen. Conventional axial (*A*) and coronal (*C*) CT images demonstrate an edematous loop of small bowel with adjacent mesenteric engorgement (*red arrows*) in the right lower quadrant. There are no definitive secondary signs of bowel ischemia/infarction such as hypoattenuating bowel wall, pneumatosis, or perforation. Proximal small bowel loops are distended and fluid-filled. Dual-energy postprocessed iodine overlay images in the axial (*B*) and coronal (*D*) planes demonstrate focal absence of color-coded iodine content within a short segment of ischemic bowel (*red arrow*). In comparison, normal well-perfused loops contain uniform bowel wall enhancement (*green arrows*).

CASE 5: CHOLELITHIASIS: CLINICAL TRANSPARENCY THROUGH INCREASED (RADI)OPACITY

On conventional CT imaging, gallstones are inconsistently radiopaque, which means that many patients with abdominal pain may warrant further imaging—ultrasound (US), magnetic resonance cholangiopancreatography (MRCP), or endoscopic retrograde cholangiopancreatography (ERCP)—to guide management.[13] At a time when emergency departments and hospital systems are strapped for resources, any functionality that makes further testing redundant is a boon. As the case of a 64-year-old patient with a history of irritable bowel syndrome nicely illustrates (Fig. 5), DECT does just that.

Unable to eat and suffering from severe right upper quadrant pain and nausea for over a day, the patient presented for emergent care because her symptoms were atypical of her chronic irritable bowel syndrome. Conventional CT imaging demonstrates gallbladder distention, pericholecystic fluid, and fat stranding, suggesting cholecystitis as the likely etiology, but unsatisfyingly, does not identify culprit gallstones. In this scenario, additional testing (at additional cost, time, and resource utilization) is often performed, beginning with right upper quadrant ultrasound to identify stones.

On conventional CT, many gallstones (aside from those that are calcified) are isoattenuating or very close in attenuation to the surrounding bile, rendering them invisible. Noncalcified gallstones, however, typically consist of cholesterol that behaves similarly to fat on dual-energy scans, demonstrating decreased attenuation at low x-ray energy and increased attenuation at high x-ray energy, relative to the surrounding bile.[1,14] This behavior can be exploited to make noncalcified gallstones visible by using virtual monoenergetic images at low keV (stones dark relative to bile) or high keV (stones bright).[14,15] Alternatively, they can be readily visualized as bright on standard VNC images (whose image content is similar to that of high keV images) or as an iodine void on the associated iodine overlay images.

Using these tools here, multiple stones can be seen layering in the dependent gallbladder and impacted within the gallbladder neck. With the causative pathology identified, DECT obviates the need for additional imaging or further delay, permitting the team to move straight to treatment.

CASE 6: RENAL LESIONS: BENIGN OR WORRISOME?

Dual-energy holds great promise as a time- and cost-saving measure when characterizing unsuspected renal lesions.[16] On encountering an indeterminate renal mass on conventional CT, the emergency radiologist often has little choice but to recommend follow-up evaluation, typically with multiphase renal mass protocol CT or MR imaging. This can prove particularly vexing when faced with multiple lesions in patients with cancer. Take the example of a 73-year-old patient with a history of invasive ductal carcinoma and melanoma, and several renal lesions detected incidentally after a fall (Fig. 6). Conventional CT can readily characterize simple cysts based on their Hounsfield Unit attenuation. Renal masses with intermediate attenuation values, however, cannot be reliably characterized on single-phase post-contrast CT scans, as their increased attenuation may be due to either mass enhancement or intrinsically hyperattenuating proteinaceous or hemorrhagic contents within a complex cyst.

DECT is helpful in this situation, as it can differentiate hyperattenuation due to iodine from non-enhancing alternatives.[16] Iodine maps remain the key tool in this differentiation. True enhancing masses or mass components contain iodine content, demonstrable on iodine maps, which disappears on VNC images.[17–19] In contrast, the serous fluid within simple cysts and the hemorrhagic or proteinaceous content within complex hyperattenuating cysts contain no iodine content. These entities remain pure grey on iodine overlay images and appear unchanged on VNC images. In this case, the simple cyst and benign hyperattenuating complex cyst contain no demonstrable iodine content, whereas the complex cystic and solid mass shows heterogeneous iodine enhancement, making it highly suspicious for malignancy. Luckily for this patient, the lesion of concern was biopsied several weeks later with pathology returning as benign fibroadipose tissue. Regardless, DECTs ability to characterize iodine content from a single post-contrast scan in such cases may render further imaging workup unnecessary. Lesions with definitive iodine content require further intervention; those without, such as incidentally detected hyperattenuating cysts, need no further evaluation.[20] When used routinely to characterize incidental renal lesions, DECT has the potential to substantially reduce patient anxiety, downstream imaging utilization, and as a consequence, radiation exposure, time burden, cost, and resource allocation.[21]

CASE 7: PYELONEPHRITIS: INCREASING DIAGNOSTIC CONFIDENCE

Some common emergency department diagnoses may have conventional CT findings that are too

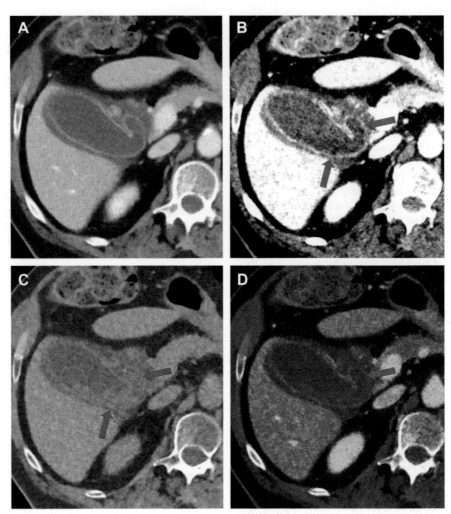

Fig. 5. Improved detection of noncalcified gallstones in a 64-year-old patient with right upper quadrant pain. Conventional axial CT image (*A*) demonstrates gallbladder distention, wall thickening with mucosal hyperemia, and pericholecystic fluid and fat-stranding, likely indicating cholecystitis. No gallstones are visible on conventional images. Axial virtual monochromatic 40 keV (*B*) and 140 keV (*C*) images demonstrate cholesterol gallstones layering within the gallbladder and within the gallbladder neck (*red arrows*), which appear dark at low keV and bright at high keV compared with the surrounding bile due to the characteristic DECT behavior of cholesterol. The iodine overlay image (*D*) nicely demonstrates the increased iodine content within the hyperemic gallbladder wall while displaying the stones as a grey void in the noise floor of the color overlay, because the underlying gray scale VNC image contains similar content to that of the high keV virtual monoenergetic image (*C*).

subtle to call, thus requiring "clinical" rather than radiological diagnosis. Consider the case of a 32-year-old woman who presented to the ED with fever/chills, hematuria, and lower back pain after being treated for presumptive urinary tract infection (UTI) 7 days prior (**Fig. 7**). The provider's index of suspicion for pyelonephritis was high, but conventional CT images appear near normal, aside from possible heterogeneity of the left renal cortex. A gambling radiologist might suggest a soft call of pyelonephritis based on these subtle findings and the clinic picture, but DECT turns this into a "slam dunk" imaging diagnosis.

DECT makes this possible by increasing conspicuity of subtle differences in iodine distribution that are challenging to detect against background parenchymal attenuation on conventional images.[20,22] In pyelonephritis, focal inflammatory infiltrates and edema hinder normal perfusion of the parenchyma by decreasing the perfusion pressure; this is the hypothesized pathophysiologic underpinning of the striated nephrogram.[23,24] DECT makes these foci of hypoperfusion more apparent, with low keV virtual monoenergetic images increasing the detection of focal renal inflammation by twofold.[25,26] Coronal iodine overlay images

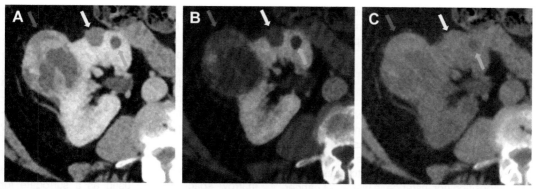

Fig. 6. Characterizing three renal lesions on a single-portal venous phase abdominal CT in a patient with a history of melanoma. Conventional CT (*A*) demonstrates three renal masses, not all of which could normally be characterized on a single-phase post-contrast scan. This can be accomplished though with the help of iodine overlay (*B*) and VNC (*C*) images. The smallest mass (*green arrows*) measures simple fluid attenuation on the conventional image, representing a simple cyst, and contains no color-coded iodine content. The largest mass (*red arrows*) contains heterogeneous soft tissue and cystic components, and is confirmed to be a heterogeneously enhancing mass due to the presence of color-coded iodine content that disappears on the VNC image. The remaining mass (*yellow arrows*) measures higher than simple fluid attenuation on the conventional image but is seen to contain no iodine content on the iodine overlay image, representing a benign hyperattenuating hemorrhagic or proteinaceous cyst.

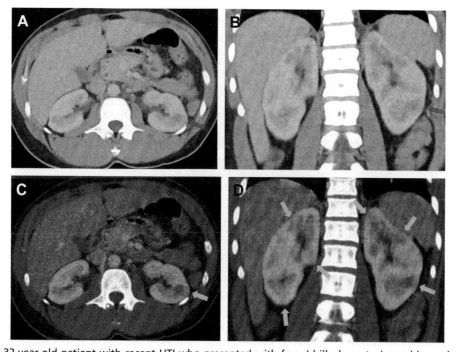

Fig. 7. A 32-year-old patient with recent UTI who presented with fever/chills, hematuria, and lower back pain. Axial (*A*) and coronal (*B*) conventional images demonstrate normal appearing corticomedullary differentiation, but possible subtle areas of decreased attenuation in the cortex of the left kidney (*red arrows*). Axial (*C*) and coronal (*D*) iodine overlay images reveal multiple regions of diminished renal cortical enhancement bilaterally (*blue arrows*), confirming pyelonephritis. The foci in the right kidney and the left upper pole are impossible to detect on the conventional images, even in retrospect.

also optimally highlight foci of cortical hypoperfusion, in this case demonstrating multiple foci in both kidneys, indicative of pyelonephritis.

CASE 8: OCCULT FRACTURES: STEALING MR IMAGINGS THUNDER

Occult fractures—those not typically visible on conventional radiographs or sometimes even CT—often require addition imaging to be detected. Without sufficient cause for suspicion such as unrelenting pain, inability to bear weight, or predisposition (for instance, a history of cancer, osteoporosis, or high-impact sports), it is all too easy in a bustling emergency room setting to forgo time- and resource-intensive MR imaging and attribute a patient's pain to muscular injury.

It is especially easy to miss a fracture diagnosis when the onset of pain is insidious and the patient denies direct trauma, as did this 79-year-old patient with a history of metastatic ovarian cancer, prior venous thromboembolism, and right hip pain for 1 week that began after awkwardly rolling into bed (**Fig. 8**). Neither radiographs nor conventional CT demonstrated a fracture line, cortical disruption, or osseous lesion to explain the presentation. So, with a history of atraumatic hip

pain and an unremarkable hip CT, should the workup end or proceed to MR imaging?

Once again, dual-energy postprocessing techniques allow the radiologist to extract additional information to guide management. In this application, three-material decomposition is used to remove the attenuation of the calcium content from the trabecular bone, leaving behind the attenuation of the underlying marrow space, which is increased by marrow space edema, hemorrhage, space occupying masses, or hematopoietic marrow.[1,6,8,27,28] An increase in the VNCa attenuation within the marrow space can be used as a surrogate for bone marrow edema on MR imaging.[27–30]

Returning to this case, the bone marrow edema overlay image clearly demonstrates asymmetrically increased marrow attenuation in the right femoral neck. Confirmatory MR imaging demonstrated a subtle fracture line, with short tau inversion recovery (STIR) images depicting marrow edema that mirrored the dual-energy edema overlay. With adequate experience in dual-energy bone marrow edema interpretation, the confirmatory MR imaging arguably becomes redundant in this scenario. Other uses of DECT marrow evaluation include identification of stress fractures and differentiation of acute from chronic vertebral compression

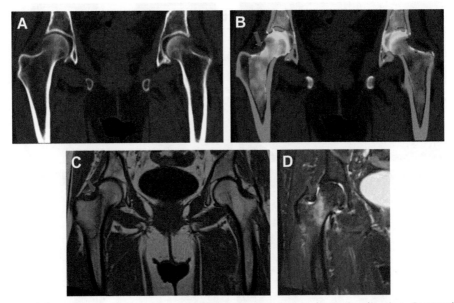

Fig. 8. Improved detection of occult fractures with DECT bone marrow edema visualization. Conventional coronal CT (*A*) in an elderly patient with right hip pain, without displaced fracture line. The bone marrow edema color overlay image (*B*) removes the attenuation of calcium from the trabecular bone and highlights the underlying marrow attenuation. Purple-encoded bone indicates typical fatty marrow as seen on the left, whereas green-encoding indicates increased marrow space attenuation from edema or hemorrhage, suggesting a non-displaced right femoral neck fracture (*red arrow*). Subsequent hip MR imaging demonstrates a T1 hypointense fracture of the right femoral neck extending into the intertrochanteric region (*C*). The STIR sequence (*D*) shows bone marrow edema in the femoral neck that mirrors the DECT bone marrow edema distribution.

fractures that might otherwise be relegated to an "age-indeterminate" characterization.

SUMMARY

In a host of applications in the emergency department, DECT affords the radiologist more information with which to make a diagnosis, without need for additional time or effort and may often reduce the need for downstream image utilization, radiation exposure, cost, and resource allocation. As demonstrated, be it through differentiating intracranial hyperattenuating foci, facilitating the identification of iodine content or detection of tissue perfusion defects, or highlighting otherwise occult pathologies, this technology can improve the certainty, accuracy, and speed of diagnosis. In doing so, not only does it make the life of a busy emergency radiologist a bit easier and more interesting, but it may also improve hospital efficiency and, more importantly, patient outcomes.

CLINICS CARE POINTS

- Postprocessing functions such as bone-subtraction and calcium overlay images aid in the identification of intracranial hemorrhage, specifically subdural hematoma and intraparenchymal hemorrhage, in patients with head trauma.

- Iodine overlay images and virtual non-contrast images have a wide range of beneficial applications in emergency imaging, including detection of active bleeding, characterizing incidental renal masses, and detection hypoperfusion in cases of bowel ischemia or pyelonephritis.

- Virtual monoenergetic images can be used to detect cholesterol gallstones that may otherwise be invisible on conventional CT in patients presenting with right upper quadrant pain concerning for biliary colic and/or cholecystitis.

- Bone marrow edema overlays can act as a surrogate for fluid-sensitive MR imaging sequences such as STIR and can help identify occult fractures.

DISCLOSURE

Dr A. Sodickson is PI of an institutional research grant from Siemens, USA on Dual Energy CT.

REFERENCES

1. Sodickson AD, Keraliya A, Czakowski B, et al. Dual energy CT in clinical routine: how it works and how it adds value. Emerg Radiol 2021;28(1):103–17.
2. Wiggins WF, Potter CA, Sodickson AD. Dual-energy CT to differentiate small foci of intracranial hemorrhage from calcium. Radiology 2020;294(1):129–38.
3. Potter CA, Sodickson AD. Dual-energy CT in emergency neuroimaging: added value and novel applications. Radiographics 2016;36(7):2186–98.
4. Tran NA, Sodickson AD, Gupta R, et al. Clinical applications of dual-energy computed tomography in neuroradiology. Semin Ultrasound CT MR 2022;43(4):280–92.
5. Hu R, Daftari Besheli L, Young J, et al. Dual-energy head CT enables accurate distinction of intraparenchymal hemorrhage from calcification in emergency department patients. Radiology 2016;280(1):177–83.
6. Yu HS, Keraliya A, Chakravarti S, et al. Multienergy computed tomography applications: trauma. Radiol Clin North Am 2023;61(1):23–35.
7. Wortman JR, Sodickson AD. Pearls, pitfalls, and problems in dual-energy computed tomography imaging of the body. Radiol Clin North Am 2018;56(4):625–40.
8. Wortman JR, Uyeda JW, Fulwadhva UP, et al. Dual-energy CT for abdominal and pelvic trauma. Radiographics 2018;38(2):586–602.
9. Fulwadhva UP, Wortman JR, Sodickson AD. Use of dual-energy CT and iodine maps in evaluation of bowel disease. Radiographics 2016;36(2):393–406.
10. Shinohara K, Asaba Y, Ishida T, et al. Nonoperative management without nasogastric tube decompression for adhesive small bowel obstruction. Am J Surg 2022;223(6):1179–82.
11. Aka AA, Wright JP, DeBeche-Adams T. Small bowel obstruction. Clin Colon Rectal Surg 2021;34(4):219–26.
12. Murray N, Darras KE, Walstra FE, et al. Dual-energy CT in evaluation of the acute abdomen. Radiographics 2019;39(1):264–86.
13. Bortoff GA, Chen MY, Ott DJ, et al. Gallbladder stones: imaging and intervention. Radiographics 2000;20(3):751–66.
14. Uyeda JW, Richardson IJ, Sodickson AD. Making the invisible visible: improving conspicuity of noncalcified gallstones using dual-energy CT. Abdom Radiol (NY) 2017;42(12):2933–9.
15. Ratanaprasatporn L, Uyeda JW, Wortman JR, et al. Multimodality imaging, including dual-energy CT, in the evaluation of gallbladder disease. Radiographics 2018;38(1):75–89.
16. Glomski SA, Wortman JR, Uyeda JW, et al. Dual energy CT for evaluation of polycystic kidneys: a multi reader study of interpretation time and diagnostic

confidence. Abdom Radiol (NY) 2018;43(12): 3418–24.

17. Brown CL, Hartman RP, Dzyubak OP, et al. Dual-energy CT iodine overlay technique for characterization of renal masses as cyst or solid: a phantom feasibility study. Eur Radiol 2009;19(5):1289–95.

18. Ascenti G, Mileto A, Krauss B, et al. Distinguishing enhancing from nonenhancing renal masses with dual-source dual-energy CT: iodine quantification versus standard enhancement measurements. Eur Radiol 2013;23(8):2288–95.

19. Chandarana H, Megibow AJ, Cohen BA, et al. Iodine quantification with dual-energy CT: phantom study and preliminary experience with renal masses. AJR Am J Roentgenol 2011;196(6):W693–700.

20. Wortman JR, Bunch PM, Fulwadhva UP, et al. Dual-energy CT of incidental findings in the abdomen: can we reduce the need for follow-up imaging? AJR Am J Roentgenol 2016;207(4):W58–68.

21. Wortman JR, Shyu JY, Fulwadhva UP, et al. Impact analysis of the routine use of dual-energy computed tomography for characterization of incidental renal lesions. J Comput Assist Tomogr 2019;43(2): 176–82.

22. Kaza RK, Ananthakrishnan L, Kambadakone A, et al. Update of dual-energy CT applications in the genitourinary tract. AJR Am J Roentgenol 2017; 208(6):1185–92.

23. Vrtiska TJ, Takahashi N, Fletcher JG, et al. Genitourinary applications of dual-energy CT. AJR Am J Roentgenol 2010;194(6):1434–42.

24. Wolin EA, Hartman DS, Olson JR. Nephrographic and pyelographic analysis of CT urography: principles, patterns, and pathophysiology. AJR Am J Roentgenol 2013;200(6):1210–4.

25. Saunders HS, Dyer RB, Shifrin RY, et al. The CT nephrogram: implications for evaluation of urinary tract disease. Radiographics 1995;15(5):1069–88.

26. Marron D, Nahum GS, Gili D, et al. Low monoenergetic DECT detection of pyelonephritis extent. Eur J Radiol 2021;142:109837.

27. Issa G, Mulligan M. Dual energy CT can aid in the emergent differentiation of acute traumatic and pathologic fractures of the pelvis and long bones. Emerg Radiol 2020;27(3):285–92.

28. Petritsch B, Kosmala A, Weng AM, et al. Vertebral Compression Fractures: Third-Generation Dual-Energy CT for Detection of Bone Marrow Edema at Visual and Quantitative Analyses. Radiology 2017;284(1):161–8.

29. Abbassi M, Jain A, Shin D, et al. Quantification of bone marrow edema using dual-energy CT at fracture sites in trauma. Emerg Radiol 2022;29(4):691–6.

30. Gosangi B, Mandell JC, Weaver MJ, et al. Bone marrow edema at dual-energy CT: A game changer in the emergency department. Radiographics 2020; 40(3):859–74.

Dual-Energy Computed Tomography and Beyond: Musculoskeletal System

Emtenen Meer, MBBS[a,b,*], Mitulkumar Patel, MD[a], Darren Chan, MBBS[a],
Adnan M. Sheikh, MD[a], Savvas Nicolaou, FRCPC[a]

KEYWORDS

- Dual-energy CT • Musculoskeletal imaging • Gout • Collagen analysis

KEY POINTS

- Dual-energy computed tomography (DECT) detects bone marrow edema associated with occult fractures, osteolytic and non-osteolytic lesions in multiple myeloma, and osteomyelitis.
- In the assessment of arthropathies, DECT allows for quantification of monosodium urate deposition (gout), evaluation for pseudogout and utilization of iodine maps to detect psoriatic arthropathy.
- DECT overcomes numerous traditional limitations of conventional computed tomography offering clinical information previously seen only on MR imaging.
- DECT collagen applications have high accuracy in detecting ligamentous injuries in the knees, ankles, feet, and hands.
- DECT provides significantly improved image quality in metal artifact studies in musculoskeletal imaging.

INTRODUCTION

Over the past decade, extensive research has been done to study dual-energy computed tomography (DECT), a tool that uses two different energy levels to provide material-specific information. Throughout recent years, DECT has proven to be an invaluable tool in radiology for its speed, reduced dose, and as an alternative to MR imaging in some instances.[1] This article discusses the novel techniques and applications that DECT has to offer in the MSK system, including the review of its most recent advances.

BASIC PRINCIPLES AND TECHNICAL CONSIDERATIONS

The basic principle of DECT or spectral imaging is to be able to characterize different materials based on the relative absorption of x-rays at different energy levels. Usually, low (eg, 80 kVp) and high (eg, 140 kVp) x-ray tube voltages are used. For this to

occur, tissue materials must be imaged simultaneously at the two energy levels. When the high and low x-ray energy spectra penetrate the tissues, Compton scatter and photoelectric effect are the two main types of interactions between photons and tissue matter. In computed tomography (CT), the attenuation of the photons mainly occurs due to the photoelectric effect, as its absorption is energy-dependent, making it critical for spectral tissue characterization.[2]

Different vendors and manufacturers achieve DECT imaging through various techniques (**Fig. 1**). A dual source with dual-detector array technique has less noise and lower risk of spatial and temporal misregistration compared with other techniques, with the downside of having a small second detector. The rapid kV-switching technique uses a single source which offers a high temporal resolution and an entire field of view but with slower acquisition time compared to dual-source CT and with the possibility of spectral overlap. Another technique is the single source

[a] Vancouver General Hospital-University of British Columbia, Vancouver, British Columbia, Canada; [b] King Faisal Specialist Hospital and Research Centre, Jeddah, Saudi Arabia
* Corresponding author. Vancouver General Hospital (VGH), 899 West 12th Avenue, Vancouver, BC V5Z 1M9.
E-mail address: Emtenan.meer@vch.ca

Radiol Clin N Am 61 (2023) 1097–1110
https://doi.org/10.1016/j.rcl.2023.05.008
0033-8389/23/© 2023 Elsevier Inc. All rights reserved.

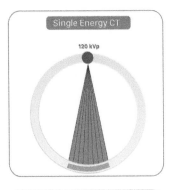 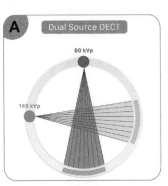

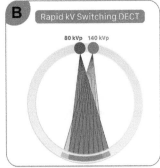 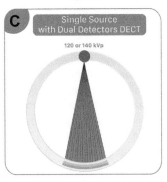

Fig. 1. DECT imaging through various techniques compared to single energy CT. (*A*) Dual source DECT, (*B*) Rapid kV switching DECT, and (*C*) Single source with dual detectors DECT.

with a dual-detector layer which has the advantage of producing an entire field of view. The disadvantage of a single-source dual-detector technique is that it reduces soft tissue contrast and has a higher radiation dose.[3]

In DECT, postprocessing is vital, and various specific algorithms are used to reconstruct images for clinical interpretation. In practice, DECT can render material-specific and energy-specific images to be highly sensitive and specific aiding the interpreting radiologist. For example, when iodine is identified, iodine-only images can be created, and iodine can be color-coded, thus making it easy to tell apart from other dense materials such as acute blood. Another example of material-specific imaging is the virtual non-calcium (VNC), where voxels containing calcium can be excluded from the images, allowing for the identification of bone marrow edema (BME). In energy-specific imaging or virtual monoenergetic imaging, DECT can simulate conventional CT by providing images that display attenuation values similar to those expected when true monoenergetic x-ray beams are emitted. A single energy can be selected, either high or low, resulting in improved signal-to-noise and contrast-to-noise ratios, respectively.[4] Material-specific display aids in material differentiation and separation, whereas energy-specific display aids in material optimization. It is worth mentioning that although two energy levels and two sources are used in DECT, the dose is not increased compared with conventional CT, which is related to the fact that the administered radiation dose is divided between the two. Regarding time, the duration of image acquisition in DECT is similar to conventional CT; however, the radiologist may require more time to interpret the additional images provided by DECT based on the pathology of interest.

ROLE IN SOFT TISSUE IMAGING
Gout

Gout is an inflammatory disease characterized by monosodium urate (MSU) crystal deposition in the soft tissues and joints. Patients can present with an attack of acute gouty arthritis. Over time, repetitive attacks may result in chronic arthropathy with the development of tophi; soft-tissue masses that form secondary to chronic granulomatous reaction to MSU crystals. The diagnosis of gout is typically based on history, clinical examination, and serum urate; however, arthrocentesis is considered the most accurate method. However, arthrocentesis can be difficult and is not applicable in many cases, such as in small joints or joints that are difficult to access.[5,6] Arthrocentesis can also have several downsides and potential complications, such as an increased risk of infection and hematoma due to its invasive nature. Imaging the suspected joints and soft tissues with radiography, ultrasound (US), CT, and MR imaging aids in the initial evaluation, differential diagnosis, and treatment follow-up with variable sensitivity and specificity.[7]

The emergence of DECT was a game changer for diagnosing gout and is now well recognized in the literature. By exploiting attenuation differences among variable materials, DECT can characterize MSU crystal deposits in the soft tissues. The reported sensitivity and specificity of DECT in gout detection are 90% to 100% and 83% to 89%, respectively.[8] With DECT gaining popularity and becoming increasingly available in many institutions, DECT serves as a less invasive alternative compared with arthrocentesis.[7]

Assessing for the presence of gout is achieved by using a two-material decomposition algorithm which will separate MSU crystals from calcium based on the atomic number. Then, MSU crystals can be color-coded, usually green, and overlaid on the grayscale images, which helps differentiate calcium from MSU deposits, and thus the diagnosis of gout can be made.[9] In addition to making the diagnosis, DECT has an excellent utility in mapping the distribution of the MSU crystals in the extremities.[10] In one study that looked at the distribution of MSU crystals using DECT, it was found that the first metatarsophalangeal (MTP) joint was the most involved, followed by the Achilles tendon, ankle joint, triceps tendon, and other MTPs, with less involvement of other assessed regions.[11]

DECT has the advantage of detecting gout in its early stages in patients who have normal urate levels. Furthermore, it can exclude the presence of gout in patients with hyperuricemia.[12] This is particularly useful in complex cases where DECT serves as a helpful diagnostic tool (Fig. 2). This has been demonstrated by a study by Nicolaou and colleagues, which reported five cases in which DECT was used to diagnose gout. In one case, DECT helped to rule out septic arthritis and malignant infiltration in a patient with chronic lymphocytic leukemia who had acute joint swelling and pain, making the diagnosis of gout, which was thought to be less likely.[13]

DECT can accurately quantify the amount of MSU deposits/tophi in patients with chronic gout using automated software. This allows for assessing the MSU deposits/tophi volume and disease burden before and after treatment, rendering it a valuable tool for follow-up.[12] The gout algorithm in DECT is not immune to artifacts. The most common artifact seen is the "nail bed artifact," which is thought to be related to similar dual-energy index values of the MSU crystal and the nail bed. Other less encountered artifacts include skin artifacts, submillimeter artifacts secondary to noise and scatter, and beam-hardening artifacts (Fig. 3).[14]

Pseudogout

Pseudogout is another inflammatory arthropathy characterized by calcium pyrophosphate dehydrate (CPPD) crystal deposition in the articular and periarticular soft tissues. Diagnosis can be suggested when chondrocalcinosis is detected on radiography or CT. Arthrocentesis can also be used to make the diagnosis.[15] In inflammatory arthropathy, the presence of articular/periarticular mineralization in the absence of MSU crystal on DECT should raise the possibility of pseudogout.[16]

In pseudogout, DECT is useful for its ability to characterize the biochemical signature of the CPPD crystals and for its ability to quantify the crystal deposits.[17] The reported sensitivity of DECT to detect CPPD crystals is 77.8% compared with that of radiography 44.4%.[18] Although DECT is not ideal for early detection of calcium pyrophosphate crystals, it is thought to have a slightly better accuracy when compared with conventional CT

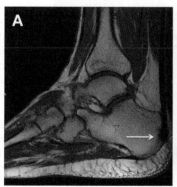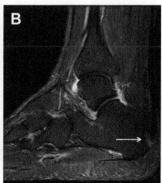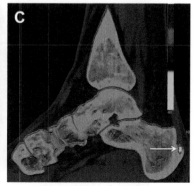

Fig. 2. DECT in a challenging case of gout. A 40-year-old man with left anterior ankle pain. Initial MR imaging was performed with (A) T1 and (B) PD fat saturated sequences showing low T1 and high PD signal intensity at the site of the Achilles attachment (arrow) suggestive of enthesitis. Four months later, (C) DECT showed a small amount of MSU deposits within the Achilles insertion (arrow).

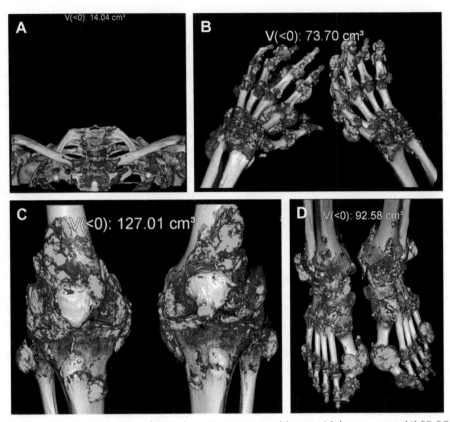

Fig. 3. Quantification and distribution of MSU deposits. A 54-year-old man with known gout. (*A*) 3D DECT images of the shoulders, (*B*) hands and wrists, (*C*) knees, and (*D*) ankles and feet show the exact distribution of the MSU deposits (color-coded *green*) in the joints as well as the MSU deposit burden per scanned region.

due to the color coding of the small structures on DECT[19,20] (**Fig. 4**).

Another benefit of DECT in the evaluation of pseudogout is collagen mapping. In the wrist, Ziegeler and colleagues studied collagen maps in patients with CPPD deposits. The study showed that DECT could detect tissue remodeling in the scapholunate (SL) ligament before the ligament eventually tears.

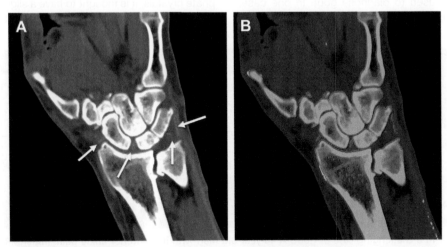

Fig. 4. Chondrocalcinosis in the knee. A 62-year-old patient with wrist injury. (*A*) Grayscale coronal image shows mineralization at the intercarpal joints and triangular fibrocartilage (*arrows*). (*B*) DECT in the same plane using the gout application shows blue foci corresponding to the mineralization, indicating chondrocalcinosis.

Their study shows that the SL ligament demonstrates high collagen density in patients with CPPD.[21] In the cervical spine, collagen mapping allows for the noninvasive quantification of CPPD in the atlantoaxial joint (AAJ). A recent study measured the mean densities of the AAJ ligaments in patients without inflammatory disease and showed that the mean collagen densities of the transverse ligament of the atlas, alar ligament, and nuchal ligament were 141.7, 117.3, and 110.6, respectively.[22]

Psoriatic Arthritis

Psoriatic arthritis is an inflammatory arthritis that affects the joints and soft tissues, particularly the small joints of the hands. On imaging, radiographs, US, and contrast-enhanced MR imaging play a vital role in the diagnosis, prognostication, and management of psoriatic arthritis.[23] The utility of DECT using iodine mapping has been recently studied, and it was found that iodine maps are comparable to contrast-enhanced MR imaging in evaluating the inflammatory lesions seen in psoriasis. This is because CT has a superior spatial resolution, which becomes especially useful in assessing small joints.[24]

Iodine maps on DECT are also a valid tool for accurately evaluating the anatomical location of inflammation in psoriasis. The most common locations for involvement in the thumb, as depicted by DECT, include the sagittal band around the metacarpophalangeal joint, the medial collateral ligament of the interphalangeal joint, and the area surrounding the extensor pollicis longus tendon.[25] In addition, a DECT scoring system for the degree of psoriatic involvement in the joint has been recently created. This scoring system determines the presence of synovitis, flexor tenosynovitis, extensor peritendonitis, and periarticular inflammation. The degree of enhancement on iodine maps is subsequently assessed, and a score of 1 to 10 is given. The scoring system allows for quantitative assessment of the therapeutic response.[26]

Collagen Analysis

Although MR imaging is considered the gold standard for assessing soft tissue injuries, MR imaging has the disadvantages of being time-consuming, expensive, and difficult to attain in an emergency setting compared with CT. On the other hand, conventional CT is not ideal for the assessment of soft tissue and ligaments. Over the past 2 decades, multiple papers have studied the utility of DECT in evaluating collagenous structures by using the tissue decomposition algorithm.[27,28] Studies have found that DECT is quick and readily available and has the added value of 3D rendering.[27]

In the knee, the anterior crucial ligament (ACL), posterior cruciate ligament (PCL), patellar, and quadriceps ligaments can be visualized on DECT.[27] Regarding the ACL, DECT was found to have a 93% accuracy rate for detecting both subacute and chronic complete ACL tears, with a sensitivity and specificity of 75% to 79% and 69% to 100%, respectively. In the acute setting, the presence of edema makes it difficult to clearly visualize the ACL.[1,29] For a higher accuracy assessment of the ACL, the knee should be looked at in the sagittal oblique plane with bone removal and soft tissue windowing.[30] In patients with knee ligament reconstruction, the collagen material decomposition application is a valuable tool for qualitative assessment of the reconstructed PCL, medial collateral ligament, lateral collateral ligament, anterolateral ligament, and medial patellofemoral ligament. However, the reconstructed ACL should be evaluated with caution on DECT.[31] Collagen analysis can also help in evaluating the meniscus in trauma cases and can show meniscal tearing, displacement, and herniation within a fracture pit (**Figs. 5** and **6**). In the ankle and foot, DECT was able to diagnose plantar plate tears, Achilles tendinopathy, and Achilles partial tears by using collagen material decomposition application which shows a decrease in collagen fibers at the site of injury.[11,32]

In the upper limb, DECT can show all the hand tendons allowing for accurate evaluation.[33] In addition, it can be used in the evaluation of ligamentous injury following penetrating trauma to the wrist, making it an MR imaging alternative for soft tissue assessment in the acute setting.[34] In the spine, the use of the VNC application with color coding has a higher diagnostic accuracy for the detection of lumbar disc herniation, the extent of disc displacement, and resultant spinal canal impingement compared with conventional CT. This makes DECT an appropriate alternative for MR imaging in claustrophobic patients and in centers where MR imaging is not readily available.[35,36]

Other Soft Tissue Applications

Other less-studied DECT applications in the soft tissues of the MSK system have been reported. By exploiting the material decomposition of fat and soft tissues in the muscles, measurement of the muscle fat fraction can be achieved using DECT, enabling quantitative assessment of fatty degeneration in the rotator cuff.[37] Fat quantification on DECT is also a reliable tool for diagnosing and monitoring therapy in patients with sarcopenia[38] (**Fig. 7**).

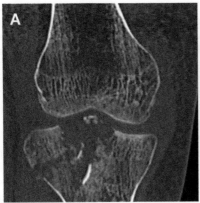
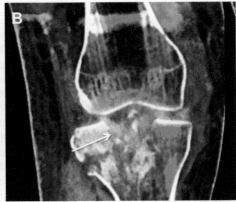

Fig. 5. Meniscal pathology on DECT. A 37-year-old patient who underwent a motor vehicle accident. Coronal images (*A*) show a tibial plateau fracture, and collagen analysis (*B*) shows herniation of the medial meniscus into the fracture cleft (*arrow*).

Pigmented villonodular synovitis or giant cell tenosynovitis is another pathology, in which DECT can aid in diagnosis. Spectral analysis with iron and calcium decomposition can help detect iron deposits in patients with knee or foot masses. The presence of iron deposits was found to correlate well with the "blooming" artifact seen on MR imaging.[39,40] DECT is also helpful in assessing soft tissue masses. A study predicts that spectral curves will be a promising tool for determining the benignity of lesions and found that an arc-shaped curve indicates the presence of abundant fat.[41] In addition, DECT is known to play a role in differentiating hyperdense blood products from calcification by using the VNC application, which becomes particularly useful in cases of trauma when patients present with a mass-like lesion.[4]

ROLE IN BONE IMAGING
Occult Hip Fractures

Conventional CT is a reasonable examination to perform in suspected occult hip fracture; however, the lack of cortical discontinuity or trabecular displacement can make it difficult for CT to delineate occult injuries and demonstrate their extent.[42] However, DECT visualization of BME may improve the depiction of subtle cortical or trabecular disruption by showing detail in areas that may otherwise be overlooked easily. DECT has been reported to have excellent accuracy in depicting occult proximal femoral fractures, with sensitivities ranging from 90% to 95%. However, the reported specificity varies among studies from as low as 40% to as high as 95%.[43,44]

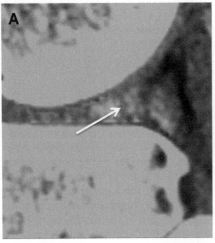
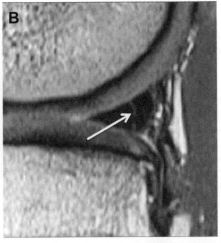

Fig. 6. Meniscal tear on DECT. A 48 year old with a twisting knee injury. (*A*) Color-coded DECT images show linear discontinuity at a cleft at the medial meniscus (*arrow*). (*B*) MR image shows a corresponding vertical tear (*arrow*)

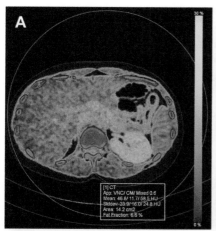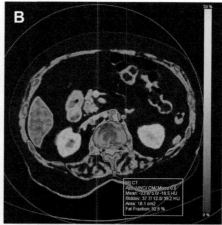

Fig. 7. Fat quantification on DECT. Fat mapping and fat friction calculations for the right paraspinal muscles at the level of L1 in two different patients. (*A*) A 30-year-old woman with a fat friction of 6.6%, compared with (*B*) a 92-year-old woman with multiple comorbidities and a fat friction of 52.5%.

An essential application of DECT in depicting proximal femoral fractures demonstrates the occult extension of a greater trochanter fracture into the intertrochanteric region.[45] A delayed diagnosis of intertrochanteric extension could lead to fracture displacement with the need for more extensive surgery, increased hospital stay, and delayed rehabilitation.[46] x-ray is the first line of investigation but has limited sensitivity to depict intertrochanteric extension, especially in osteopenia. MR imaging is the favored modality to show intertrochanteric extension, although it is often difficult to visualize the medial femoral cortex clearly.[47] DECT can aid in diagnosing intertrochanteric extension by demonstrating the extension of BME into this region, even in the absence of trabecular displacement, while allowing clear visualization of the cortical bone[42] (**Fig. 8**).

Osteoporotic Vertebral Compression Fractures

When the axial load and bending forces surpass the inherent strength of the vertebra, it can lead to osteoporotic vertebral compression fractures.[42,48] If an early fracture goes undiagnosed, it can result in progressive vertebral collapse with the potential for extensive pain and disability.[42,49] Occult vertebral compression fractures may not be readily apparent at radiography or CT. MR imaging shows abnormal signal intensity at the fracture site, and a fracture line can sometimes be visualized.[42] DECT can show BME at the site of the occult vertebral body fracture similar to MR imaging (**Fig. 9**). Correlation with images obtained with the bone window setting may show subtle compression of a vertebral endplate or a cortical step-off. DECT can help differentiate a chronic

fracture deformity without BME from an acute fracture with BME, just like MR imaging. DECT has shown excellent promise in helping identify osteoporotic vertebral compression fractures, with a sensitivity ranging from 85% to 90% and a specificity of over 95%.[42,50,51]

Periprosthetic Fracture

Periprosthetic fractures occur in 4.1% of primary total hip arthroplasties. Delayed intervention could lead to poor outcomes with increased morbidity.[42,52] Although radiographs are the primary imaging modality to help assess periprosthetic fractures, subtle nondisplaced fracture lines around the components may be challenging to. MR imaging shows susceptibility artifacts due to the metallic implants, although titanium implants and metal artifact reduction (MAR) techniques can overcome this limitation. Conventional CT is also limited by beam hardening and streak artifacts from the prosthesis, but DECT can help identify subtle periprosthetic fractures by depicting BME in adjacent periprosthetic regions. It is essential to differentiate a periprosthetic fracture with an intact prosthesis (Vancouver type B1) from a fracture causing traumatic loosening (Vancouver type B2), as the former is treated with fixation alone. In contrast, traumatic loosening is usually treated with revision arthroplasty.[42,53]

Pathologic Fractures

A pathologic fracture occurs when there is a fracture through a lesion, which may be a benign tumor, malignant neoplasm, or osteomyelitis.[42] The affected bone may be weakened by trabecular destruction caused by the lesion and upregulation

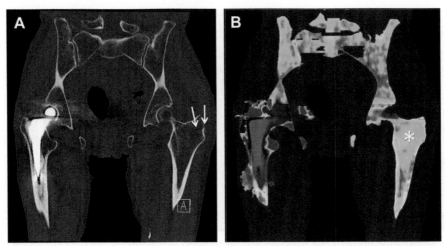

Fig. 8. DECT in occult hip fracture. A 73-year woman with a history of a fall. (A) Coronal CT pelvis shows non-displaced fracture of the left femoral greater trochanter (arrows). (B) DECT color map shows bone marrow edema extending through the intertrochanteric region (asterisk) with no definitive medial cortical breach identified on the grayscale image suggestive of intertrochanteric extension.

of osteoclast differentiation. Diagnosing pathologic fractures has long been challenging for radiologists, and MR imaging is the most common imaging examination performed to differentiate pathologic from non-pathologic fractures.[42,54] However, because MR imaging is not readily available in emergency settings, DECT can help characterize pathologic fractures. It can also depict BME associated with malignant lesions and help differentiate from the linear pattern of BME associated with a fracture (**Fig. 10**). One crucial potential pitfall of DECT is that acute hemorrhage into bones in a traumatic fracture may be falsely identified as a pathologic fracture. In the authors' experience, pathologic fractures show a relatively larger area of abnormality at DECT compared with the severity of the fracture. The absence of trabecular or cortical disruption at a focal point and contiguous involvement of the bone help differentiate

metastatic bone involvement from simple fractures.[42]

Multiple Myeloma

Plasma cell disorders pose a heterogeneous group of diseases with several patterns and degree of bone involvement. Multiple myeloma (MM) is a disorder characterized by uncontrolled clonal proliferation of malignant plasma cells, mainly in the bone marrow (BM).[55] It is the most frequent primary BM disorder in adults and causes around 1% of all neoplastic diseases. Bone involvement is the most persistent manifestation of MM and is responsible for a major part of morbidity and mortality associated with the disease.[55,56]

On imaging, x-rays, CT and MR imaging play a pivotal role in diagnosing the disease, prognosis,

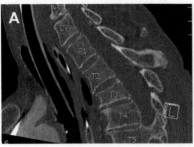
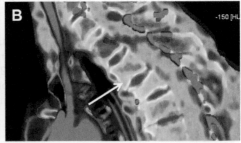

Fig. 9. DECT in osteoporotic vertebral fracture. An 83-year-old woman with a history of fall. (A) Sagittal CT image shows suspicious non-displaced fracture through anteroinferior T2 vertebral body with no significant loss of vertebral body height or bony retropulsion. There is also an acute wedge compression fracture of the body of T3 with 50% height loss. (B) DECT color maps show significant bone marrow edema in the anteroinferior T2 body (arrow).

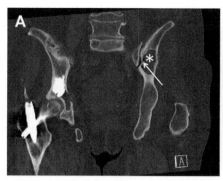
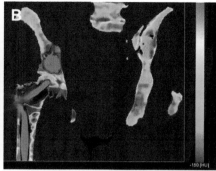

Fig. 10. Pathologic fracture on DECT. A 48-year-old woman with iliac bone metastatic lesion from thyroid cancer. (A) Coronal images show an iliac bone lytic lesion (*asterisk*) with a pathologic fracture (*arrow*) that extends into the sacroiliac joint with gas bubbles within the lesion and in sacroiliac bone. (B) DECT color maps demonstrate bone marrow edema relatively larger than the linear fracture area.

and management. The results of DECT using VNC are comparable to MR imaging in evaluating BM infiltration in MM (**Fig. 11**).[55] DECT can aid in detecting non-osteolytic BM infiltration of the spine and pelvis in patients with myeloma. BM infiltration can be qualitatively assessed using color-coded maps and quantitatively analyzed using Hounsfield unit measurements based on the region of interest (ROI). With MR imaging as a gold standard of reference, the use of the dual-energy VNC technique offers excellent diagnostic performance (sensitivity 93.3% and specificity 92.4% for the depiction of BM infiltration with an area under the receiver operating characteristic curve of 0.978 and a cutoff value of −44.9 HU).[55] Dual-energy VNC application may have a role in depicting non-osteolytic BM infiltration in MM. It can serve as a backup imaging modality for patients with contraindications for MR imaging and/or fluorodeoxyglucose PET/CT.[55]

Osteomyelitis

The incidence of pyogenic osteomyelitis has recently increased, resulting in significant morbidity.[57,58] Imaging is usually required to determine the extent of tissue destruction in spondylodiscitis.[59] MR imaging accurately detects inflammatory BM lesions, destruction of the endplate and disc, and soft-tissue abscesses. Soft-tissue inflammation of the disc is the hallmark of the disease on imaging, that is, fluid-in-disc sign. Also, T1 typically reveals a loss of fat signal and a loss of endplate definition. The use of gadolinium further increases diagnostic accuracy with contrast-enhancement of inflammatory lesions. However, early imaging may be nonspecific for spondylodiscitis due to similarities with Modic I subchondral reactive edema.[57,60]

Although CT allows the detection of endplate destruction, it is not well suited for identifying soft-tissue involvement. Nevertheless, DECT visualizes

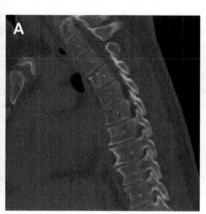
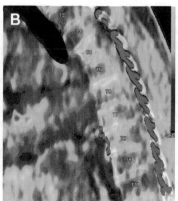
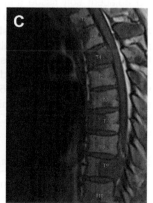

Fig. 11. DECT in multiple myeloma. A 36-year-old man with multiple myeloma (A) sagittal CT lumbar spine images are inconspicuous. (B) Color-coded dual-energy CT images show BM lesions comparable to (C) T1-weighted MR image.

connective tissue components by exploiting collagen's spectral properties.[2,57] DECT collagen mapping indicates severely altered connective tissue components with the destruction of the disc. Hence, DECT has added value compared with conventional CT for diagnosing spondylodiscitis, especially when MR imaging is unavailable or contraindicated, for example, in claustrophobia.[57,61]

Role in Metal Artifact Reduction

An innovative application of the DECT is the MAR algorithm that functions through the implementation of the specific postprocessing for energy, which allows for creating a virtual monochromatic energy spectrum.[62,63] In cases with metallic implants, the metal artifacts reduce the diagnostic quality of conventional CT images. This limits the assessment of the implant integrity and evaluation of periprosthetic anatomical structures, increasing the risk of missing relevant findings.[62] The main mechanisms that create metal artifacts are photon starvation and beam hardening, scattering, partial volume effects, undersampling, and patient motion. DECT uses virtual monochromatic images (VMIs) by setting the different peak settings of kilovolts (photon energy) allowing users to freely select the optimal energy for maximum diagnostic image utility (usually between 40 and 140 keV).[62,64]

The hypothesis is that these monochromatic images are created once the data derived from higher (typically 140 kV) and lower beams (80–100 kV) have been processed. Moreover, the DECT workstation allows the image energy level to be adjusted to optimize the balance between soft tissue detail and artifact reduction. Compared with conventional CT, DECT demonstrates decreased susceptibility to beam-hardening artifacts, provides better quality, and enhances the visualization of the periprosthetic cortex, medullary bone trabeculation, and adjacent soft tissue (**Fig. 12**). These advantages are obtained without an increase in the total radiation dose.[65–67] Some studies have shown that the higher the energy levels of VMI, the greater the ability to reduce the effects of beam hardening. Bamberg and Zhou considered monochromatic energies with values between 95 and 150 keV to be more effective. They have also shown that the higher the energy values set, the more the tissue contrast is reduced.[62]

Role in Computed Tomography Arthrography

Even though CT arthrography has been widely used in clinical practice since nearly the advent of CT, more research is still needed for optimization of this technique. The reported scan parameters differ by institution and radiologist, with most using a technique with 120 or 140 kVp tube energy and tube currents ranging from 125 to 200 mAs.[68] Subhas and colleagues performed a study attempting to optimize the single-energy CT arthrography technique and determine if DECT provides any additional benefit, specifically to identify and quantify iodine in cartilage. The result showed that iodine sensitivity (ie, change in attenuation per unit change in iodinated contrast concentration) increases as the tube voltage decreases, with 80 kVp having the highest sensitivity. The 80 kVp level was ~75% more sensitive to iodine than 120 kVp, ~50% more sensitive than linearly mixed DECT, and ~100% more sensitive than 140 kVp.[68] Usually, radiologists avoid using lower kVp, believing there will be more scatter and more noise. This is true if the tube current is kept constant; however, noise can be reduced if the tube current is increased. Likewise, although an increase in tube current can lead to an increase in dose when tube voltage is kept constant, the dose can be reduced by decreasing the tube voltage. Therefore, it is possible to deliver the same dose using different tube voltages by appropriately varying the tube currents.[68] The noise is nearly identical in the dose-matched single-energy CT techniques using different tube voltages and a dose-matched DECT technique. This allows us to select the optimal technique for the tissues being imaged, which is often cartilage in the case of CT arthrography. Subsequently, it was confirmed that the CT dose index (CTDI) values measured and calculated using a dosimeter matched very closely to the CTDI values displayed on the scanner. Hence, clinically, the CTDI values provided by the scanner can be used as a quick and easy method of comparing doses between techniques without the need to conduct dosimetry.[68–70]

DECT is a promising imaging modality for virtual unenhanced CT (VUCT) in single-contrast CT scanning. VUCT created from DECT has already been proven to have diagnostic value in abdominal and genitourinary imaging by identifying various lesions with fewer scans and lower radiation exposure.[71–73] Materials with a large atomic number, such as iodine, show higher attenuation on CT at low tube voltage settings. This characteristic is valuable when iodine needs to be differentiated from other materials, such as bone, renal stones, calcium plaques, hemorrhage, and instrumentation.[71,74] The HU ratio of a material at different tube voltages can be used to differentiate the composition of mixtures which can be achieved by DECT arthrography using this equation: mean HU at 80 kVp/mean HU at 140 kVp.[71]

Subhas and colleagues reported that the saturation of CT numbers (3071 HU) at 80 kVp occurs

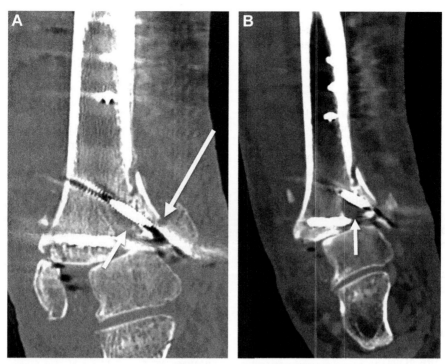

Fig. 12. Metal artifact reduction. A 50 year old with hardware failure with fracture. (*A*) Coronal CT of the leg shows the distal fibular metallic plate (*long arrow*), with possible loosening (*short arrow*). (*B*) Coronal CT in higher kV value better depicts the loosening around the plate (*short arrow*).

at 31% iodinated contrast material concentration and revealed that the saturation is limited by the lower 80 kVp saturation point, as with the DECT technique, which uses both 80 and 140 kVp.[71] The contrast material concentration higher than 31% could not be used in DECT arthrography for VUCT applications. Theoretically, the HU of iodine contrast mixture with a concentration over 30% should be 3071 on CT at 80 kVp. Moreover, the HU of contrast material at a concentration over 50% and 65% should be 3071 on CT at 120 and 140 kVp, respectively. However, when CT arthrography is performed in humans with a more concentrated iodinated contrast material, the HU shows variable values in a different ROI. The heterogeneity of HU is probably due to the heterogeneous mixing of synovial fluid and the contrast material or heterogeneous soft tissue content, such as synovium, in the selected ROI.[71]

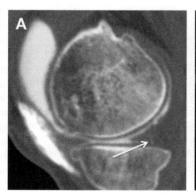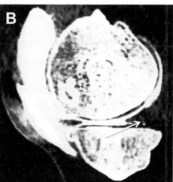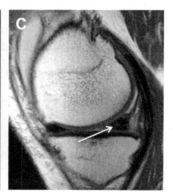

Fig. 13. DECT arthrography. A 43-year-old man with knee pain. (*A*) DECT arthrography shows iodinated contrast within the joint space with faint cleft of iodinated material extending into posterior horn of the meniscus (*arrow*). (*B*) Iodine map shows color-coded image with better delineation of the contrast material and meniscal tear (*arrow*). (*C*) MR image confirms the presence of small meniscal tear in the posterior horn (*arrow*).

DECT arthrography may be helpful for the preoperative diagnostic workup of intra-articular lesions and surgical planning regarding bone morphology (**Fig. 13**).[71]

SUMMARY

In conclusion, DECT is a powerful and versatile imaging technique that has made significant advances in MSK imaging in recent years. Its ability to produce detailed images with comparable radiation to conventional CT makes it a valuable tool to every radiologist, especially as an alternative to MR imaging in the acute setting. The MSK system places significant value on DECT for imaging crystal arthropathy, identifying fractures, and minimizing metal artifacts. In the future, DECT is predicted to have a significant role in patients with psoriatic arthritis and in aiding the differential diagnosis of soft tissue masses. As this technology continues to improve and new techniques are developed, DECT will likely become an even more valuable tool for clinicians and patients.

CLINICS CARE POINTS

- The gout application increases both the sensitivity and specifity for diagnosing gout on CT, and aids in the quantification of gout burden, in mapping MSU crystal distribution and in monitoring treatment response.

- Collagen analysis has a high accuracy for detecting soft tissue injuries when MRI is difficult to attain, however, in the acute setting, assessment may be limited due to the presence of soft tissue edema.

- The rate of detection of occult and microtrabicular fractures on CT improves by supplementing grey-scale CT images with virtual non-calcium application images.

- Metal artifact reduction algorithms can overcome the limitations produced by beam hardening artifacts produced by metallic hardware, and hence betters assessment for hardware integrity.

DISCLOSURES

S. Nicolaou has a Master research agreement with Siemens Healthineers.

REFERENCES

1. Fickert S, Niks M, Dinter DJ, et al. Assessment of the diagnostic value of dual-energy CT and MRI in the detection of iatrogenically induced injuries of anterior cruciate ligament in a porcine model. Skeletal Radiol 2012;42(3):411–7.

2. Nicolaou S, Liang T, Murphy DT, et al. Dual-energy CT: A promising new technique for assessment of the musculoskeletal system. Am J Roentgenol 2012;199(5_supplement). https://doi.org/10.2214/ajr.12.9117.

3. Mallinson PI, Coupal TM, McLaughlin PD, et al. Dual-energy CT for the musculoskeletal system. Radiology 2016;281(3):690–707.

4. Gibney B, Redmond CE, Byrne D, et al. A review of the applications of dual-energy CT in acute neuroimaging. Can Assoc Radiol J 2020;71(3):253–65.

5. Tashakkor AY, Wang JT, Tso D, et al. Dual-energy computed tomography: A VALID tool in the assessment of gout? Int J Clin Rheumatol 2012;7(1):73–9.

6. Kravchenko D, Karakostas P, Kuetting D, et al. The role of dual energy computed tomography in the differentiation of acute gout flares and acute calcium pyrophosphate crystal arthritis. Clin Rheumatol 2021;41(1):223–33.

7. Weaver JS, Vina ER, Munk PL, et al. Gouty Arthropathy: Review of clinical manifestations and treatment, with emphasis on imaging. J Clin Med 2021;11(1):166.

8. Wong WD, Shah S, Murray N, et al. Advanced musculoskeletal applications of dual-energy computed tomography. Radiol Clin 2018;56(4):587–600.

9. Chou H, Chin TY, Peh WC. Dual-energy CT in gout - A review of current concepts and applications. Journal of Medical Radiation Sciences 2017;64(1):41–51.

10. Sanghavi PS, Jankharia BG. Applications of dual energy CT in clinical practice: A pictorial essay. Indian J Radiol Imag 2019;29(03):289–98.

11. Mallinson PI, Stevens C, Reisinger C, et al. Achilles tendinopathy and partial tear diagnosis using dual-energy computed tomography collagen material decomposition application. J Comput Assist Tomogr 2013;37(3):475–7.

12. Desai MA, Peterson JJ, Garner HW, et al. Clinical utility of dual-energy CT for evaluation of Tophaceous Gout. Radiographics 2011;31(5):1365–75.

13. Nicolaou S, Yong-Hing CJ, Galea-Soler S, et al. Dual-energy CT as a potential new diagnostic tool in the management of gout in the acute setting. Am J Roentgenol 2010;194(4):1072–8.

14. Mallinson PI, Coupal T, Reisinger C, et al. Artifacts in dual-energy CT gout protocol: A review of 50 suspected cases with an artifact identification guide. Am J Roentgenol 2014;203(1). https://doi.org/10.2214/ajr.13.11396.

15. Rosenthal AK, Ryan LM. Nonpharmacologic and pharmacologic management of CPP Crystal Arthritis and BCP Arthropathy and periarticular syndromes. Rheum Dis Clin N Am 2014;40(2):343–56.

16. Rajiah P, Sundaram M, Subhas N. Dual-energy CT in musculoskeletal imaging: What is the role beyond gout? Am J Roentgenol 2019;213(3):493–505.

17. Pascart T, Norberciak L, Legrand J, et al. Dual-energy computed tomography in calcium pyrophosphate deposition: Initial clinical experience. Osteoarthritis Cartilage 2019;27(9):1309–14.

18. Tanikawa H, Ogawa R, Okuma K, et al. Detection of calcium pyrophosphate dihydrate crystals in knee meniscus by dual-energy computed tomography. J Orthop Surg Res 2018;13(1). https://doi.org/10.1186/s13018-018-0787-0.

19. Budzik JF, Marzin C, Legrand J, et al. Can dual-energy computed tomography be used to identify early calcium crystal deposition in the knees of patients with calcium pyrophosphate deposition? Arthritis Rheumatol 2021;73(4):687–92.

20. Tedeschi SK, Solomon DH, Yoshida K, et al. A prospective study of dual-energy CT scanning, US and X-ray in acute calcium pyrophosphate crystal arthritis. Rheumatology 2019;59(4):900–3.

21. Ziegeler K, Richter S-T, Hermann S, et al. Dual-energy CT collagen density mapping of wrist ligaments reveals tissue remodeling in CPPD patients: First results from a clinical cohort. Skeletal Radiol 2020;50(2):417–23.

22. Wittig TM, Ziegeler K, Kreutzinger V, et al. Dual-energy computed tomography collagen density mapping of the cranio-cervical ligaments—a retrospective feasibility study. Diagnostics 2022;12(12):2966.

23. Fassio A, Matzneller P, Idolazzi L. Recent advances in imaging for diagnosis, monitoring, and prognosis of psoriatic arthritis. Front Med 2020;7. https://doi.org/10.3389/fmed.2020.551684.

24. Fukuda T, Umezawa Y, Asahina A, et al. Dual Energy CT iodine map for delineating inflammation of inflammatory arthritis. Eur Radiol 2017;27(12):5034–40.

25. Ogiwara S, Fukuda T, Kawakami R, et al. Anatomical analysis of inflammation in hand psoriatic arthritis by dual-energy CT iodine map. European Journal of Radiology Open 2021;8:100383.

26. Kayama R, Fukuda T, Ogiwara S, et al. Quantitative analysis of therapeutic response in psoriatic arthritis of digital joints with dual-energy CT iodine maps. Sci Rep 2020;10(1). https://doi.org/10.1038/s41598-020-58235-9.

27. Sun C, Miao F, Wang X, et al. An initial qualitative study of dual-energy CT in the knee ligaments. Surg Radiol Anat 2008;30(5):443–7.

28. Alabsi H, Alreshoodi S, Low E, et al. Advancements in dual-energy CT applications for Musculoskeletal Imaging. Current Radiology Reports 2017;5(11). https://doi.org/10.1007/s40134-017-0249-1.

29. Peltola EK, Koskinen SK. Dual-energy computed tomography of cruciate ligament injuries in acute knee trauma. Skeletal Radiol 2015;44(9):1295–301.

30. Bai R, Li X, Li R, et al. Optimization of low-dose scan parameters in dual-energy computed tomography for displaying the anterior cruciate ligament. J Int Med Res 2020;48(7). https://doi.org/10.1177/0300060520927874. 030006052092787.

31. Jeon JY, Lee S-W, Jeong YM, et al. The utility of dual-energy CT collagen material decomposition technique for the visualization of tendon grafts after knee ligament reconstruction. Eur J Radiol 2019;116:225–30.

32. Stevens CJ, Murphy DT, Korzan JR, et al. Plantar plate tear diagnosis using dual-energy computed tomography collagen material decomposition application. J Comput Assist Tomogr 2013;37(3):478–80.

33. Deng K, Sun C, Liu C, et al. Initial experience with visualizing hand and foot tendons by dual-energy computed tomography. Clin Imag 2009;33(5):384–9.

34. Persson A, Jackowski C, Engström E, et al. Advances of dual source, dual-energy imaging in postmortem CT. Eur J Radiol 2008;68(3):446–55.

35. Booz C, Nöske J, Martin SS, et al. Virtual noncalcium dual-energy CT: Detection of Lumbar Disk Herniation in comparison with standard gray-scale CT. Radiology 2019;290(2):446–55.

36. Schömig F, Pumberger M, Palmowski Y, et al. Vertebral disk morphology of the lumbar spine: A retrospective analysis of collagen-sensitive mapping using dual-energy computed tomography. Skeletal Radiol 2020;50(7):1359–67.

37. Baillargeon AM, Baffour FI, Yu L, et al. Fat quantification of the rotator cuff musculature using dual-energy CT–a pilot study. Eur J Radiol 2020;130:109145.

38. Molwitz I, Leiderer M, McDonough R, et al. Skeletal muscle fat quantification by dual-energy computed tomography in comparison with 3T mr imaging. Eur Radiol 2021;31(10):7529–39.

39. Becce F, Federau C, Letovanec I, et al. Dual-energy computed tomography molecular imaging of pigmented villonodular synovitis. Rheumatology 2014;54(3):457.

40. Aggarwal A, Singbal SB, Yiew DS, et al. Pigmented villonodular synovitis. J Clin Rheumatol 2019;1. https://doi.org/10.1097/00124743-900000000-99087.

41. Sun X, Shao X, Chen H. The value of energy spectral CT in the differential diagnosis between benign and malignant soft tissue masses of the musculoskeletal system. Eur J Radiol 2015;84(6):1105–8.

42. Gosangi B, Mandell JC, Weaver MJ, et al. Bone marrow edema at dual-energy CT: A game changer in the emergency department. Radiographics 2020;40(3):859–74.

43. Reddy T, McLaughlin PD, Mallinson PI, et al. Detection of occult, undisplaced hip fractures with a dual-energy CT algorithm targeted to detection of bone marrow edema. Emerg Radiol 2014;22(1):25–9.

44. Kellock TT, Nicolaou S, Kim SS, et al. Detection of bone marrow edema in nondisplaced hip fractures:

Utility of a virtual noncalcium dual-energy CT application. Radiology 2017;284(3):798–805.

45. Kim SJ, Park BM, Yang KH, et al. Isolated fractures of the greater trochanter report of 6 cases. Yonsei Med J 1988;29(4):379.

46. Chana R, Noorani A, Ashwood N, et al. The role of MRI in the diagnosis of proximal femoral fractures in the elderly. Injury 2006;37(2):185–9.

47. Kim S-J, Ahn J, Kim HK, et al. Is magnetic resonance imaging necessary in isolated greater trochanter fracture? A systemic review and pooled analysis. BMC Muscoskel Disord 2015;16(1). https://doi.org/10.1186/s12891-015-0857-y.

48. Papaioannou A, Watts NB, Kendler DL, et al. Diagnosis and management of vertebral fractures in elderly adults. Am J Med 2002;113(3):220–8.

49. Kurtz S, Ong K, Lau E, et al. Projections of primary and revision hip and knee arthroplasty in the United States from 2005 to 2030. J Bone Joint Surg 2007; 89(4):780–5.

50. Karaca L, Yuceler Z, Kantarci M, et al. The feasibility of dual-energy CT in differentiation of vertebral compression fractures. The British Journal of Radiology 2016;89(1057):20150300.

51. Kaup M, Wichmann JL, Scholtz J-E, et al. Dual-energy CT–based display of bone marrow edema in osteoporotic vertebral compression fractures: Impact on diagnostic accuracy of radiologists with varying levels of experience in correlation to Mr Imaging. Radiology 2016;280(2):510–9.

52. Griffiths EJ, Cash DJW, Kalra S, et al. Time to surgery and 30-day morbidity and mortality of periprosthetic hip fractures. Injury 2013;44(12):1949–52. https://doi.org/10.1016/j.injury.2013.03.008.

53. Marshall RA, Weaver MJ, Sodickson A, et al. Periprosthetic femoral fractures in the emergency department: What the Orthopedic Surgeon wants to know. Radiographics 2017;37(4):1202–17.

54. Fayad LM, Kamel IR, Kawamoto S, et al. Distinguishing stress fractures from pathologic fractures: A multimodality approach. Skeletal Radiol 2005;34(5): 245–59.

55. Kosmala A, Weng AM, Heidemeier A, et al. Multiple Myeloma and Dual-Energy CT: Diagnostic Accuracy of Virtual Noncalcium Technique for Detection of Bone Marrow Infiltration of the Spine and Pelvis. Radiology 2018;286(1):205–13.

56. Dimopoulos M, Terpos E, Comenzo RL, et al. International Myeloma Working Group Consensus statement and guidelines regarding the current role of imaging techniques in the diagnosis and monitoring of multiple myeloma. Leukemia 2009;23(9):1545–56.

57. Eurorad.org. Eurorad. https://www.eurorad.org/case/16622. Accessed January 10, 2023.

58. Kehrer M, Pedersen C, Jensen TG, et al. Increasing incidence of pyogenic spondylodiscitis: A 14-year population-based study. J Infect 2014;68(4):313–20.

59. Esendagli-Yilmaz G, Uluoglu O. Pathologic basis of pyogenic, nonpyogenic, and other spondylitis and discitis. Neuroimaging Clin 2015;25(2):159–61.

60. Tali ET. Spinal infections. Eur J Radiol 2004;50(2): 120–33.

61. Czuczman GJ, Marrero DE, Huang AJ, et al. Diagnostic yield of repeat CT-guided biopsy for suspected infectious spondylodiscitis. Skeletal Radiol 2018;47(10):1403–10.

62. Simonetti I, Verde F, Palumbo L, et al. Dual energy computed tomography evaluation of skeletal traumas. Eur J Radiol 2021;134:109456.

63. Aran S, Daftari Besheli L, Karcaaltincaba M, et al. Applications of dual-energy CT in emergency radiology. Am J Roentgenol 2014;202(4). https://doi.org/10.2214/ajr.13.11682.

64. Wellenberg RHH, Hakvoort ET, Slump CH, et al. Metal artifact reduction techniques in musculoskeletal CT-imaging. Eur J Radiol 2018;107:60–9.

65. Carotti M, Salaffi F, Beci G, et al. The application of dual-energy computed tomography in the diagnosis of musculoskeletal disorders: A review of current concepts and applications. La Radiologia Medica 2019;124(11):1175–83.

66. Lee YH, Park KK, Song H-T, et al. Metal artefact reduction in Gemstone Spectral Imaging dual-energy CT with and without metal artefact reduction software. Eur Radiol 2012;22(6):1331–40.

67. Bamberg F, Dierks A, Nikolaou K, et al. Metal artifact reduction by dual energy computed tomography using monoenergetic extrapolation. Eur Radiol 2011; 21(7):1424–9.

68. Subhas N, Freire M, Primak AN, et al. CT arthrography: In vitro evaluation of single and dual energy for optimization of technique. Skeletal Radiol 2010; 39(10):1025–31.

69. Reiser M, Karpf PM, Bernett P. Diagnosis of chondromalacia patellae using CT arthrography. Eur J Radiol 1982;2(3):181–6.

70. De Filippo M, Bertellini A, Pogliacomi F, et al. Multidetector computed tomography arthrography of the knee: Diagnostic accuracy and indications. Clin Imag 2009;33(6):493.

71. Chai JW, Choi J-A, Choi J-Y, et al. Visualization of joint and bone using dual-energy CT arthrography with contrast subtraction: In vitro feasibility study using porcine joints. Skeletal Radiol 2014;43(5):673–8.

72. Graser A, Johnson TR, Chandarana H, et al. Dual Energy CT: Preliminary observations and potential clinical applications in the abdomen. Eur Radiol 2008;19(1):13–23.

73. Fletcher JG, Takahashi N, Hartman R, et al. Dual-energy and dual-source CT: Is there a role in the abdomen and pelvis? Radiol Clin 2009;47(1):41–57.

74. Johnson TR, Krauß B, Sedlmair M, et al. Material differentiation by dual energy CT: Initial experience. Eur Radiol 2006;17(6):1510–7.

Photon Counting Computed Tomography– Applications

Ludovica Lofino, MD[a,*], Daniele Marin, MD[b]

KEYWORDS

- Computed tomography • Photon-counting detector CT • Multi-energy imaging

KEY POINTS

- Understanding how photon counting detector computed tomography works and how it differs from energy-integrating detector systems.
- Getting an overview of the limitations of modern CT systems and how photon counting CT could help overcome such limitations.
- Delving into each subspecialty of diagnostic imaging to understand the wide array of advantages that photon counting CT can have for patient management.

INTRODUCTION

In recent years, medical imaging has gone through significant advancements that have revolutionized diagnostic capabilities, enabling healthcare professionals to visualize anatomical structures and detect alterations with unmatched precision. Among the remarkable breakthroughs in this field, photon counting computed tomography (PCCT) has emerged as a transformative technology, offering new possibilities for better patient care and smoother department workflow.

PCCT utilizes an advanced detector technology that can directly convert photons into an electrical signal without having to transform them into visible light, thus providing information on the energy of the single photon. Furthermore, by eliminating the conversion into visible light, PCCT detectors do not require interpixel reflectors improving geometric dose efficiency and spatial resolution, with effective pixel size as small as 0.2 mm for the ultra-high-resolution mode (UHR) and 0.4 mm for the multi-energy mode (as opposed to 0.6 mm of conventional energy-integrating detector CT (EID CT) systems). Because PCCT can provide information on the energy of the individual photons,

energy thresholds can be defined so that two energy bins can be created (low and high energy). For both noncontrast and contrast-enhanced scans, a lower energy threshold can be used to eliminate electronic noise; whereas the higher energy threshold is used in contrast-enhanced scans to create multi-energy and material classification images: virtual monoenergetic images (VMI), virtual noncontrast images (VNC), and iodine maps.[1]

Because these multi-energy images can be created with the same tube current (120 kV or 140 kV for most adult clinical applications), patients of every size can benefit from the advantages of this new technology with no deterioration in image quality, thus overcoming previous limitations of dual-energy CT (DECT) for clinical applications in larger patients.

CLINICAL APPLICATIONS OF PHOTON COUNTING COMPUTED TOMOGRAPHY

Chest Imaging

Photon counting technology has demonstrated great potential in the field of chest imaging, especially for lesion detection and dose reduction in cancer screening. The optimization of radiation

a Duke University Medical Center, Durham, NC, USA; b Radiology, Duke University Medical Center, Durham, NC, USA
* Corresponding author. Department of Radiology, 2301 Erwin Road, Duke Hospital North, Durham, NC 27710.
E-mail address: ludovica.lofino@duke.edu

Radiol Clin N Am 61 (2023) 1111–1115
https://doi.org/10.1016/j.rcl.2023.06.004
0033-8389/23/© 2023 Elsevier Inc. All rights reserved.

radiologic.theclinics.com

exposure through PCCT could help reduce potential risks associated with repeated screenings while still being diagnostically accurate.

In a preclinical investigation, the performance of PCCT was evaluated in the detection and quantification of small lung nodules ranging from 3 to 12 mm, and compared against conventional EID CT. The results of the study indicated that PCCT, with its ultra-high resolution (UHR) acquisitions, exhibited a markedly reduced absolute percent error (4.8% error) when measuring the volume of lung nodules in comparison to conventional EID CT (12.6% error).[2]

In the context of lung cancer screening, PCCT has exhibited notable advancements in image quality and reduced noise levels, with a lower radiation dose.[3] A study showed that PCCT has also demonstrated superior capabilities in visualizing pulmonary emphysema and delineating lung nodule borders when compared to conventional EID CT. Consequently, the integration of PCCT in low-dose lung cancer screening protocols holds promise for enhancing diagnostic accuracy, facilitating early detection while keeping patient dose optimized.[4]

Cardiovascular Imaging

The multi-energy techniques of PCCT play a crucial role in cardiovascular imaging, where benefits include tissue characterization, iodine distribution and perfusion, and reduction of beam-hardening artifacts (such as those associated with calcium blooming). Furthermore, due to its Ultra-High-Resolution technology, small vessels can be identified and analyzed with unprecedented precision.

PCCT helps with the accurate assessment of luminal stenosis particularly in the presence of dense calcifications and metallic stents, thereby facilitating accurate characterization of atherosclerotic plaques and guiding a more precise patient management.[5] This was further investigated by a study that compared the quality of coronary CT angiography (CCTA) of PCCT and EID CT and found that PCCT had higher image quality and improved diagnostic confidence.[6] Another important implication of PCCT in CT angiography is the possibility to use VMI images at low keV levels to enhance iodine attenuation and have a better resolution of small vascular structures. This could also provide a way to administer lower doses of iodinated contrast media to patients.[3]

Gastrointestinal Imaging

With its ultra-high resolution and high contrast-to-noise ratio, together with its multi-energy capabilities, PCCT emerges as a valuable tool in gastrointestinal imaging across different clinical scenarios. Its applications extend to the evaluation of gastrointestinal cancers as well as inflammatory diseases, presenting new possibilities for improved diagnostic accuracy and streamlined workflow. Higher spatial resolution up to 0.2 mm can help in the detection of liver tumors, such as hepatocellular carcinoma (HCC) or intrahepatic cholangiocarcinoma (ICC), as well as pancreatic tumors, such as ductal adenocarcinoma (PDAC) or neuroendocrine tumor (NET) (**Fig. 1**). Furthermore, with PCCT it is possible to acquire spectral images at 0.4 mm, thus pairing two important tools that can help detect smaller tumors in earlier stages.

Recent studies have focused on the utilization of PCCT in the quantification of liver fat, representing yet another noteworthy advancement. Magnetic resonance imaging (MRI) stands as the most accurate tool for the precise diagnosis of hepatic steatosis. Nonetheless, this imaging modality has limitations, including time-consuming acquisition, substantial costs, and the requirement for patient compliance.[7] PCCT is a promising alternative to MR imaging in the assessment of hepatic steatosis, offering advantages in terms of efficiency and feasibility. In a recent study, the fat fraction analysis conducted on a population of obese patients demonstrated promising accuracy for PCCT, which could be a valuable tool for opportunistic screening.[8]

PCCT also holds significant potential in the context of inflammatory bowel diseases (IBD), such as Crohn's disease or ulcerative colitis. Given the relatively younger age of incidence in patients with this condition, it becomes even more important to keep radiation dose as low as possible while still ensuring diagnostic efficacy. PCCT can help provide better visualization of small structures in the mesentery (such as vasa recta) and enhance subtle bowel wall enhancement in the early phases of bowel edema, while still having a lower radiation dose than conventional EID systems.[9,10]

Genitourinary Imaging

PCCT technology enables the acquisition of spectral data during each examination, allowing for convenient post-processing and analysis of Virtual Noncontrast (VNC) images, iodine maps, and virtual monoenergetic images (VMI) even after the patient has left the scanner. This could prove beneficial in the characterization of incidental renal masses, eliminating the need for multiple follow-up scans and providing a more efficient less

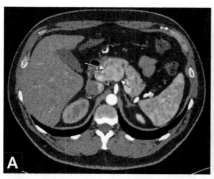 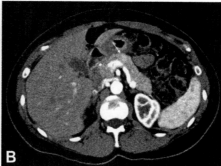

Fig. 1. Images show the axial plane of an arterial phase abdominal CT. (*A*) A 51-year-old man (body mass index of 32.5 kg/m²) with a large mass in the pancreatic head (*arrows*). (*B*) A 45-year-old woman (body mass index of 26 kg/m²) with a small hyperenhancing mass in the pancreatic body (*arrow*).

nvasive approach to diagnosis and monitoring. VNC images, in particular, have proven to be significantly accurate when comparing them to true noncontrast (TNC) images.[11] Having accurate Hounsfield Unit (HU) measurements in VNC images is critical not only to help characterize incidental findings but also to give departments the necessary confidence to start replacing TNC images, with greater impact on the ability to reduce radiation dose. PCCT has also demonstrated promising potential in the field of renal stone imaging and management. A study on 30 patients with renal stones showed that PCCT had better detection and characterization of small stones (<3 mm) compared to dual-energy EID-CT.[12] This was confirmed by another study, which also showed that PCCT had lower radiation dose, of up to 30%.[13]

Musculoskeletal Imaging

PCCT has emerged as a powerful tool in musculoskeletal radiology, offering enhanced tissue characterization and improved diagnostic accuracy. Its applications extend to various musculoskeletal conditions, including bone and soft tissue disorders as well as oncologic pathologies, particularly for screening and monitoring of multiple myeloma and detection of bone lesions. A pilot study showed that when comparing PCCT to EID CT in the context of multiple myeloma screening, PCCT had a lower radiation dose (up to 83%) with equal or even higher image quality.[14] Another study on 27 dose-matched patients with multiple myeloma showed that PCCT performed better when detecting lytic lesions and pathologic fractures.[15]

PCCT could also improve the detection of bone metastases. A study on patients with breast cancer and bone metastases found that PCCT had higher sensitivity and specificity for detecting bone metastases when compared to conventional EID systems, with better visualization of lesion margins and content.[16] PCCT also showed less metal artifacts than EID CT, substantially improving diagnostic confidence of periprosthetic fractures and implant loosening, especially in the spine.[17]

Pediatric Imaging

A significant challenge in pediatric imaging is ensuring adequate image quality while minimizing radiation dose as much as possible because of the higher sensitivity to radiation exposure. This is particularly important because of the additional need to visualize smaller structures in children compared to adults. PCCT has shown equal or superior image quality than conventional EID CT, with lower radiation exposure.[18] This could overcome this significant challenge in various contexts of pediatric imaging, ranging from musculoskeletal to chest and cardiovascular (**Fig. 2**).

Another important implication of PCCT is the possibility of using multi-energy datasets to enhance otherwise non-diagnostic scans and to reduce the amount of contrast media that these patients receive. This can be achieved while keeping a high-pitch mode, which is a great limitation of conventional EID systems, thus making examinations even more diagnostically efficient.[19]

Neuroradiology

Neuroradiology is another field that could experience significant advancements with the implementation of PCCT. This is because of three distinct aspects that could revolutionize the field and overcome previous limitations: reduced noise levels, enhanced spatial resolution, and the utilization of multi-energy material decomposition techniques.

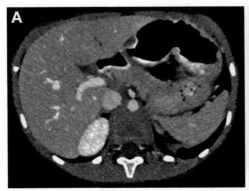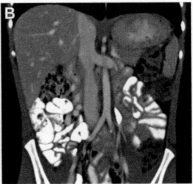

Fig. 2. Axial (*A*) and coronal (*B*) planes of a low-dose contrast-enhanced abdominal CT scan of a 5-year-old boy with suspected bowel obstruction (total $CTDI_{vol}$ = 3.25 mGy).

Firstly, due to its higher soft-tissue contrast and lower noise magnitude, PCCT has shown greater gray matter (GM)–white matter (WM) contrast when compared to conventional EID CT both *ex-vivo* and *in-vivo*. This could be highly relevant to assess subtle GM alteration in the setting of acute stroke, demyelinating diseases, and brain edema.[20] Furthermore, the superior spatial resolution of PCCT could help in the visualization of small structures, such as in temporal bone imaging. A recent study showed that temporal bone CT scans on a PCCT had superior spatial resolution and better visualization of critical structures of the inner ear when compared to conventional EID CT. This was achieved with a significant reduction in radiation exposure as well.[21]

Finally, calcium removal software based on material decomposition could help make more accurate measurements of carotid artery stenosis, which could help patient management in many critical scenarios.[1]

SUMMARY

Photon counting CT technology has the potential to transform clinical practice, leading to improved patient care, enhanced disease management, and a more precise approach to healthcare with lower risks associated with radiation exposure.

The possibility of overcoming patient size and age limitations when addressing certain diseases could expand patient care to a much larger population, and the potential of opportunistic screening, together with a convenient yet precise post-processing analysis of incidental findings may improve and streamline workflow in a clinical setting where radiology departments have become increasingly busy due to the ever-growing demand of examinations. The evidence gained thus far is definitely compelling, however, due to the limited number of studies conducted

and the inclusion of a small patient sample, this field remains largely unexplored, and many questions still need to be answered.

CLINICS CARE POINTS

- A new modality of imaging that offers higher resolution, lower noise and better spectral separation, together with an implementation of faster and easier multi-energy reconstructions.

DISCLOSURE

The authors have nothing to disclose.

REFERENCES

1. Nehra AK, Rajendran K, Baffour FI, et al. Seeing more with less: clinical benefits of photon-counting detector CT. Radiographics 2023;43(5):e220158.
2. Zhou W, Montoya J, Gutjahr R, et al. Lung nodule volume quantification and shape differentiation with an ultra-high resolution technique on a photon-counting detector computed tomography system. J Med Imaging 2017;4(4):043502.
3. Si-Mohamed SA, Miailhes J, Rodesch P-A, et al. Spectral photon-counting CT technology in chest imaging. J Clin Med 2021;10(24). https://doi.org/10.3390/jcm10245757.
4. Inoue A, Johnson TF, Walkoff LA, et al. Lung cancer screening using clinical photon-counting detector computed tomography and energy-integrating-detector computed tomography: a prospective patient study. J Comput Assist Tomogr 2023;47(2):229–35.
5. Sandfort V, Persson M, Pourmorteza A, et al. Spectral photon-counting CT in cardiovascular imaging. J Cardiovasc Comput Tomogr 2021;15(3):218–25.

6. Si-Mohamed SA, Boccalini S, Lacombe H, et al. Coronary CT angiography with photon-counting CT: first-in-human results. Radiology 2022;303(2): 303–13.

7. Reeder SB, Hu HH, Sirlin CB. Proton density fat-fraction: a standardized mr-based biomarker of tissue fat concentration. J Magn Reson Imaging 2012;36(5):1011–4.

8. Schwartz FR, Ashton J, Wildman-Tobriner B, et al. Liver fat quantification in photon counting CT in head to head comparison with clinical MRI - First experience. Eur J Radiol 2023;161:110734.

9. Schwartz FR, Samei E, Marin D. Exploiting the potential of photon-counting CT in abdominal imaging. Invest Radiol 2023. https://doi.org/10.1097/RLI. 0000000000000949.

10. Decker JA, Bette S, Lubina N, et al. Low-dose CT of the abdomen: Initial experience on a novel photon-counting detector CT and comparison with energy-integrating detector CT. Eur J Radiol 2022;148: 110181.

11. Mergen V, Racine D, Jungblut L, et al. Virtual non-contrast abdominal imaging with photon-counting detector CT. Radiology 2022;305(1):107–15.

12. Marcus RP, Fletcher JG, Ferrero A, et al. Detection and characterization of renal stones by using photon-counting-based CT. Radiology 2018;289(2): 436–42.

13. Niehoff JH, Carmichael AF, Woeltjen MM, et al. Clinical low dose photon counting CT for the detection of urolithiasis: evaluation of image quality and radiation dose. Tomography 2022;8(4):1666–75.

14. Schwartz FR, Vinson EN, Spritzer CE, et al. Prospective multireader evaluation of photon-counting CT for multiple myeloma screening. Radiol Imaging Cancer 2022;4(6):e220073.

15. Baffour FI, Huber NR, Ferrero A, et al. Photon-counting detector CT with deep learning noise reduction to detect multiple myeloma. Radiology 2023; 306(1):229–36.

16. Wehrse E, Sawall S, Klein L, et al. Potential of ultra-high-resolution photon-counting CT of bone metastases: initial experiences in breast cancer patients. NPJ Breast Cancer 2021;7(1):3.

17. Zhou W, Bartlett DJ, Diehn FE, et al. Reduction of metal artifacts and improvement in dose efficiency using photon-counting detector computed tomography and tin filtration. Invest Radiol 2019;54(4):204–11.

18. Graafen D, Emrich T, Halfmann MC, et al. Dose reduction and image quality in photon-counting detector high-resolution computed tomography of the chest: routine clinical data. J Thorac Imaging 2022;37(5):315–22.

19. Cao J, Bache S, Schwartz FR, et al. Pediatric applications of photon-counting detector CT. AJR Am J Roentgenol 2023;220(4):580–9.

20. Pourmorteza A, Symons R, Reich DS, et al. Photon-counting CT of the brain: in vivo human results and image-quality assessment. AJNR Am J Neuroradiol 2017;38(12):2257–63.

21. Benson JC, Rajendran K, Lane JI, et al. A new frontier in temporal bone imaging: photon-counting detector CT demonstrates superior visualization of critical anatomic structures at reduced radiation dose. AJNR Am J Neuroradiol 2022; 43(4):579–84.

Moving?

Make sure your subscription moves with you!

To notify us of your new address, find your **Clinics Account Number** (located on your mailing label above your name), and contact customer service at:

Email: journalscustomerservice-usa@elsevier.com

800-654-2452 (subscribers in the U.S. & Canada)
314-447-8871 (subscribers outside of the U.S. & Canada)

Fax number: 314-447-8029

Elsevier Health Sciences Division
Subscription Customer Service
3251 Riverport Lane
Maryland Heights, MO 63043

*To ensure uninterrupted delivery of your subscription,
please notify us at least 4 weeks in advance of move.

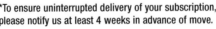
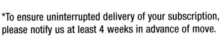

Printed and bound by CPI Group (UK) Ltd, Croydon, CR0 4YY

08/05/2025

01864749-0020